FIRST AID

FOR THE®
USMLE
STEP 3

TAO LE, MD

Fellow in Allergy and Clinical Immunology
Department of Medicine
Johns Hopkins University

VIKAS BHUSHAN, MD

Diagnostic Radiologist

MURTUZA M. AHMED, MD

Fellow in Pulmonary, Critical Care, and Sleep Medicine
Department of Medicine
University of Pennsylvania

PATRICK O'CONNELL, MD

Clinician Educator
Apple Hill Internal Medicine

McGraw-Hill
MEDICAL PUBLISHING DIVISION

New York / Chicago / San Francisco / Lisbon / London / Madrid / Mexico City
Milan / New Delhi / San Juan / Seoul / Singapore / Sydney / Toronto

The **McGraw-Hill** Companies

First Aid for the® USMLE Step 3

5 6 7 8 9 0 QPD/QPD 0 9 8 7 6

NOTICE

Medicine is an ever-changing science. As new research and clinical experience broaden our knowledge, changes in treatment and drug therapy are required. The authors and the publisher of this work have checked with sources believed to be reliable in their efforts to provide information that is complete and generally in accord with the standards accepted at the time of publication. However, in view of the possibility of human error or changes in medical sciences, neither the authors nor the publisher nor any other party who has been involved in the preparation or publication of this work warrants that the information contained herein is in every respect accurate or complete, and they disclaim all responsibility for any errors or omissions or for the results obtained from use of the information contained in this work. Readers are encouraged to confirm the information contained herein with other sources. For example and in particular, readers are advised to check the product information sheet included in the package of each drug they plan to administer to be certain that the information contained in this work is accurate and that changes have not been made in the recommended dose or in the contraindications for administration. This recommendation is of particular importance in connection with new or infrequently used drugs.

ISBN 0-07-142183-1

This book was set in Electra LH by Rainbow Graphics.
The editor was Catherine A. Johnson.
Project management was provided by Rainbow Graphics.
The production supervisor was Phil Galea.
The designer was Marsha Cohen/Parallelogram.
Quebecor World Dubuque was printer and binder.

This book is printed on acid-free paper.

To the contributors to this and future editions, who took time to share their experience, advice, and humor for the benefit of students.

and

To our families, friends, and loved ones, who endured and assisted in the task of assembling this guide.

CONTENTS

SECTION III	HIGH-YIELD CCS CASES	259

AUTHORS

Murtuza M. Ahmed, MD

Fellow in Pulmonary, Critical Care, and Sleep Medicine
Department of Medicine
University of Pennsylvania
Pulmonary

Ghazaleh Aram, MD

Resident in Internal Medicine
Department of Medicine
Johns Hopkins Bayview Medical Center
Ambulatory Medicine; Ethics and Statistics; Gastroenterology

Fadi Abu Shahin, MD

Resident in Obstetrics and Gynecology
Deparment of Obstetrics and Gynecology
Northwestern University
High-Yield CCS Cases

Charles Bergstrom, MD

Resident in Pediatrics
Department of Pediatrics
University of California, San Francisco
Pediatrics

Kevin Chan, MD

Resident in Internal Medicine
Department of Medicine
University of California, Los Angeles
Endocrinology; Hematology; Musculoskeletal; Nephrology

Dickson Cheung, MD

Assistant Residency Director of Emergency Medicine
Department of Emergency Medicine
Johns Hopkins Bayview Medical Center
Emergency Medicine

Anisa Cott, MD

Chief Resident in Psychiatry
Department of Psychiatry
Johns Hopkins University
Psychiatry

Alireza Khazaeizadeh, MD

Associate Professor
Department of Biochemistry
St. Luke's University School of Medicine
High-Yield CCS Cases

Flora Kisuule, MD

Instructor of Medicine
Department of Medicine
Johns Hopkins Bayview Medical Center
High-Yield CCS Cases

Monika Korff, MD

Fellow in Allergy and Clinical Immunology
Department of Medicine
Johns Hopkins University
Infectious Disease; Oncology

Patrick O'Connell, MD

Clinician Educator
Apple Hill Internal Medicine
Cardiology

Michael Rafii, MD

Resident in Neurology
Department of Neurology
Johns Hopkins University
Neurology

Charles Rose, MD

Former Instructor
Department of Nuclear Medicine
University Hospital
High-Yield CCS Cases

Bahar Sedarati, MD

Associate Professor
Department of Pathology
St. Luke's University School of Medicine
High-Yield CCS Cases

Mae Sheikh-Ali, MD

Resident in Internal Medicine
Department of Medicine
Drexel University
High-Yield CCS Cases

Véronique Taché, MD

Resident in Obstetrics and Gynecology
Department of Obstetrics and Gynecology
University of California, Davis
Gynecology; Obstetrics

With *First Aid for the*® *USMLE Step 3*, we continue our commitment to providing residents and international medical graduates with the most useful and up-to-date preparation guides for the USMLE exams. This new addition to the First Aid series represents a thorough review in many ways and includes the following:

- An exam preparation guide for the computerized USMLE Step 3 with test-taking strategies for the new FRED format.
- A high-yield guide to the CCS that includes invaluable tips and shortcuts.
- A review of hundreds of high-yield Step 3 topics with an emphasis on management.
- One hundred minicases with presentations and management similar to CCS cases.

We invite you to share your thoughts and ideas to help us improve *First Aid for the*® *USMLE Step 3*. See How to Contribute, p. xiii.

	Baltimore	Tao Le
	Los Angeles	Vikas Bhushan
	Philadelphia	Murtuza M. Ahmed
December 2004	*York, PA*	Patrick O'Connell

ACKNOWLEDGMENTS

This has been a collaborative project from the start. We gratefully acknowledge the thoughtful comments, corrections, and advice of the residents, international medical graduates, and faculty who have supported the authors in the development of *First Aid for the® USMLE Step 3*.

For support and encouragement throughout the process, we are grateful to Thao Pham and Selina Bush.

Thanks to Aiham Al Ashhab, M.D., Michele Bergstrom, Pete Bergstrom, Kim Bergstrom, Joseph Boselli, M.D., Godelinde Degroot, Rita El-Hajj, M.D., Jodi Friedman, M.D., L. David Martin, M.D., Howard Miller, M.D., Clara Paik, M.D., Akram Shhadeh, M.D., Nawras Shukeir, M.D., and Allan Tunkel, M.D., for their support to the authors during the manuscript preparation process.

Thanks to our publisher, McGraw-Hill, for the valuable assistance of their staff. For enthusiasm, support, and commitment to this challenging project, thanks to our editor, Catherine Johnson. For outstanding editorial work, we thank Andrea Fellows. A special thanks to David Hommel (Rainbow Graphics) for remarkable production work.

Baltimore	Tao Le
Los Angeles	Vikas Bhushan
Philadelphia	Murtuza M. Ahmed
York, PA	Patrick O'Connell

HOW TO CONTRIBUTE

To continue to produce a high-yield review source for the USMLE Step 3 exam, you are invited to submit any suggestions or corrections. We also offer **paid internships** in medical education and publishing ranging from three months to one year (see next page for details).

Please send us your suggestions for

- Study and test-taking strategies for the computerized USMLE Step 3.
- New facts, mnemonics, diagrams, and illustrations.
- CCS-style cases.
- Low-yield topics to delete.

For each entry incorporated into the next edition, you will receive a $10 gift certificate, as well as personal acknowledgment in the next edition. Diagrams, tables, partial entries, updates, corrections, and study hints are also appreciated, and significant contributions will be compensated at the discretion of the authors. Also let us know about material in this edition that you feel is low yield and should be deleted.

The preferred way to submit entries, suggestions, or corrections is via electronic mail. Please include name, address, school affiliation, phone number, and e-mail address (if different from the address of origin). If there are multiple entries, please consolidate into a single e-mail or file attachment. Please send submissions to:

firstaidteam@yahoo.com

Otherwise, please send entries, neatly written or typed or on disk (Microsoft Word), to:

First Aid for the USMLE Step 3
P.O. Box 27
Woodstock, MD 21163-9982
Attention: Contributions

NOTE TO CONTRIBUTORS

All entries become property of the authors and are subject to editing and reviewing. Please verify all data and spellings carefully. In the event that similar or duplicate entries are received, only the first entry received will be used. Include a reference to a standard textbook to facilitate verification of the fact. Please follow the style, punctuation, and format of this edition if possible.

INTERNSHIP OPPORTUNITIES

The author team is pleased to offer part-time and full-time paid internships in medical education and publishing to motivated physicians. Internships may range from three months (e.g., a summer) up to a full year. Participants will have an opportunity to author, edit, and earn academic credit on a wide variety of projects, including the popular First Aid series. Writing/editing experience, familiarity with Microsoft Word, and Internet access are desired. For more information, e-mail a résumé or a short description of your experience along with a cover letter to the authors at their e-mail address above.

Guide to the USMLE Step 3

For house officers, the USMLE Step 3 is the last step to becoming a licensed physician. For international medical graduates (IMGs) applying for residency training in the United States, this is an opportunity to strengthen the residency application and obtain an H1B visa. Regardless of who you are, **do not** make the mistake of assuming that Step 3 is just like Step 2. Whereas Step 2 focuses on clinical diagnosis, disease pathogenesis, and basic management, Step 3 emphasizes initial and **long-term** management of **common** clinical problems in **outpatient** settings. Indeed, part of the exam includes **computerized patient simulations** in addition to the traditional multiple-choice questions.

Step 3 is not a retread of Step 2.

In this section, we will talk more about Step 3 and will provide you with proven approaches to conquering the exam. For a high-yield guide to the Computer-Based Clinical Simulations (CCS), go to **Section I Supplement: Guide to the CCS.** For a detailed description of Step 3, visit **www.usmle.org** or refer to the *USMLE Step 3 Content Description and Sample Test Materials* booklet that you will receive upon registering for the exam.

How Is Step 3 Structured?

The Step 3 exam is a two-day computer-based test (CBT) administered by Prometric, Inc. The USMLE is now using new testing software called **FRED.** FRED is different from the Step 1 and Step 2 exams you took in that you can now **highlight** and **strike out** test choices as well as make **brief notes** to yourself.

Day 1 includes seven 60-minute blocks of 48 multiple-choice questions for a total of 336 questions over seven hours. You get at least 45 minutes of break time and 15 minutes for an optional tutorial. During the time allotted for each block, you can answer test questions in any order as well as review responses and change answers. Examinees cannot go back and change answers from previous blocks. Once an examinee finishes a block, he or she must click on a screen icon to continue to the next block. Time not used during a testing block will be added to your overall break time, but it cannot be used to complete other testing blocks. Expect to spend up to nine hours at the test center.

Day 2 consists of four 30-minute blocks of 36 questions for a total of 144 questions. You also get **nine interactive case simulations** over four hours using the Primum CCS format.

What Is Step 3 Like?

Even if you're familiar with the CBT and the Prometric test centers, FRED is a new testing format that you should access from the USMLE CD-ROM or Web site and try out prior to the exam. In addition, there is the CCS format, which definitely requires practice.

If you familiarize yourself with the FRED testing interface ahead of time, you can skip the 15-minute tutorial offered on exam day and add those minutes to your allotted break time of 45 minutes.

For security reasons, examinees are not allowed to bring personal electronic equipment into the testing area, including digital watches, watches with computer communication and/or memory capability, cellular telephones, and electronic paging devices. Food and beverages are also prohibited. Examinees are given laminated writing surfaces for note taking that must be returned after the examination. The testing centers are monitored by audio and video surveillance equipment.

You should become familiar with a typical question screen (download the software to run sample test materials at www.usmle.org/step3). A window to the left displays all the questions in the block and shows you the unanswered questions (marked with an "*i*"). Some questions will contain figures or color illustrations adjacent to the question. Although the contrast and brightness of the screen can be adjusted, there are no other ways to manipulate the picture (e.g., zooming, panning). Larger images are accessed with an "**exhibit**" button. The examinee can also call up a window displaying normal **lab** values. You may mark questions to review at a later time by clicking the checkmark at the top of the screen. The **annotation** feature functions like the provided erasable dryboards and allows you to jot down notes during the exam. Play with the **highlighting/strike-through** and annotation features with the vignettes and multiple choices.

Do a few practice blocks to get a feel for what tools actually help you process questions more efficiently and accurately. If you find that you are not using the marking, annotation, or highlighting tools, then keyboard shortcuts can save you time over using a mouse.

The Primum CCS software is a patient simulation in which you are **completely** in charge of the patient's management regardless of the setting. You obtain a selected history and physical, develop a short differential, order diagnostics, and implement treatment and monitoring. CCS features **simulated time** (the case can play out over hours, days, or months), **different locations** from outpatient to ER to ICU settings, **free-text** entry of orders (no multiple choice here!), and patient response to your actions over simulated time (patients can get well, worsen, or even die depending on your actions or inaction). Please see **Section I Supplement: Guide to the CCS** for a practical guide to acing the CCS.

For diehard test takers, the USMLE also offers an opportunity to take a simulated test, or "Practice Session," at a Prometric center in the United States or Canada for about $50. You may register for a practice session online at the USMLE Web site.

What Types of Questions Are Asked?

Virtually all questions on Step 3 are vignette-based. A substantial amount of extraneous information may be given, or a clinical scenario may be followed by a question that could be answered without actually reading the case. It is your job to determine which information is superfluous and which is pertinent to the case at hand. There are three question formats:

- **Single items.** This is the **most frequent** question type. It consists of the traditional single-best-answer question with four to five choices.
- **Multiple-item sets.** This consists of a clinical vignette followed by two to three questions regarding that case. The questions can be answered **independently** of each other. Again, there is only one best answer.
- **Cases.** This is a clinical vignette followed by two to five questions. You ac-

Keyboard shortcuts:

A–E–Letter choices.

Enter or Spacebar–Move to the next question.

Esc–Exit pop-up Lab and Exhibit windows.

Alt-T–Countdown and time-elapsed clocks for current session and overall test.

For long vignettes, skip to the question stem first, and then read the case.

tually receive additional information as you answer questions, so it is important that you answer questions sequentially without skipping.

The questions will be organized by clinical **settings,** including an outpatient clinic, an inpatient hospital, and an emergency department. According to the USMLE, the clinical care **situations** you will encounter in these settings include the following:

- Initial workup—20–30%.
- Continued care—**50–60%.**
- Urgent intervention—25–25%.

The clinical **tasks** that you will be tested on are as follows:

- History and physical—8–12%.
- Diagnostic studies—8–12%.
- Diagnosis—8–12%.
- Prognosis—8–12%.
- Applying basic concepts—8–12%.
- Managing patients—**39–55%.**
    - Health maintenance—5–9%.
    - Clinical intervention—18–22%.
    - Clinical therapeutics—12–16%.
    - Legal and ethical issues—4–8%.

Remember that Step 3 tends to focus on outpatient continuing management scenarios.

There are a few things to keep in mind when approaching these vignette questions.

- Note the age and race of the patient in each clinical scenario. When ethnicity is given, it is often relevant. Know these well (see high-yield facts), especially for more common diagnoses.
- Be able to recognize key facts that distinguish major diagnoses.
- Questions often describe clinical findings instead of naming eponyms (e.g., they cite "audible hip click" instead of "positive Ortolani's sign").

How Are the Scores Reported?

Like the Step 1 and 2 score reports, your Step 3 report includes your pass/fail status, two numeric scores, and a performance profile organized by discipline and disease process. The first score is a three-digit scaled score based on a predefined proficiency standard. A three-digit score of **184** is required for passing as of fall 2004. The second score scale, the two-digit score, defines 75 as the minimum passing score (equivalent to a score of 184 on the first scale). This score is not a percentile. A score of 82 is equivalent to a score of 200 on the first scale. Approximately **95%** of graduates from U.S. and Canadian medical schools pass Step 3 on their first try (see Table 1). Approximately **two-thirds of IMGs** pass on their first try.

Check the USMLE Web site for the latest passing requirements.

How Do I Register to Take the Exam?

To register for the exam in the United States and Canada, apply online at the Federation of State Medical Boards (FSMB) Web site (**www.fsmb.org**). A printable version of the application is also available on this site. Note that some states require you to apply for licensure when you register for Step 3. A list of those states is on the FSMB Web site. The registration fee varies and was $610 in 2004.

Table 1.   Recent Step 3 Examinee Results

	2001		2002	
	# TESTED	% PASSING	# TESTED	% PASSING
U.S./Canadian Schools (MD/DO)				
First-time exams	13,249	94%	15,554	95%
Repeat exams	1,131	56%	1,351	65%
Total U.S./Canadian	14,380	91%	16,905	92%
Non-U.S./Canadian Schools				
First-time exams	5,381	61%	6,857	66%
Repeat exams	4,961	40%	5,658	50%
Total non-U.S./Canadian	10,342	51%	12,515	59%

Source: www.usmle.org.

Once you have received your orange scheduling permit, decide when and where you would like to take the exam. For a list of Prometric locations nearest you, visit **www.prometric.com.** Call Prometric's toll-free number (1-800-619-5327) or visit **www.prometric.com** to arrange a time to take the exam.

Your orange scheduling permit will contain the following important information:

- USMLE identification number.
- The eligibility period in which you may take the exam.
- Your "scheduling number," which you will need to make your exam appointment with Prometric.
- Your "Candidate Identification Number," or CIN, which you must enter at your Prometric workstation in order to access the exam.

Prometric has no access to the codes and will not be able to supply these numbers. **Do not lose your permit!** You will not be allowed to take Step 3 unless you present your permit along with an unexpired, government-issued photo identification that contains your signature (e.g., driver's license, passport). Make sure the name on your photo ID exactly matches the name that appears on your scheduling permit.

Because the exam is scheduled on a "first-come, first-served" basis, call Prometric as soon as you receive your scheduling permit!

What If I Need to Reschedule the Exam?

You can change your date and/or center within your three-month period without charge by contacting Prometric. If space is available, you may reschedule up to five days before your test date. If you need to reschedule outside your initial three-month period, you can apply for a single three-month extension (e.g., April/May/June can be extended through July/August/September) after your eligibility period has begun (go to **www.nbme.org** for more information).

For other rescheduling needs, you must submit a new application along with another application fee.

What About Time?

Time is of special interest on the CBT exam. The computer will keep track of how much time has elapsed. However, the computer will show you only how much time you have remaining in a given block (unless you look at the full clock with Alt-T). Therefore, it is up to you to determine if you are pacing yourself properly. Note that on **Day 1** you have approximately **75 seconds** per multiple-choice question, but on **Day 2** you have only **50 seconds** per question. If you recognize that a question is not solvable in a reasonable period of time, move on after making an educated guess; there are **no penalties** for wrong answers.

It should be noted that 45 minutes is allowed for break time. However, you can elect not to use all of your break time, or you can gain extra break time either by skipping the tutorial or by finishing a block ahead of the allotted time. The computer **will not warn you** if you are spending more than your allotted break time.

If I Leave During the Exam, What Happens to My Score?

You are considered to have started the exam once you have entered your CIN onto the computer screen. In order to receive an official score, you must finish the entire exam. This means that you must start and either finish or run out of time for each block of the exam. If you do not complete all the blocks, your exam will be documented as an incomplete attempt on your USMLE score transcript, but no actual score will be reported.

The exam ends when all blocks have been completed or time has expired. As you leave the testing center, you will receive a written test-completion notice to document your completion of the exam.

How Long Will I Have to Wait Before I Get My Scores?

The USMLE typically reports scores three to four weeks after the examinee's test date. However, during peak times, score reports may take **up to six weeks.** Official information concerning the time required for score reporting is posted on the USMLE Web site.

▶ USMLE/NBME RESOURCES

We strongly encourage you to use the free materials provided by the testing agencies and to study the following NBME publications:

- **USMLE Bulletin of Information.** This publication provides you with nuts-and-bolts details about the exam (included on the USMLE Web site; free to all examinees).
- **USMLE Step 3 Content Description and Sample Test Materials.** This is a hard copy of test questions and test content also found on the CD-ROM.
- **NBME Test Delivery Software (FRED) and Tutorial.** This includes 168 valuable practice questions. The questions are available on the USMLE CD-ROM and Web site. Make sure you are using the new FRED version and not the older Prometric version.

- **USMLE Web site (www.usmle.org).** In addition to allowing you to become familiar with the CBT format, the sample items on the USMLE Web site provide the only questions that are available directly from the test makers. Student feedback varies as to the similarity of these questions to those on the actual exam, but they are nonetheless worthwhile to know.

▶ TESTING AGENCIES

National Board of Medical Examiners (NBME)
Department of Licensing Examination Services
3750 Market Street
Philadelphia, PA 19104-3102
215-590-9500
www.nbme.org

Educational Commission for Foreign Medical Graduates (ECFMG)
3624 Market Street, Fourth Floor
Philadelphia, PA 19104-2685
215-386-5900
Fax: 215-386-9196
www.ecfmg.org

Federation of State Medical Boards (FSMB)
P. O. Box 619850
Dallas, TX 75261-9850
817-868-4000
Fax: 817-868-4099
www.fsmb.org

USMLE Secretariat
3750 Market Street
Philadelphia, PA 19104-3190
215-590-9700
www.usmle.org

Guide to the CCS

► **INTRODUCTION**

The Primum CCS is a computerized patient simulation that is administered on the second day of Step 3. You will be given nine cases over four hours and will have up to 25 minutes per case. Like the rest of the Step 3 exam, the CCS is meant to test your ability to properly diagnose and manage common conditions in various patient-care settings. Many of the conditions are obvious or easily diagnosed. Clinical problems range from acute to chronic and from mundane to life-threatening. A case may last from a few minutes to a few months in terms of **simulated time,** even though you have only 25 minutes of **real time** per case. Regardless of where the patient is during the case (i.e., office, ER, or ICU), you are the patient's **primary** physician and have **complete** responsibility for care.

The focus is management, management, management. You will see few diagnostic zebras in the CCS.

► **WHAT IS THE CCS LIKE?**

For the CCS, there is **no substitute** for trying out the cases on the USMLE CD-ROM or downloading the software from the USMLE Web site. If you spend at least a few hours doing the sample cases and familiarizing yourself with the interface, you **will do better** on the actual exam, regardless of your prior computer experience.

Do all the sample CCS cases prior to the actual exam.

For each case, you will be presented with a chief complaint, vital signs, and the history of present illness (HPI). At that point, you will initiate patient management, continue care, and advance the case taking one of the following four types of actions that are represented on the computer screen.

1. Get Interval History or Physical Exam

You can get a focused or full physical exam. You can also get interval history to see how a patient is doing. Getting interval history or doing a physical exam will **automatically** advance the clock in simulated time.

Quick tips and shortcuts:

- If the vital signs are unstable, you may be forced to write some orders (e.g., IV fluids, oxygen, type and crossmatch) even **before** doing the exam.
- Keep the physical exam **focused.** A full physical and exam is often wasteful and can cost you valuable simulated time in an emergency situation. You can always do additional physical exam components as necessary.

2. Write Order or Review Chart

You can manage the patient by typing orders. You can order tests, monitoring, treatments, procedures, consultations, and counseling in your management of the patient. The order sheet format is free-text entry, so you need to type whatever you want. The computer has a 12,000-term vocabulary for approximately 2,500 orders or actions. If you order a medication, you also need to specify the **route** and **frequency.** If the patient comes into the case with preexisting medications, they will appear on the order sheet with an order time of "Day 1 @00:00." The medications will continue unless you decide to cancel them. Unlike interval history or PE, you must **manually** advance simulated time to see the results or your orders (see below).

The orders require free-text entry. There is no multiple choice here!

Quick tips and shortcuts:

- As long as the computer can recognize the **first three characters** of your order, it can provide a list of orders to choose from.
- Simply type the test, therapy, or procedure you want. Don't type any verbs like "get," "administer," or "do."
- Do the sample cases to get a sense of the common abbreviations the computer will recognize (e.g., CBC, CXR, ECG).
- Familiarize yourself with routes and dosing frequencies for common medications. You do not need to know dosages or drip rates.
- Don't ever assume that other health care staff or consultants will write orders for you. Even routine actions such as IV fluids, oxygen, monitoring, and diabetic diet have to be ordered by you. If a patient is preop, don't forget NPO, type and crossmatch, and antibiotics.
- You can always change your mind and cancel an order as long as the clock has not been advanced.
- Review any preexisting medications on the order sheet. Sometimes the patient's problem is due to a preexisting medication **side effect** or a drug-drug interaction!

3. Obtain Results or See Patient Later

To see how the case evolves after you have entered your orders, you have to advance the clock. You can specify a time to see the patient either in the future or when the next results become available. When you advance the clock, you may receive messages from the patient, the patient's family, or the health care staff updating you on the patient's status prior to the specified time or result availability. If you stop a clock advance to a future time (such as a follow-up appointment) to review results from previous orders, that future time appointment will be canceled.

Quick tips and shortcuts:

- Before advancing the clock, ask yourself whether the patient should be okay during that time period.
- Before advancing the clock, ask yourself whether the patient is in the appropriate location or should be transferred to a new location.
- If you receive an update while the clock is advancing, especially if the patient is **worsening,** you should review your current management.

4. Change Location

According to the USMLE, you have an outpatient office with admitting privileges to a 400-bed tertiary-care facility. As in real life, the patient typically presents to you in an office or ER setting. Once you've done all you can, you can transfer the patient to another setting to receive appropriate care. This may include the **ward** or **ICU.** Note that the ICU represents all types of ICUs, including medical, surgical, pediatric, obstetrics, neonatal, and so on. When appropriate, the patient may be discharged **home** with follow-up.

Quick tips and shortcuts:

- Always ask yourself if the patient is in the right location for optimal management.
- Remember that you remain the **primary physician** wherever the patient goes.

- When changing locations (and especially when discharging the patient), discontinue any orders that are no longer needed.
- Anyone discharged home requires a follow-up appointment.
- Before discharging a patient, think about whether the patient needs any health maintenance or counseling.

Wherever the patient goes, you go!

Finishing the Case

The case ends when you have used your allotted 25 minutes. If the measurement objectives for the case have been met, the computer may ask you to exit it early. Toward the end of a case, you will be given a warning that the case will end. You are given an opportunity to cancel orders as well as write some short-term orders. You will be asked for a final diagnosis before exiting.

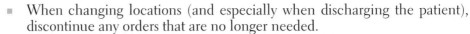

▶ HOW IS THE CCS GRADED?

You will be graded by a scoring algorithm based on generally accepted practices of care. It allows for wide variation and recognizes that there may be more than one appropriate way to approach a case. In general, you **gain** points for appropriate management actions and **lose** points for actions that are not indicated or that can harm your patient. These actions are worth **different** points such that key actions (e.g., emergent needle thoracostomy for a patient with tension pneumothorax) will earn you big points, and very inappropriate actions (e.g., liver biopsy for a patient with an ear infection) will lose you big points. Note that you may not get full credit for correct actions if you perform them **out of sequence** or **after an inappropriate delay** in simulated time. **Unnecessary and excessive orders** (even if there is no risk to the patient) will cost you points. The bottom line is that the CCS tends to reward **thorough but efficient** medicine.

The final diagnosis and reasons for consultation do not count toward your score!

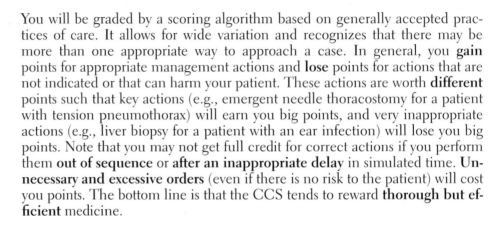

▶ HIGH-YIELD STRATEGIES FOR THE CCS

As mentioned before, it is key that you do the available practice CCS cases prior to the exam. Make sure that you do both outpatient and inpatient cases. Try different abbreviations to get a feel for the vocabulary when you write orders. Try using different approaches to the same case to see how the computer reacts. Read through the 100 cases in **Section III: High-Yield Cases.** They will show you how clinical conditions can present and play out as a CCS case. Remember that the computer wants you to do the **right things** at the **right times** with **minimum waste** and **unnecessary risk** to the patient. When taking the exam, also keep the following in mind:

- **Read through the HPI carefully.** Use it to develop a short differential that will direct your physical exam and initial management. Often, the diagnosis is apparent before you even do the physical. Jot down pertinent positives and negative so that you don't have to come back and review the chart. Keep in mind any drug allergies.
- **Any unstable patient needs immediate management.** If the vital signs are unstable, you may want to do some basic management such as IV fluids and oxygen before doing your physical exam. With unstable patients, you should be ordering tests that will give you fast results in identifying and managing the underlying condition.
- **Consultants are rarely helpful.** You will get some points for calling a consultant for an indicated procedure (e.g., a surgeon for an appendectomy).

Otherwise, consultants will offer little in the way of diagnostic or management help.

- **Don't forget health maintenance, education, and counseling.** After treating a patient's tension pneumothorax, counsel the patient about smoking cessation if the HPI mentions that he is an active smoker.
- **Don't treat just the patient.** The computer will not let you treat a patient's family or sexual partner, but it does allow you to provide education or counseling. If a female patient is of childbearing age, check a pregnancy test prior to starting a potentially teratogenic treatment.
- **Sometimes the patient will worsen despite good care.** And sometimes the patient will improve with poor management. If the case is not going your way, reassess your approach to make sure you're not missing anything. If you are confident about your diagnosis and management, then stop second-guessing. Sometimes the computer tests your ability to handle difficult clinical situations.

A worsening patient may reflect the testing goals of the case rather than an error on your part.

SECTION II

Database of
High-Yield Facts

SECTION II

Ambulatory Medicine

► EAR, NOSE, AND THROAT (ENT)

Hearing Loss

Common in the elderly. Distinguish conductive from sensorineural hearing loss:

- **Weber test:** Hold a vibrating tuning fork in the middle of the patient's forehead and ask in which ear it sounds louder. With conductive hearing loss, the sound will be louder in the diseased ear. With sensorineural hearing loss, it will be louder in the normal ear.
- **Rinne test:** Place a vibrating tuning fork against the patient's mastoid bone and, once it is no longer audible, immediately reposition it near the external meatus. In a normal person, the vibration will be audible. With sensorineural hearing loss, air conduction will be audible longer than bone conduction; with conductive hearing loss, the opposite will be the case.

Major causes of hearing loss are as follows:

- **External canal: Cerumen impaction, foreign bodies** in the ear canal, otitis externa, new growth/mass.
- **Internal canal:** Otitis media, barotraumas, perforation of the tympanic membrane.
- **Other:**
  - Drug-induced loss **(aminoglycosides).**
  - **Noise-induced** loss.
  - **Presbycusis** (age-related hearing loss).
  - **Otosclerosis:** Progressive fixation of the stapes → bilateral progressive **conductive hearing loss.** Begins in the second or third decade of life and may advance in pregnancy. **Exam is normal. Surgery** with stapedectomy or stapedotomy yields excellent results.

Otosclerosis is the most common cause of conductive hearing loss in young adults.

Mastoiditis

If otitis media infection extends to the bone, it may affect the **temporal bone** behind the ear, resulting in **pain, tenderness,** and **swelling** over the mastoid (see Figure 2.1-1). Treat initially with **empiric broad-spectrum antibiotics;** then use narrow-spectrum antibiotics based on culture results. Complications include **hearing loss, labyrinthitis,** and **facial nerve palsy.**

Cholesteatoma

A **cholesteatoma** forms when squamous epithelium is abnormally trapped in the middle ear, usually as a result of chronic otitis media or tympanic membrane perforation. It appears as a mass of **keratinaceous debris** that may erode bone and promote infection. Complications include facial **paralysis** caused by CN VII involvement, **meningitis,** and **brain abscess.**

Allergic Rhinitis

Affects up to 20% of the adult population. May be associated with **asthma.**

Symptoms

- **Congestion, rhinorrhea,** sneezing, irritation of the eyes, **postnasal drip.**
- Associated with environmental allergen exposure and with sensitivity to pollens, animal dander, dust mites, and mold spores. May be seasonal.

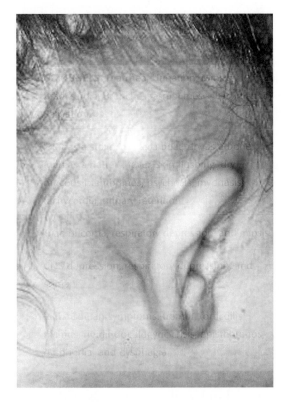

FIGURE 2.1-1. Acute mastoiditis.

Postauricular swelling and redness in a young girl with acute mastoiditis. (Courtesy of Robin Cotton, MD. Reproduced, with permission, from Harrison's Online, www.AccessMedicine.com, © 2004 McGraw-Hill.)

EXAM

Exam reveals edematous, pale mucosa.

DIAGNOSIS

- Often based on clinical impression given the signs and symptoms.
- Testing confirms the specific **IgE** antibody to the allergen.
- Skin testing to a standard panel of antigens or blood testing to look for specific IgE antibodies via radioallergosorbent test (**RAST**).

TREATMENT

- **Allergen avoidance:** Use dust-mite-proof covers on bedding and remove carpeting; keep the home dry; avoid pets.
- **Drugs:**
  - **Antihistamines (diphenhydramine, fexofenadine):** Block the effects of histamine released by mast cells.
  - **Sympathomimetics (pseudoephedrine):** α-adrenergic agonist effects → vasoconstriction.
  - **Intranasal anticholinergics (ipratropium):** Reduce mucous membrane secretions.
  - **Intranasal corticosteroids:** Anti-inflammatory property → excellent symptom control.
- **Immunotherapy ("allergy shots").** Slow to work, but useful for difficult-to-control symptoms.

Epistaxis

Bleeding from the nose or nasopharynx. Roughly **90%** are **anterior** nasal septum bleeds (at Kiesselbach's plexus). The main cause is local trauma 2° to **digital manipulation.** May also be due to nasal mucosa dryness, nasal septal deviation, antiplatelet medications, bone abnormality in the nares, rhinitis, and bleeding diathesis.

SYMPTOMS

- **Posterior bleeds:** More brisk and less common; blood is swallowed and may not be seen.
- **Anterior bleeds:** Usually less severe; bleeding is visible as it exits the nares.

TREATMENT

- Direct **pressure;** topical **nasal vasoconstrictors** (phenylephrine or oxymetazoline).
- If bleeding does not stop, **cauterize** with silver nitrate or insert **nasal packing** (with antibiotics to prevent infection, covering for S. *aureus*).
- Type and screen; IV access.

Sialadenitis and Sialolithiasis

- **Sialadenitis:** Inflammation of the salivary glands, usually affecting the **parotid** or **submandibular** gland. Presents with acute swelling of the gland and ↑ **pain and swelling with meals.** Usually occurs in the setting of **dehydration** or **chronic illness.** When caused by bacterial infection, **S.** *aureus* is the most common organism. Viral causes include EBV, coxsackievirus, and parainfluenza. Treat with **antibiotics, hydration, warm compresses,** lemon drops, and massage of the gland.
- **Sialolithiasis:** Calculus formation in Wharton's duct (drains the submandibular gland) and Stensen's duct (drains the parotid gland).

Hoarseness

A term used loosely to describe any alterations in a patient's normal voice; more correctly called **dysphonia.** If it persists for more than a few weeks, an otolaryngologist should be seen for direct visualization of the larynx. Common causes include **laryngitis,** benign lesions (polyps, nodules), cancer, hypothyroidism, **allergic rhinitis,** and chronic sinusitis. Think of recent events such as neck trauma, intubation, or voice abuse.

EXAM

Conduct a neuro exam and an ENT exam for clues. Obtain direct laryngeal view if symptom duration is greater than a few weeks. Check **TSH.**

TREATMENT

- Depends on the etiology. If GERD, give proton pump inhibitors. Eliminate inciting agents (e.g., inhalational exposure, tobacco).
- **Surgery** for appropriate malignancies.

Leukoplakia

Any **white lesion** of the **oral cavity** that cannot be removed by rubbing the mucosal surface. Can occur in response to **chronic irritation** and can represent either **dysplasia** or early invasive **squamous cell carcinoma.**

If a patient is hoarse in the morning and then improves, think of GERD with reflux laryngeal irritation.

▶ DERMATOLOGY

Atopic Dermatitis (Eczema)

Pruritic, **lichenified** eruptions, classically in the **antecubital fossa.** Also appear on the neck, face, wrists, and upper trunk. Characterized by ↑ serum **IgE** and repeated skin infections. Patients have a personal or family history of allergic manifestations (e.g., asthma, allergic rhinitis). Episodes tend to recur with remissions from adolescence to the 20s.

SYMPTOMS/EXAM

Severe itching, with distribution generally in the face, neck, upper trunk, and bends of the elbows and knees. Skin is **dry, leathery,** and lichenified (see Figures 2.1-2 and 2.1-3). Usually worse in the winter and in low-humidity conditions.

DIFFERENTIAL

Seborrheic dermatitis, contact dermatitis, impetigo.

TREATMENT

Keep skin moisturized. **Steroid cream** should be used sparingly and should be tapered off when flares resolve. The first-line steroid-sparing agent is **tacrolimus** ointment.

Contact Dermatitis

Caused by **exposure to certain substances** in the environment. These allergens may → acute, subacute, or chronic eczematous inflammation.

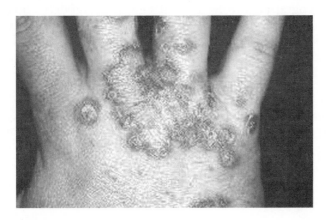

FIGURE 2.1-2. Atopic dermatitis.

Lichenified plaques, erosions, and fissures are characteristic of atopic dermatitis. (Courtesy of James J. Nordlund, MD. Reproduced, with permission, from Harrison's Online, www.AccessMedicine.com, © 2004 McGraw-Hill.)

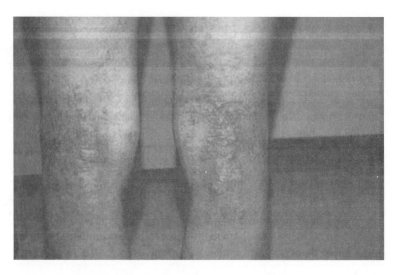

FIGURE 2.1-3. Atopic dermatitis (eczema).

(Reproduced, with permission, from Bondi EE, Jegasothy BV, Lazarus GS [eds]. *Dermatology: Diagnosis & Therapy.* Stamford, CT: Appleton & Lange, 1991.)

SYMPTOMS

Presents with itching, burning, and an **intensely pruritic** rash.

EXAM

- **Acute:** Presents with vesicles, weeping erosions where vesicles have ruptured, crusting, and excoriations. The pattern of lesions often reflects the mechanism of exposure (look for line of vesicles, lesions under a watchband, etc.; see Figure 2.1-4).
- **Chronic:** Hyperkeratosis, lichenification.

DIAGNOSIS

Usually a **clinical diagnosis** that is made in the setting of a possible exposure; consider the **geographic** involvement of a given region of the body that was in contact with the irritating substance. In the case of leather, patch testing can be used to elicit the reaction with the exact agent that caused the dermatitis. Consider the occupation of the individual and the exposure area of the body to see if they suggest a diagnosis.

Common causes of contact dermatitis include leather, nickel (earrings, watches, necklaces), and poison ivy.

TREATMENT

Cold compresses and oatmeal baths help soothe the area. **Topical steroids.** A short course of oral steroids may be needed if a large region of the body is involved. **Avoid causative agent.**

Psoriasis

A common, **idiopathic,** benign skin disease characterized by **erythematous plaques** with sharply defined margins. It is generally chronic with a probable **genetic predisposition.**

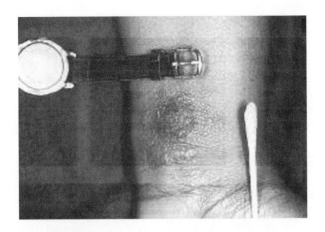

FIGURE 2.1-4. Contact dermatitis.

The erythematous, edematous base of the eruption corresponds to the posterior surface of the watch. (Courtesy of the Department of Dermatology, Wilford Hall USAF Medical Center and Brooke Army Medical Center, San Antonio, TX. Reproduced, with permission, from Harrison's Online, www.AccessMedicine.com, © 2004 McGraw-Hill.)

SYMPTOMS/EXAM

Well-demarcated **silvery, scaly plaques** (most common type) on the knees, elbows, and scalp (see Figure 2.1-5). Nails show **pitting and onycholysis** (see Figure 2.1-6).

TREATMENT

- **Limited disease: Topical steroids,** occlusive dressings, topical vitamin D analogs, topical retinoids.
- **Generalized disease** (> 30% of the body): **UVB** light exposure three times a week; **PUVA** (psoralen and UVA) if UVB does not work. Methotrexate may also be used.

Erythema Nodosum (EN)

An inflammatory lesion that is more common in **women** and is often associated with other conditions, such as **infections or sarcoid.**

SYMPTOMS

Lesions may be preceded by **fever, malaise,** and **arthralgia.** Recent upper respiratory illness or diarrheal illness may suggest a cause. Lesions are **painful.**

EXAM

Deep-seated, poorly demarcated, **painful red nodules** without ulceration on the **extensor surfaces of the lower legs** (see Figure 2.1-7).

DIFFERENTIAL

- Cellulitis, trauma, thrombophlebitis.
- EN itself has a differential diagnosis; although it is often **idiopathic,** it can also be 2° to **sarcoidosis, inflammatory bowel disease,** or infections such as *Streptococcus,* **coccidioidomycosis,** or **TB.**

Psoriatic arthritis characteristically involves the distal interphalangeal joints.

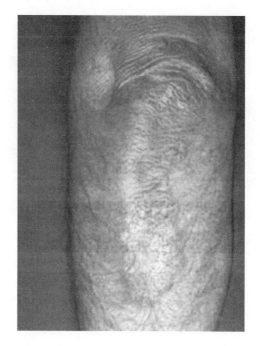

FIGURE 2.1-5. Psoriasis.

A scaly, erythematous, silvery plaque can be seen on the elbow. (Reproduced, with permission, from CMDT Online, www.AccessMedicine.com, © 2004 McGraw-Hill.)

DIAGNOSIS

Look for the underlying cause; check CXR, PPD, and ASO titer at two- to four-week intervals. If no cause is found, only a small percentage go on to develop sarcoidosis.

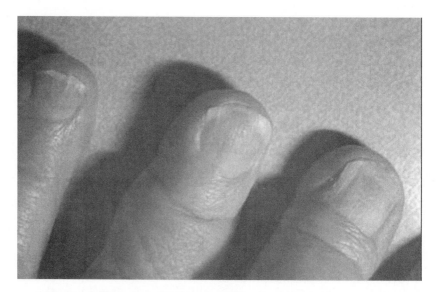

FIGURE 2.1-6. Pitting and onycholysis.

Associated with psoriasis. (Reproduced, with permission, from CMDT Online, www.AccessMedicine.com, © 2004 McGraw-Hill.)

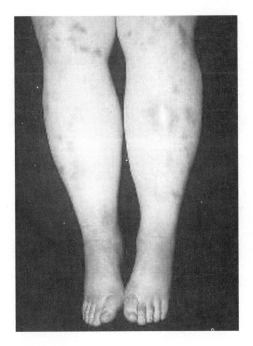

FIGURE 2.1-7. Erythema nodosum.

Multiple painful nodules can be seen with overlying erythematous, warm, and shiny skin. (Courtesy of GlaxoWellcome Pharmaceuticals. Adapted, with permission, from Harrison's Online, www.AccessMedicine.com, © 2004 McGraw-Hill.)

TREATMENT

Treat the underlying disease. EN is usually **self-limited,** but **NSAIDs** are helpful for pain. In more persistent cases, **potassium iodide** drops and corticosteroids may be considered.

Rosacea

Occurs in patients 30–60 years of age. More common in people with **fair skin,** those with **light hair and eyes,** and those who have frequent flushing.

SYMPTOMS

Recurrent **flushing** may be elicited by spicy foods, alcohol, or emotional reactions.

EXAM

Erythema and **inflammatory papules** of the cheeks, forehead, nose, and chin (see Figure 2.1-8). **Mimics acne.** Rhinophyma (thickened, lumpy skin on the nose) occurs late in the course of the disease (see Figure 2.1-9).

DIFFERENTIAL

The absence of comedones in rosacea and the patient's age help distinguish the condition from acne.

TREATMENT

- **Initial therapy:** The goal is to **control rather than cure** the chronic disease. Use mild cleansers (Dove, Cetaphil) to **keep the area clean.** Ben-

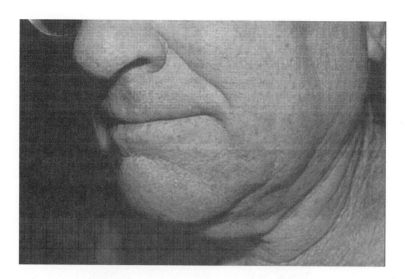

FIGURE 2.1-8. Rosacea.

Note erythema and small pustules as well as the absence of comedones. (Reproduced, with permission, from CMDT Online, www.AccessMedicine.com, © 2004 McGraw-Hill.)

zoyl peroxide. **Metronidazole** topical gel is commonly used with or without oral antibiotics as the initial therapy.

- **Persistent symptoms:** Oral **antibiotics** (tetracycline, minocycline), **tretinoin cream.** For maintenance, topical metronidazole may be used once daily. For management of flushing, **clonidine** or β-blockers sometimes work well.

- Consider referral for surgical evaluation if rhinophyma is present and is not responding to treatment.

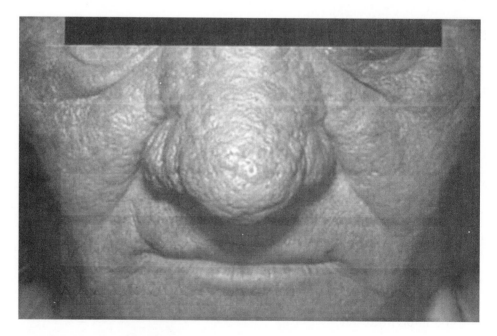

FIGURE 2.1-9. Rhinophyma.

(Reproduced, with permission, from CMDT Online, www.AccessMedicine.com, © 2004 McGraw-Hill.)

Erythema Multiforme (EM)

An acute inflammatory disease that is sometimes recurrent. EM is probably a distinct disease entity from Stevens-Johnson syndrome and toxic epidermal necrolysis. Many causative factors are linked with EM, such as **infectious agents** (especially **HSV** and **Mycoplasma**), drugs, connective tissue diseases, physical agents, x-ray therapy, pregnancy, and internal malignancies.

SYMPTOMS

May be preceded by **malaise, fever,** or itching and burning at the site where the eruptions will occur.

EXAM

Target lesions and papules, typically on the back of **hands** and on the **palms, soles,** and limbs (see Figure 2.1-10). Recur in crops for 2–3 weeks.

DIAGNOSIS

Typically a **clinical** diagnosis. **Biopsy** can help with uncertain cases.

TREATMENT

Mild cases are not treated. If many target lesions are present, patients usually respond well to **prednisone** for 1–3 weeks. **Azathioprine** has been helpful in cases that are unresponsive to other treatments. **Levamisole** has also been successfully used in patients with chronic or recurring oral lesions. When HSV causes recurrent EM, maintenance **acyclovir** or valacyclovir can reduce recurrences of both.

Pemphigus Vulgaris

A rare **autoimmune** disease that → **blistering** as autoantibodies destroy intracellular adhesions between epithelial cells in the skin. Pemphigus vulgaris is the most common subtype of pemphigus.

SYMPTOMS/EXAM

Flaccid bullae and erosions where bullae have been unroofed (see Figure 2.1-11). Oral lesions usually occur before the skin lesions. If it is not treated early, the disease usually generalizes and can affect the esophagus as well. A ⊕ **Nikolsky** sign is elicited when gentle lateral traction on the skin separates the epidermis from the underlying tissue.

DIAGNOSIS

Skin biopsy shows **acantholysis** (separation of epidermal cells from each other); immunofluorescence shows antibodies in the epidermis.

TREATMENT

Corticosteroids and immunosuppressive agents.

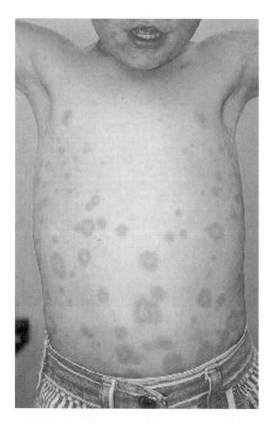

FIGURE 2.1-10. Erythema multiforme.

Symmetric distribution of target macules. (Courtesy of Michael Redman, PA-C. Reproduced, with permission, from Harrison's Online, www.AccessMedicine.com, © 2004 McGraw-Hill.)

▶ **GENITOURINARY**

Urinary Incontinence

Constant or intermittent involuntary passage of urine, more commonly occurring in the **elderly**. May be due to an **upper motor neuron** problem (hyperreflexia and spasticity), a **lower motor neuron** problem (flaccidity and overflow), or bladder dysfunction (overactive detrusor, loss of pelvic support).

Sympathomimetics favor **S**torage.

DIAGNOSIS

- **Urge incontinence:** A sudden, intense urge to void resulting from involuntary detrusor contraction.
    - Idiopathic, but may worsen in the setting of a mass, stone, or infection, all of which irritate the bladder.
    - There may also be a behavioral component in which the trigger to void is linked with circumstances such as entering the home or walking past a bathroom.
- **Overflow incontinence:** ↑ Intraurethral pressure or ↓ bladder tone prevent complete bladder emptying. Commonly 2° to BPH, diabetic neuropathy, or mechanical derangement from prior surgery.
- **Stress incontinence:** Leakage of urine in the setting of maneuvers that ↑ intra-abdominal pressure, such as laughing, sneezing, or coughing. If a

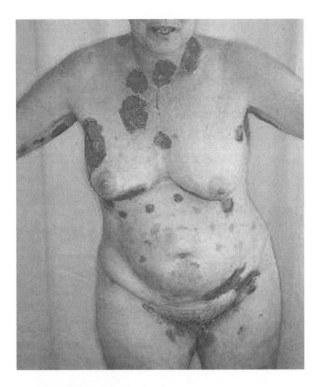

FIGURE 2.1-11. Pemphigus vulgaris.

Vesiculobullous lesions and erosions of pemphigus vulgaris are seen throughout the chest and abdomen. (Courtesy of James J. Nordlund, MD. Reproduced, with permission, from Harrison's Online, www.AccessMedicine.com, © 2004 McGraw-Hill.)

young outpatient woman complains of incontinence, **stress incontinence** is the most likely cause.

- **New-onset incontinence:** Consider drugs, UTI, and stool impaction. May also be an early sign of depression or delirium.

TREATMENT

- **Urge incontinence:** Key is to keep the bladder volume low (frequent toileting) and anticipate the need to go to the bathroom. Behavioral training may also help—e.g., resisting the immediate urge to rush to the bathroom and waiting for the detrusor contraction to stop.
- **Overflow incontinence:** Avoid antihistamines, cold medications, and decongestants. Frequent toileting. May require surgical correction of obstructing lesions such as an enlarged prostate.
- **Stress incontinence:** Pelvic floor muscle exercises (Kegel), biofeedback, and methods to ↓ abdominal pressure.

Palpable bladder after voiding → overflow incontinence.

Erectile Dysfunction (ED)

Inability to achieve or maintain an erection sufficient to effect penetration and ejaculation. Affects 30 million men. Associated with age; some degree of ED is seen in 40% of 40-year-olds and in 70% of 70-year-olds.

EXAM

Look for exam findings suggesting an organic cause—e.g., small testes, evidence of Peyronie's, perineal sensation/cremaster reflex, evidence of peripheral neuropathy, or galactorrhea. Assess peripheral pulses; look for skin atrophy, hair loss, and low skin temperature.

DIFFERENTIAL

- **Psychological:**
    - Symptoms often have a sudden onset.
    - Patients are unable to sustain or sometimes even obtain an erection.
    - Patients have normal nocturnal penile tumescence (those with organic causes do not).
- **Organic:**
    - **Endocrine:** Hypothyroidism or thyrotoxicosis, pituitary or gonadal disorder, ↑ prolactin.
    - **Vascular disease:** Atherosclerosis of penile arteries or venous leaks.
    - **Neurologic disease:** Stroke, temporal lobe seizure, multiple sclerosis, spinal surgery, neuropathy.
- **Exogenous:** Drugs that cause ED include β-blockers, clonidine, CNS depressants, anticholinergics, and TCAs.

Diabetes mellitus may lead to both vascular and neurologic causes of ED.

DIAGNOSIS

Assess TSH, prolactin, and testosterone; order a fasting glucose to assess for diabetes.

TREATMENT

- **Phosphodiesterase-5a (PDE-5a) inhibitors (sildenafil [Viagra], tadalafil, vardenafil):** Inhibit cGMP-specific phosphodiesterase type 5a, improving relaxation of smooth muscle in the corpora cavernosa.
    - Side effects include flushing, headache, and ↓ BP.
    - Patients cannot be on nitrates or α-blockers and use PDE-5a inhibitors.
- Testosterone for hypogonadism.
- Behavioral treatment for depression and anxiety.
- Vascular surgery may be an option if indicated.

Benign Prostatic Hypertrophy (BPH)

Hyperplasia of the prostate → bladder outlet obstruction. Occurrence ↑ with age. Common in patients > 45 years of age.

SYMPTOMS

Frequency, urgency, nocturia, ↓ force and size of stream, and incomplete emptying → overflow incontinence.

EXAM

Presents with a firm, rubbery, smooth surface (as opposed to the rock-hard areas that suggest prostate cancer).

DIAGNOSIS

Appropriate history and exam. Check UA for infection or hematuria, both of which should prompt further evaluation. PSA is ↑ in up to 50% of patients but is not diagnostically useful.

- α-blockers (**terazosin**), 5α-reductase inhibitors (**finasteride**).
- Avoid anticholinergics, antihistamines, or narcotics.
- If refractory to meds, consider surgery such as transurethral resection of the prostate (**TURP**). Open procedure if gland size is > 75 g.

COMPLICATIONS

Acute urinary retention 2° to necrosis and edema of a small part of the prostate; UTIs from incomplete emptying.

Workup of Prostatic Nodules and Abnormal PSA

Significant controversy surrounds prostate cancer screening, with different groups offering different recommendations ranging from no screening to a yearly rectal exam and PSA testing. If an abnormality is found on exam, proceed to prostatic biopsy. The PSA may be used as a marker to follow the response to prostate cancer treatment.

▶ CANCER SCREENING

Table 2.1-1 outlines recommended guidelines for the screening of common forms of cancer.

Table 2.1-1. Recommended Cancer Screening Guidelines

TYPE OF CANCER	RECOMMENDATIONS
Cervical cancer	An annual Pap smear is recommended starting at age 18 or at the onset of sexual activity. After three normal Pap smears, the screening interval can be ↑ to every three years.
Breast cancer	Monthly self-examination and an annual exam by a physician. Mammography should be conducted every year after age 40–50 (may start earlier if there is a positive family history at a young age).
Colon cancer	Hemoccult annually (especially in patients > 50 years old); flex sigmoidoscopy (every 3–5 years in those > 50) or colonoscopy (every 10 years in those > 50). If a first-degree relative has colon cancer, begin screening at age 40 or when the patient is 10 years younger than the age at which that relative was diagnosed, whichever comes first.
Prostate cancer	Controversial. Some groups recommend no screening; others recommend a yearly rectal exam and PSA beginning at age 45 for African-Americans and for patients with a strong family history, and beginning at age 50 for all others.

Table 2.1-2 lists indications for adult immunizations.

Table 2.1-2. Indications for Immunization in Adults

IMMUNIZATION	INDICATION/RECOMMENDATION
Tetanus	Give 1° series in childhood, then boosters every 10 years.
Hepatitis B	Administer to all young adults and to patients at ↑ risk (e.g., IV drug users, health care providers, those with chronic liver disease).
Pneumococcal	Give to those > 65 years or to any patient at ↑ risk (e.g., splenectomy, HIV, or immunocompromised patients on chemo or posttransplant).
Influenza	Give annually for all patients > 50 years and to high-risk patients.
Hepatitis A	Give to those traveling to endemic areas, those with chronic liver disease (hepatitis B or C), and IV drug abusers.
Smallpox	Currently recommended only for individuals working in laboratories in which they are exposed to the virus.
Meningococcal	Not recommended for routine use. Used in outbreaks. There is an ↑ risk of disease in college students, but the vaccine is only suggested and is not mandatory in this group.

Cardiovascular

Most common in patients with a history of long-standing hypertension, cocaine use, or aortic root disease such as Marfan's syndrome or Takayasu's arteritis.

SYMPTOMS

- Sudden-onset severe chest pain, sometimes radiating to the back.
- May present with neurologic symptoms from occlusion of vessels supplying the brain or spinal cord.

EXAM

Look for any of the following: aortic regurgitation, **asymmetric pulses,** neurologic findings.

DIFFERENTIAL

MI, pulmonary embolus, pneumothorax.

DIAGNOSIS

Requires a high index of suspicion. CXR has low sensitivity but may show a widened mediastinum or a hazy aortic knob. **CT scan with IV contrast** is diagnostic and shows the extent of dissection. Transesophageal echocardiography (TEE) is highly sensitive and specific.

TREATMENT

- **Initial medical stabilization:** Aggressive **HR and BP control** with β-blockers first (typically IV propranolol), followed by IV nitroprusside if needed.
- **Ascending dissection (type A): Emergency surgical repair.**
- **Descending dissection (distal to the left subclavian artery—type B):** Medical management unless there is intractable pain, progressive dissection, or vascular occlusion of aortic branches.

Always think about dissection in patients with chest pain!

COMPLICATIONS

Aortic rupture, acute aortic regurgitation, tamponade, neurologic impairment, limb or mesenteric ischemia, renal ischemia.

One of the major contributors to atherosclerotic vascular disease. An ↑ LDL and a low concentration of HDL are the 1° contributors.

SYMPTOMS

Asymptomatic unless the patient develops ischemia (e.g., angina, stroke, claudication) or unless severe hypertriglyceridemia → pancreatitis.

EXAM

- Look for evidence of atherosclerosis—e.g., carotid, subclavian, and other bruits; diminished pulses; ischemic foot ulcers.

- Look for **xanthomas** (lipid depositions) over the tendons, above the upper eyelid, and on the palms.

DIFFERENTIAL

Hypercholesterolemia can be idiopathic, genetic, or 2° to other diseases, such as diabetes, nephrotic syndrome, and hypothyroidism.

DIAGNOSIS

- Based on a lipid panel. A full fasting lipid panel consists of total cholesterol, HDL, LDL, and triglycerides.
- Because triglycerides rise following a meal, only total cholesterol and HDL can be measured after a meal. Triglycerides and LDL can be measured only when fasting.
- LDL is not measured directly; it is **calculated** on the basis of total cholesterol, HDL, and triglycerides. **High triglycerides** (> 400) make LDL calculation unreliable.
- Look for other contributing conditions. **Check glucose and TSH;** check body weight; consider nephrotic syndrome.

TREATMENT

Treatment is aimed at preventing pancreatitis when triglycerides are very high as well as at preventing atherosclerotic disease (see Table 2.2-1).

- **Triglycerides:** If > 500, recommend dietary modification (↓ total fat and ↓ saturated fat) and aerobic exercise, and begin medication (fibrate or nicotinic acid). At lower levels, treatment can begin with diet and exercise, and medication can be added as needed. **Treat diabetes** if present.
- **LDL:** In patients with **diabetes or CAD, the goal LDL is < 100.** The mainstay of treatment is diet, exercise, and a **statin.** LDL control is the 1° cholesterol-related goal in patients with CAD or diabetes.
- **HDL:** Can be modestly ↑ with fibrate or nicotinic acid.

Table 2.2-1. Mechanisms and Side Effects of Cholesterol-Lowering Medications

MEDICATION	PRIMARY EFFECT	SIDE EFFECT	COMMENTS
HMG-CoA reductase inhibitors ("statins")	↓ LDL	Hepatitis, myositis.	Potent LDL-lowering medication.
Cholesterol absorption inhibitors (ezetimibe)	↓ LDL		Introduced in 2003; its role in therapy is being defined.
Fibrates (gemfibrozil)	↓ triglycerides, slightly ↑ HDL	Potentiates myositis with statins.	
Bile acid–binding resins	↓ LDL	Bloating and cramping.	Most patients cannot tolerate GI side effects.
Nicotinic acid (niacin)	↓ LDL, ↑ HDL	Hepatitis, flushing.	Aspirin before dose ↓ flushing.

▶ CORONARY ARTERY DISEASE (CAD)

Atherosclerotic occlusion of the coronary arteries. **Major risk factors** are age, family history, smoking, diabetes, hypertension, and high cholesterol.

SYMPTOMS

- **Asymptomatic.**
- **Stable angina:** Chest tightness/pain or shortness of breath with a consistent amount of exertion; relief with rest or nitroglycerin. Reflects a stable, flow-limiting plaque.
- **Unstable angina (acute coronary syndrome):** Chest tightness/pain and/or shortness of breath, typically at rest, that does not improve with nitroglycerin. Reflects a plaque that has ruptured with formation of a clot in the lumen of the blood vessel.

EXAM

- Exam can be normal when the patient is asymptomatic.
- Look for signs of heart failure ($\uparrow$ JVD, bibasilar crackles, lower extremity edema) from prior MI.
- Look for vascular disease elsewhere—e.g., bruits, asymmetric pulses, and lower extremity ischemic ulcers.

DIFFERENTIAL

See the differential for MI below.

DIAGNOSIS

- **Stress testing:** Exercise or dobutamine to $\uparrow$ HR; ECG, echocardiogram, or radionuclide to assess perfusion (see the section on stress testing below).
- **Cardiac catheterization:** Defines the location and severity of lesions.

TREATMENT

- **To slow progression: Control diabetes, $\downarrow$ BP, $\downarrow$ cholesterol (goal low-density cholesterol < 100), stop smoking.**
- **To prevent angina:** β-blockers $\downarrow$ BP and $\downarrow$ cardiac workload, which will $\downarrow$ exertional angina. If symptoms arise on a β-blocker, a long-acting nitrate or calcium channel blocker can be added.
- **To prevent MI: Aspirin;** clopidogrel for aspirin-sensitive patients.

▶ ENDOCARDITIS

Inflammation of the heart valves; can be infectious or noninfectious. Infectious endocarditis is commonly seen in IV drug abusers and in those with valvular lesions or prosthetic heart valves.

SYMPTOMS

- **Acute endocarditis:** Fever, rigors, heart failure from valve destruction, symptoms related to systemic emboli (neurologic impairment, back pain, pulmonary symptoms).
- **Subacute bacterial endocarditis:** Weeks to months of fever, malaise, and weight loss. Also presents with symptoms of systemic emboli.
- **Noninfectious endocarditis:** Generally asymptomatic. Can cause heart failure by destroying valves.

EXAM

New **murmur.** Findings associated with emboli include focal neurologic deficits and tenderness to percussion over the spine. With infectious endocarditis, look at the fingers and toes for deep-seated, painful nodules (**Osler's nodes** = "Ouch"ler's nodes) and small skin infarctions (**Janeway lesions**). Retinal exudates are called **Roth's spots.**

DIFFERENTIAL

The differential diagnosis of endocarditis is outlined below and in Table 2.2-2.

- **Differential of a vegetation found on echocardiography:** Infectious endocarditis, nonbacterial thrombotic endocarditis (NBTE, or marantic endocarditis), verrucous endocarditis (or Libman-Sacks endocarditis), valve degeneration.
- **Differential of bacteremia:** Infectious endocarditis, infected hardware (e.g., from a central line), abscess, osteomyelitis.

DIAGNOSIS

- The discovery of noninfectious endocarditis is usually an incidental finding on echocardiography. It may be found during the workup of systemic emboli.
- Infectious endocarditis is diagnosed by a combination of lab and clinical data. If suspicious, obtain **three sets of blood cultures** and an echocardiogram. If the transthoracic echocardiogram is $\ominus$, proceed to **TEE** (more sensitive). $\oplus$ blood cultures and echocardiogram findings diagnose endocarditis.

Any patient with S. aureus bacteremia should be evaluated for endocarditis with echocardiography.

TREATMENT

- **Prolonged antibiotics,** generally for 4–6 weeks. Begin empiric therapy with gentamicin and antistaphylococcal penicillin (**oxacillin or nafcillin**). If there is a risk of methicillin-resistant S. *aureus*, use vancomycin instead of oxacillin/nafcillin.
- **Valve replacement** for fungal endocarditis, **heart failure** from valve destruction, valve ring abscess, or systemic emboli despite adequate antibiotic therapy.

Table 2.2-2. Causes of Endocarditis

ACUTE	SUBACUTE	CULTURE NEGATIVE	NBTE (MARANTIC ENDOCARDITIS)	VERRUCOUS ENDOCARDITIS (LIBMAN-SACKS)
Most commonly S. aureus.	Viridans streptococci, Enterococcus, S. epidermidis, gram-negative rods, Candida.	HACEK organisms,[a] Coxiella burnetii, noncandidal fungi.	Thrombus formation on valve seen in many cancers.	Seen in lupus; vegetation composed of fibrin, platelets, immune complexes, and inflammatory cells.

[a]**HACEK** = **H**aemophilus aphrophilus and **H.** parainfluenzae, **A**ctinobacillus actinomycetemcomitans, **C**ardiobacterium hominis, **E**ikenella corrodens, **K**ingella kingae.

- Following treatment for infectious endocarditis, patients should receive endocarditis prophylaxis.
- **NBTE:** Treat the underlying disorder. Heparin is useful in the short term.
- **Verrucous:** No treatment is required. Patients should receive endocarditis prophylaxis (see below).

COMPLICATIONS

Spinal osteomyelitis, valve destruction and heart failure, embolic stroke.

PREVENTION

Give endocarditis prophylaxis to patients who are undergoing procedures associated with a risk of bacteremia (see Table 2.2-3) and have any of the following risk factors:

- **Prosthetic valves** (mechanical or bioprosthetic).
- Prior bacterial endocarditis.
- Acquired valve dysfunction.
- Most congenital heart abnormalities.
- Hypertrophic cardiomyopathy.
- **Mitral valve prolapse with mitral regurgitation.**

Prophylaxis regimens are as follows:

- **Amoxicillin** (clindamycin if penicillin allergy) one hour before the procedure.
- If the patient is undergoing a GI or GU procedure and has a high-risk valve lesion (e.g., a prosthetic valve, prior endocarditis, or congenital heart abnormalities that cause cyanosis), cover *Enterococcus* with IV ampicillin and gentamicin.

Table 2.2-3. **Selected Procedures Carrying a Risk of Bacteremia**

Dental:
- **Extractions**
- Oral surgery
- Any procedure below the gum line

Pulmonary:
- Tonsillectomy and adenoidectomy
- Surgical operations of the respiratory mucosa (includes **biopsies**)

GI:
- Sclerotherapy of esophageal varices
- Esophageal dilation
- Biliary procedures
- Surgical procedures involving the mucosa (includes **biopsies**)

GU:
- Cystoscopy
- Prostate surgery

Inability of the heart to pump adequate blood to meet the needs of the body. Can be categorized in different ways. One such categorization is as follows:

- Systolic dysfunction.
- Diastolic dysfunction.
- Valvular dysfunction.
- Arrhythmia causing heart failure.

Systolic Heart Failure

Weakened pumping function of the heart muscle. Common causes include **ischemic heart disease, long-standing hypertension,** and viral or idiopathic cardiomyopathy in younger patients.

SYMPTOMS

- Poor exercise tolerance, dyspnea on exertion, easy fatigability.
- If patients are volume overloaded, they may present with **orthopnea, paroxysmal nocturnal dyspnea,** and ankle swelling.

EXAM

- Bibasilar crackles.
- Diffuse PMI that is displaced to the left (reflects cardiomegaly).
- **S3 gallop.**
- ↑ JVD (normal is about 0–2 cm vertical elevation above the sternomanubrial junction).
- Lower extremity edema.

DIFFERENTIAL

- Deconditioning.
- Lung disease (e.g., COPD).
- Heart failure of other types (e.g., diastolic dysfunction).
- Other causes of edema (e.g., low albumin and nephrotic syndrome).

DIAGNOSIS

History and exam are suggestive, but determination of the ejection fraction via an imaging study is the definitive diagnosis:

- **Echocardiogram.**
- Radionuclide imaging (e.g., thallium).
- **Look for the cause of the low ejection fraction:** Perform a stress test or cardiac catheterization to look for CAD; test for TSH levels and for HIV. Look for a history of alcohol use or exposure to offending medications such as **doxorubicin;** may perform myocardial biopsy.

TREATMENT

- **Maintenance medications:**
  - β-blockers: Metoprolol, atenolol, others.
  - **Afterload reduction:** Ideally an **ACEI** or an angiotensin receptor blocker (ARB).

ACEIs, ARBs, and spironolactone all cause hyperkalemia.

Ventricular tachycardia is a common cause of death in patients with a ↓ ejection fraction.

- Spironolactone if the patient's potassium can tolerate it.
- Digoxin is falling out of favor because it has toxicities and does not improve mortality.
- **Exacerbations: Loop diuretics** such as furosemide when the patient is volume overloaded.
- **Other:**
  - **Automatic implantable cardiac defibrillator (AICD):** Associated with ↓ mortality from ventricular tachycardia, but very expensive.
  - Treat the cause of the systolic heart failure, such as CAD.

Diastolic Heart Failure

During diastole, the heart is **stiff** (↓ compliance) and does not relax well, resulting in ↑ diastolic filling pressure. **Hypertension with ventricular hypertrophy** is the most common cause; uncommon causes include infiltrative diseases such as amyloidosis and sarcoidosis.

SYMPTOMS

The same as those for systolic heart failure.

EXAM

Similar to that for systolic failure. Listen for an **S4** rather than an S3.

DIFFERENTIAL

The same as that for systolic heart failure.

Active ischemia can acutely worsen diastolic dysfunction, so treat any coexisting CAD!

DIAGNOSIS

Presents with symptoms of heart failure with a normal ejection fraction on echocardiogram. Echo usually shows ventricular hypertrophy.

TREATMENT

- Control hypertension.
- Give diuretics to control volume overload, but **avoid overdiuresis,** which ↓ preload and therefore cardiac output.

Valvular Causes of Heart Failure

- Right-sided valvular lesions do not typically cause heart failure.
- In left-sided valvular lesions, aortic stenosis or aortic regurgitation and mitral stenosis or mitral regurgitation can each cause symptoms of heart failure.
- See the section on valvular disease for more detail.

Arrhythmia Causing Heart Failure

This cause of heart failure is generally apparent from palpitations or ECG. Rhythms that can cause symptoms of heart failure include **atrial fibrillation** and bradyarrhythmias. Others present abruptly with palpitations, shortness of breath, or even syncope.

One of the major contributors to cardiovascular disease; more common with increasing age and in blacks.

SYMPTOMS

Asymptomatic unless severe. If severe, patients may complain of chest tightness, shortness of breath, headache, or visual disturbances.

EXAM

BP > 140/90. A displaced PMI or an **S4** indicates LVH. Fundi show **AV nicking** and "copper-wire" changes to the arterioles. Listen for bruits, which indicate peripheral vascular disease. In severe hypertension, look for papilledema and retinal hemorrhages.

DIFFERENTIAL

Most cases are essential hypertension, but consider causes of 2° hypertension:

- **Endocrine causes:** Cushing's syndrome, Conn's syndrome (aldosterone-producing tumor), hyperthyroidism.
- Chronic renal failure.
- Renal artery stenosis (listen for abdominal bruit).
- **Young patients: Fibromuscular dysplasia** of the renal arteries, aortic coarctation.
- **Medications:** OCPs, NSAIDs.

DIAGNOSIS

BP > 140/90 on two separate occasions (elevation of **either** systolic or diastolic BP). A systolic BP of 120–139 or a diastolic BP of 80–89 is considered "prehypertension" and predicts the development of hypertension.

TREATMENT

- **Goal:** BP < 140/90. In diabetics and those with renal insufficiency, the goal is < 130/80.
- **Interventions:**
  - **Step 1—lifestyle modification:** Weight loss, exercise, ↓ sodium intake.
  - **Step 2—medications: Begin with a thiazide** unless there is an indication for another class (see Table 2.2-4).
- Control other cardiovascular risk factors, such as diabetes, smoking, and high cholesterol.

COMPLICATIONS

Long-standing hypertension contributes to renal failure, heart failure (systolic and diastolic), CAD, peripheral vascular disease, and stroke.

▶ **MYOCARDIAL INFARCTION (MI)**

Sudden rupture of an atherosclerotic plaque with partial or complete occlusion of the coronary artery. Less commonly from coronary vasospasm seen with cocaine.

Table 2.2-4. Antihypertensive Medications

Commonly Used Classes	Optimal Use	Main Side Effects
Thiazide diuretics	First-line treatment if no indication for other agents.	↓ excretion of calcium and uric acid.
β-blockers	Low ejection fraction, **angina.**	Bradycardia, erectile dysfunction, bronchospasm in asthmatics.
ACEIs	Low ejection fraction, chronic kidney disease, diabetes with **microalbuminuria.**	**Cough,** angioedema, hyperkalemia.
ARBs	Same as ACEIs; cough with ACEI.	Hyperkalemia.
Calcium channel blockers	Second-line agent.	Lower extremity edema.

Diabetics, women, and older men often present with dyspnea, diaphoresis, and nausea rather than with chest pain.

Low blood pressure with bradycardia and clear lungs indicates right ventricular infarction with sinus node ischemia.

Symptoms

The classic symptom of **crushing substernal chest pressure** radiating to the jaw or left shoulder applies mainly to middle-aged men; older men, women, and diabetics often present with nonspecific symptoms such as dyspnea, nausea, and diaphoresis.

Exam

- Diaphoresis.
- Bibasilar crackles or a new S3 indicates a low ejection fraction. Low blood pressure suggests cardiogenic shock.

Differential

- **Always think of** pneumothorax, pulmonary embolus, and aortic dissection.
- **Others:** Esophageal spasm, peptic ulcer, cholecystitis, bronchospasm, pneumonia, costochondritis, pericarditis.

Diagnosis

- Look for other causes of chest pain—take a history! Check CXR, check BP in both arms, and ask about pain radiating to the back.
- **ECG:** Look for > 1-mm **ST-segment elevation** in contiguous leads (see Figure 2.2-1) or a **new left bundle branch block.**
- **Serial cardiac enzymes:** Evaluate CK, CK-MB, and **troponin.** All begin to rise within a few hours. Troponin is nearly 100% specific for myocardial injury (also expect it to be ⊕ with myocarditis, cardiac contusion, etc.).
- ⊕ **cardiac enzymes with a nondiagnostic ECG:** Called "non-ST-elevation MI," or NSTEMI. Indicates that the ruptured plaque did not completely occlude the coronary lumen but that myocardium is dying nonetheless.

Treatment

- **ST-elevation MI (STEMI):**
  - **Immediately:** Aspirin, IV β-blocker (↓ HR to 60 if BP will tolerate), O_2, heparin. If the patient is still in pain, give IV morphine or nitrates.

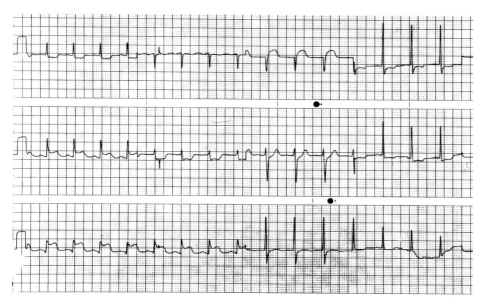

FIGURE 2.2-1. Myocardial infarction.

(Reproduced, with permission, from Stobo JD et al. *The Principles and Practice of Medicine*, 23rd ed. Stamford, CT: Appleton & Lange, 1996:20, Fig. 1-3-3-A.)

- **As soon as possible:** Revascularize. Cardiac catheterization with **angioplasty** when available, or thrombolytics if angioplasty is not available.
- **Within the first day:** Begin oral β-blockers, ACEIs (if BP tolerates). The role of empiric statin use is unclear, but it is probably beneficial.
- **Long term:** Treat CAD with aspirin, β-blockers, and statins (if LDL > 100). If ejection fraction is low, treat systolic dysfunction with an ACEI or ARB and spironolactone.
- NSTEMI—a bit more complicated:
  - **Immediately:** As above for immediate treatment of STEMI, except that low-molecular-weight heparin (enoxaparin) is preferred over unfractionated heparin.
  - **Glycoprotein IIb/IIIa inhibitors** (e.g., eptifibatide or abciximab) should be given to all patients who will undergo catheterization or who are at high risk as suggested by ongoing pain, stuttering chest pain, or ST depression with pain.
  - **As soon as possible:** Revascularize with **angioplasty.** If this is not possible, **do not give thrombolytics!** If the patient will not go to bypass surgery, give clopidogrel.
  - **Long term:** As above.

COMPLICATIONS

- If a patient suddenly becomes short of breath, think of papillary muscle rupture → sudden mitral regurgitation, ventricular wall rupture → left-to-right shunt (ruptured ventricular septum), or cardiac tamponade (free wall rupture).
- If chest pain recurs, think about reocclusion or pericarditis.
- Ventricular arrhythmias are a serious risk in the post-MI period.

Absolute contraindications to thrombolytics:

- *Internal bleeding*
- *An ischemic stroke within the past year*
- *A hemorrhagic stroke at any time*
- *Aortic dissection*
- *Intracranial neoplasm*

Inflammation of the pericardial sac. The many causes include viral infection, mediastinal radiation, MI, cancer, rheumatologic diseases (**SLE**), and idiopathic pericarditis.

SYMPTOMS

Positional chest pain that is often improved by sitting up. If a large effusion is present, the patient may be short of breath.

EXAM

Exam may reveal a pericardial friction rub.

DIFFERENTIAL

Myocardial ischemia, aortic dissection, pneumonia, pulmonary embolism, pneumothorax.

DIAGNOSIS

Finding ST-segment elevation in numerous ECG leads will help distinguish pericarditis from MI.

- **Diffuse ST-segment elevation** on ECG (see Figure 2.2-2).
- Echocardiogram may reveal an associated effusion.
- Search for an underlying cause—take a history for viral illness, radiation exposure, and malignancy. Check antinuclear antibodies, PPD, blood cultures if febrile, and renal function.

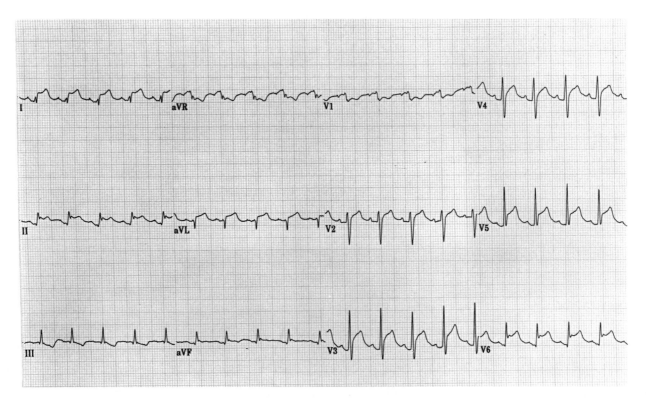

FIGURE 2.2-2. Pericarditis.

(Reproduced, with permission, from Stobo J et al. *The Principles and Practice of Medicine*, 23rd ed. Stamford, CT: Appleton & Lange, 1996:20, Fig. 1-3-2A.)

- When possible, treat the underlying disorder, such as SLE or advanced renal failure.
- For viral or idiopathic pericarditis, give NSAIDs or aspirin. Avoid NSAIDs in post-MI pericarditis because they may interfere with scar formation.

COMPLICATIONS

Patients can develop a clinically significant pericardial effusion and **tamponade**.

▶ PERIPHERAL VASCULAR DISEASE

Atherosclerotic disease of vessels other than the coronary arteries. Risk factors are similar to those for CAD: **smoking**, diabetes, hypercholesterolemia, hypertension, and increasing age.

SYMPTOMS

Depends on the organ affected:

- **Mesenteric ischemia:** Postprandial abdominal pain and food avoidance.
- **Lower extremity:** Claudication, ulceration.
- **Kidneys:** Usually asymptomatic, but may present with difficult-to-control hypertension.
- **CNS:** Stroke and TIA (see the Neurology chapter).

EXAM

- **Mesenteric disease:** No specific findings. The patient may be thin because of weight loss from avoiding food.
- **Lower extremity disease:** Ulcers, diminished pulses, skin atrophy and loss of hair, and **bruits** over affected vessels (abdominal, femoral, popliteal).
- **Renal artery stenosis:** Listen for **bruit during systole and diastole** (highly specific).

DIFFERENTIAL

- **Abdominal pain:** Stable symptoms can mimic PUD or biliary colic. If the colon is predominantly involved, episodes of pain and bloody stool can look like infectious colitis.
- **Lower extremities: Spinal stenosis** can produce lower extremity discomfort similar to claudication. Claudication improves with standing still, but spinal stenosis classically improves with **sitting** (lumbar flexion improves spinal stenosis symptoms).

DIAGNOSIS

- **Mesenteric disease:** A diagnosis of exclusion. Angiography reveals lesions.
- **Lower extremity disease: Ankle-brachial index** (compares BP in the lower and upper extremity), Doppler ultrasound. Angiography or MRA is used in preparation for revascularization but is generally not used for diagnosis.
- **Renal artery stenosis:** Angiography, MRA, or ultrasound with Doppler flow (technically difficult).

Acute vessel occlusion from an embolus or an in situ thrombus presents with sudden pain (abdominal or extremity) and is an emergency.

TREATMENT

- Control risk factors, especially smoking.
- **Mesenteric disease:** Surgical revascularization or angioplasty.
- **Lower extremity disease:** Exercise to improve functional capacity, surgical revascularization, and sometimes angioplasty. Cilostazol is moderately useful (improves pain-free walking distance 50%); while pentoxifylline has marginal benefit.
- **Renal artery stenosis:** Surgery or angioplasty might be useful.

▶ STRESS TESTING

Indications for stress testing are as follows (not a comprehensive list):

- **Diagnosis** of CAD/evaluation of symptoms.
- Preoperative evaluation.
- Risk assessment in patients with known disease.
- Decision making about the need for revascularization.

Contraindications (not a comprehensive list) include the following:

- Severe aortic stenosis.
- Unstable coronary syndrome.
- Decompensated heart failure.

Testing consists of a stressing modality and an evaluating modality (see Tables 2.2-5 and 2.2-6).

- The stressor can be walking on a treadmill or IV dobutamine.
- Evaluating modalities are ECG, echocardiogram, and nuclear imaging such as thallium.
- An additional testing method is adenosine or dipyridamole with nuclear imaging. Adenosine and dipyridamole dilate the coronary arteries, but areas with plaque cannot vasodilate. These agents thus ↑ blood flow in healthy arteries but cause no change in diseased arteries, creating a differential flow that is detected on nuclear imaging.

Table 2.2-5.   Stressing Modalities in Cardiac Testing

STRESSING MODALITY	PROS	CONS
Treadmill	Good for patients who can walk.	
Dobutamine	Good for patients who cannot exercise.	
Adenosine or dipyridamole (with nuclear imaging)	Good for patients who cannot exercise.	Can cause bronchospasm—be cautious in patients with COPD.

Table 2.2-6.   **Evaluating Modalities in Cardiac Testing**

EVALUATING MODALITY	PROS	CONS
ECG	Inexpensive.	Cannot localize the lesion; cannot use with baseline ST-segment abnormalities or left bundle branch block.
Echocardiogram	Good in patients with left bundle branch block; cheaper than nuclear imaging.	Technically limited echo images or resting wall motion abnormalities can limit usefulness.
Radionuclide tracer (thallium or technetium)	Localizes ischemia; localizes infarcted tissue.	Expensive.

► CARDIAC TAMPONADE

Small-volume fluid collections can cause symptoms if they accumulate quickly. Gradually developing collections can accumulate 1–2 L before causing symptoms. Common causes include pericarditis with effusion, ventricular free wall rupture, aortic dissection extending to the aortic root, and trauma.

SYMPTOMS

- Shortness of breath, syncope.
- Symptoms associated with the underlying process, such as chest pain with an MI.

EXAM

↑ **JVP is found in nearly 100% of patients.** Also presents with hypotension, tachycardia, **pulsus paradoxus** (a drop in systolic BP during inspiration > 10 mmHg), and muffled heart sounds.

DIFFERENTIAL

- **Acute development:** Pulmonary embolus, MI, tension pneumothorax.
- **Gradual development:** Heart failure, lung disease.

DIAGNOSIS

CXR may show a large cardiac silhouette if there is a large-volume effusion; ECG may show low voltage. **Echocardiogram** shows effusion and may show right atrial or right ventricular dynamic collapse in diastole.

TREATMENT

If there is hemodynamic compromise, treat with IV fluids and urgent **pericardiocentesis.** For recurrent effusions, a pericardial window may be needed.

Think of tamponade in any patient with pulseless electrical activity.

All valve lesions need endocarditis prophylaxis except mitral valve prolapse.

Table 2.2-7 describes the clinical characteristics and treatment of common valvular lesions.

Table 2.2-7. Presentation and Treatment of Select Valvular Lesions

LESION	SYMPTOMS	EXAM	TREATMENT	COMMENTS
Mitral stenosis	Symptoms of heart failure, hemoptysis.	Diastolic murmur, opening snap.	HR control, balloon valvuloplasty, valve replacement.	Usually caused by **rheumatic fever.**
Mitral regurgitation	Usually asymptomatic unless severe or acute; then symptoms of heart failure.	**Blowing** systolic murmur at the apex, **radiating to the axilla.**	If acute, usually needs surgery. For chronic mitral regurgitation, repair or replace the valve when symptomatic or if the ejection fraction is falling.	Long-standing regurgitation dilates the atrium, ↑ the chance of atrial fibrillation.
Mitral valve prolapse	Asymptomatic.	Midsystolic click; also murmur if mitral regurgitation is present.	Endocarditis prophylaxis only with mitral regurgitation.	Questionable association with palpitations and panic attacks.
Aortic stenosis	Chest pain, syncope, heart failure.	Harsh systolic murmur radiating to the carotids. **Small and slow carotid upstroke** (parvus et tardus) with severe stenosis.	**Avoid overdiuresis; avoid vasodilators** such as nitrates and ACEIs. Surgery for all symptomatic patients.	Once symptoms appear, mortality is 50% at three years.
Aortic regurgitation	Usually asymptomatic until advanced; then symptoms of heart failure.	**Wide pulse pressure.** Soft, high-pitched diastolic murmur.	**Afterload reduction** with ACEIs, hydralazine. Valve replacement if symptomatic or ↓ ejection fraction.	Many cases are associated with aortic root disease, dissection, syphilis, ankylosing spondylitis, and Marfan's.

CARDIOVASCULAR

HIGH-YIELD FACTS

Emergency Medicine

Determine which toxin the patient was exposed to and by what means—i.e., through ingestion (most common), inhalation, injection, or absorption. Determine how much exposure was involved and when; ascertain if any other substances were involved. Ask about symptoms and determine if the exposure was intentional.

EXAM/DIAGNOSIS

Vitals signs give clues to the type of ingestion:

- **Hyperthermia:** Thyroid medication, nicotine, aspirin, anticholinergics, amphetamines, PCP, cocaine, SSRIs, neuroleptics.
- **Hypothermia:** Carbon monoxide, alcohol, sedative-hypnotics, barbiturates.
- **Tachycardia:** Cocaine, amphetamines, PCP, thyroid medication, anticholinergics, TCAs.
- **Bradycardia:** β-blockers, calcium channel blockers, clonidine, digitalis, opioids.
- **Tachypnea:** Salicylates, organophosphates.
- **Hypertension:** Amphetamines, cocaine, PCP, anticholinergics.
- **Hypotension:** Sedative-hypnotics, organophosphates, alcohols, opioids, digitalis, β-blockers, calcium channel blockers, TCAs.

Other diagnostic clues based on symptoms and signs are as follows:

- **Breath odor:**
  - **Bitter almonds:** Cyanide.
  - **Violets:** Turpentine.
  - **Mothballs:** Camphor, naphthalene.
  - **Garlic:** Organophosphates.
  - **Pear:** Chloral hydrate.
- **Pupils:**
  - **Constricted:** Follow the mnemonic **COPS**—Clonidine, Opiates, Pontine bleed, Sedative-hypnotics.
  - **Dilated:** Amphetamines, anticholinergics, cocaine.
- **Pulmonary edema:** Opioids, salicylates, toxic inhalations (chlorine, nitric oxide, phosgene), cocaine, organophosphates, ethylene glycol.
- **Bowel sounds:**
  - ↑: Opiate withdrawal, sympathomimetics.
  - ↓: Anticholinergics, opiate toxicity.
- **Skin findings:**
  - **Needle tracks:** Opioids.
  - **Diaphoresis:** Salicylates, organophosphates, sympathomimetics.
  - **Jaundice:** Acetaminophen (after liver failure), mushroom poisoning.
  - **Alopecia:** Arsenic, thallium, chemotherapeutic agents.
  - **Cyanosis:** Drugs causing methemoglobinemia (e.g., nitrates/nitrites, "caine" anesthetics, aniline dyes, chlorates, dapsone, sulfonamides).

Table 2.3-1 gives symptoms and signs associated with common toxin-induced syndromes ("toxidromes").

Table 2.3-1. Common "Toxidromes"

	SYMPTOMS/SIGNS	EXAMPLES
Cholinergics	**DUMBBELS: D**iarrhea, **U**rination, **M**iosis, **B**radycardia, **B**ronchospasm, **E**mesis, **L**acrimation, **S**alivation.	Organophosphates, pilocarpine, pyridostigmine, muscarine-containing mushrooms.
Anticholinergics	"Hot as a stove, red as a beet, dry as a bone, mad as a hatter": fever, skin flushing, dry mucous membranes, psychosis, mydriasis, tachycardia, urinary retention.	Heterocyclic antidepressants, atropine, scopolamine, antihistamines, Jimson weed.
Opioids	Triad of coma, respiratory depression, and miosis.	Morphine, oxycodone, heroin.
Sedative-hypnotics	CNS depression, respiratory depression, and coma.	Alcohol, barbiturates, benzodiazepines.
Extrapyramidal	Parkinsonian symptoms: tremor, torticollis, trismus, rigidity, oculogyric crisis, opisthotonos, dysphonia, and dysphagia.	Phenothiazines, haloperidol, metoclopramide.

TREATMENT

- Elimination:
  - **Activated charcoal:** First-line treatment. Administer in a dose of 1 g/kg. Avoid multiple doses of cathartics (e.g., sorbitol), especially in young children.
  - **Whole bowel irrigation** (e.g., polyethylene glycol with electrolytes to wash toxins from the GI tract): Useful for ingestions of lithium, iron, heavy metals, sustained-released drugs, and body packers (e.g., cocaine).
- Removal of unabsorbed toxin:
  - **Emesis:** Ipecac in adults (30 cc) and children (15 cc).
    - **Indications:** The patient is awake; the ingestion was recent (< 30–60 minutes); the ingestion was moderately or highly toxic.
    - **Contraindications:** Altered mental status, ↓ or absent gag reflex, caustic agents (to prevent reinjury of the esophagus on emesis), agents that are easily aspirated, nontoxic ingestion.
  - **Gastric lavage:**
    - **Indications:** Known or suspected serious ingestion; recent ingestion (< 30–60 minutes); the patient is awake and cooperative or intubated; the patient can be placed in the left lateral decubitus position.
    - **Contraindications:** Same as those with emetics.
- Removal of absorbed toxin:
  - **Alkalization methods:** Involve mixing D_5W with 2–3 amps of $NaHCO_3$.
    - Alkalinization of blood improves clearance of heterocyclic antidepressants.
    - Alkalinization of urine to pH > 8 ionizes weak acids into ionized molecules, thus ↑ excretion of salicylates, phenobarbital, and chlorpropamide.

- **Charcoal hemoperfusion:** ↑ absorption of toxic substances in the blood by filtering blood from a shunt through a column of activated charcoal. Particularly useful for aminophylline, barbiturates, carbamazepine, and digoxin.
- **Hemodialysis:** Filters **small, ionized molecules** such as salicylates, theophylline, methanol, lithium, barbiturates, and ethylene glycol.

Substance-specific antidotes are outlined in Table 2.3-2. Drug withdrawal treatments are delineated in Table 2.3-3.

Diagnose and treat the victim's physical and emotional injuries. Collect legal evidence; document your findings carefully and completely.

- **Where and when** did the assault occur?
- What happened **during the assault?** Determine the following:
    - **Number** of assailants.
    - Use of force, weapons, objects, or restraints.
    - **Orifices** penetrated.
    - Use of alcohol or drugs.
- What happened **after the assault?**
    - Did the patient **bathe, defecate, urinate, brush teeth,** or **change clothes?**
    - Are there any specific symptoms or pains?
- Has the patient had **sexual intercourse in the last 72 hours?**
- Determine the **risk of pregnancy.** Last menstrual period? Any birth control?

EXAM

General trauma and pelvic exam (see the trauma discussion below).

DIAGNOSIS

- Medically indicated tests:
    - Pregnancy test.
    - Culture for gonorrhea and chlamydia.
    - Serology for syphilis.
    - Hepatitis B and C testing.
    - HIV testing.
- **Evidence collection:** Must pass through an unbroken **chain of evidence.**
    - Debris and dried secretions from skin.
    - Combed and plucked head and pubic hairs.
    - Fingernail scraping and clipped fingernails.
    - Saliva sample.
    - Oral, anal, and vaginal smears.
    - Blood sample.
    - Nasal mucus sample.

TREATMENT

- Treat traumatic injuries.
- **Infection prevention:**
    - Gonorrhea, chlamydia, trichomonas, bacterial vaginosis.
    - Hepatitis B and HIV prophylaxis.
- **Pregnancy prevention:** Two Ovral tablets PO stat and in 12 hours.
- Counseling.

Table 2.3-2. **Specific Antidotes**

Toxin	Antidote
Acetaminophen	N-acetylcysteine
Anticholinesterases/ organophosphates	Atropine, pralidoxime
Antimuscarinics, anticholinergics	Physostigmine
Arsenic, mercury, lead	British anti-Lewisite (BAL): dimercaprol + 2,3-dimercaptosuccinic acid
Atropine	Physostigmine
Benzodiazepine	Flumazenil
β-blockers	Glucagon
Carbon monoxide	O_2
Cyanide	Amyl nitrite pearls, sodium nitrite, sodium thiosulfate
Digoxin	Digitalis Fab fragments
Ethylene glycol, methanol	Fomepizole; alternatively, ethanol drip
Heparin	Protamine sulfate
Iron	Deferoxamine
Isoniazid (INH)	Pyridoxine (vitamin B_6)
Lead	Calcium disodium edetate (EDTA)
Nitrites	Methylene blue
Opioids	Naloxone
Phenothiazines	Diphenhydramine, benztropine
Salicylates	Sodium bicarbonate, dialysis
TCAs	Sodium bicarbonate
Warfarin	Vitamin K, fresh frozen plasma

HIGH-YIELD FACTS

EMERGENCY MEDICINE

Table 2.3-3. Drug Withdrawal Syndromes and Treatment

DRUG	WITHDRAWAL SYMPTOMS	TREATMENT
Alcohol	Tremor, tachycardia, hypertension, agitation, seizures, hallucinations, **DTs** (autonomic instability, including tachycardia, hypertension, and delirium) within 2–7 days. Mortality is 15–20%.	Benzodiazepines; haloperidol for hallucinations. Thiamine, folate, and multivitamin replacement—i.e., **banana bag** (does not affect withdrawal but may prevent Wernicke's encephalopathy).
Barbiturates	Anxiety, seizures, delirium, tremor, cardiac and respiratory depression.	Benzodiazepines.
Benzodiazepines	Rebound anxiety, seizures, tremor. May lead to **DTs.**	Benzodiazepines.
Cocaine and amphetamines	Depression, hyperphagia, hypersomnolence (washout syndrome).	Supportive treatment. Avoid β-blockers in cocaine users (→ uninhibited α-cardiac stimulation with cocaine use).
Opioids	Anxiety, insomnia, **flulike symptoms,** sweating, piloerection, fever, rhinorrhea, nausea, stomach cramps, diarrhea, mydriasis.	Symptom management. Clonidine and/or buprenorphine for moderate withdrawal; methadone for severe symptoms.

▶ **TRAUMA**

Begin with the ABCs and 1° survey; then progress to resuscitation and the 2° survey (see below).

ABCs AND 1° Survey

Always do the trauma algorithm in order.

Initiate trauma treatment as follows:

- **A:** Airway maintenance with cervical spine control.
- **B:** Breathing with ventilation.
- **C:** Circulation with hemorrhage control.
- **D:** Disability—brief neurologic examination:
  - **AVPU system: A**—Alert; **V**—responds to Vocal stimuli; **P**—responds to Painful stimuli; **U**—Unresponsive.
  - **Glasgow Coma Scale (GCS):** Based on the **best** response of E + V + M (see Figure 2.3-1).
  - **Other neurologic exam:** Examine for unequal pupils, depressed skull fracture, focal weakness, and posturing.
- **E:** Exposure/Environmental control—completely undress the patient, but prevent hypothermia.
- **Resuscitation.**
  - **IV access:** Think **short and fat** IV lines—e.g., two large-bore, 18-gauge antecubital lines.
  - Estimate and replace fluid and blood losses.

The maximum score on the GCS is 15; the lowest score is 3.

Eye Opening (E)	Verbal Response (V)	Motor Response (M)
4 Spontaneous	**5** Oriented	**6** Obeys commands
3 Responds to voice	**4** Confused speech	**5** Localizes pain
2 Responds to pain	**3** Inappropriate speech	**4** Withdraws to pain
1 No response	**2** Incomprehensible	**3** Abnormal flexion
	1 No response	**2** Abnormal extension
		1 No response

FIGURE 2.3-1. Scoring of the Glasgow Coma Scale.

THE 2° Survey

The 2° **survey**—total patient evaluation—proceeds as follows:

- **AMPLE** history: **A**llergies, **M**edications, **P**ast medical history, **L**ast meal eaten, **E**vents/Environment related to the injury.
- **Organ system assessment and management:**
    - **Head and skull:**
        - **Assessment:** Inspect for trauma, pupils, and LOC. Inspect for hemorrhage around the mastoid (**Battle's sign**), eyes (**raccoon's eyes**), and tympanic membrane (all are indicative of a basilar skull fracture). Inspect the nose for CSF leakage and for unstable airway due to facial fractures.
        - **Management:** Maintain airway; continue oxygenation and ventilation. Obtain a CT of the head and face if indicated; intubate if necessary. If the GCS is < 8, intubate!
    - **Neck:**
        - **Assessment:** Look for trauma; palpate for midline tenderness/deformity and tracheal deformity.
        - **Management:** Maintain in-line immobilization and protection with a hard cervical collar. Obtain cervical spine radiographs as needed.
    - **Chest:**
        - **Assessment:** Inspect for irregular or paradoxical breathing patterns from multiple rib fractures—i.e., **flail chest.** Listen for equal and bilateral breath sounds (if not found, suspect **pneumothorax**) and clear heart sounds (if muffled and accompanied by JVD, suspect **cardiac tamponade**).
        - **Management:** Tube thoracostomy if pneumothorax (needle thoracostomy if tension pneumothorax); pericardiocentesis if cardiac tamponade.
    - **Abdomen:**
        - **Assessment:** Inspect the anterior and posterior abdomen for signs of trauma. Palpate the pelvis for tenderness. Obtain a pelvic x-ray; arrange for an abdominal ultrasound/abdominal CT if indicated.
        - **Management:** Transfer to an OR in the presence of a penetrating wound to the abdomen deeper than the fascia or with any significant bleeding or bowel injury.
    - **Perineum/rectum/vagina:** Assess for trauma, including urethral bleeding. Check for prostate position, rectal tone, and rectal blood. If the patient is female, check for vaginal trauma and blood in the vaginal vault.

GCS < 8–intubate!

The spleen is the most commonly injured solid organ in blunt abdominal trauma.

- **Musculoskeletal:**
  - **Assessment:** Look for evidence of trauma, including contusions, lacerations, and deformities. Inspect the extremities for tenderness, crepitus, abnormal range of motion, and sensation.
  - **Management:** Obtain radiographs as needed. Maintain immobilization of the patient's thoracic and lumbar spine. Apply a splint as indicated. Open fractures and suspected compartment syndromes require urgent orthopedic consultation. Administer tetanus immunization as required.

▶ COMMON DYSRHYTHMIAS

See Figures 2.3-2 through 2.3-13 for a variety of board-testable dysrhythmias.

▶ ADVANCED CARDIAC LIFE SUPPORT (ACLS)

Start with **CPR** and **determine rhythm.**

> **ACLS steps—ABCDEF**
>
> **A**irway
> **B**reathing
> **C**irculation
> **D**rugs
> **E**lectricity (shock)
> **F**luids

Ventricular Fibrillation (VF)/Pulseless Ventricular Tachycardia (VT)

- **Shock** three times up to 360 J.
- Then **epinephrine** (up to 3x) → shock → vasopressin → shock.
- Amiodarone, lidocaine, magnesium, or procainamide may be tried. Shock after each dose.

Pulseless Electrical Activity (PEA)

- Identify and treat underlying causes:
  - **The 5 H's:** Hypovolemia, Hypoxia, H^+ acidosis, Hyper-/Hypokalemia, Hypothermia.
  - **The 5 T's:** "Tablets" (drug OD), cardiac Tamponade, Tension pneumothorax, Thrombosis—coronary, Thrombosis—PE.
- Epinephrine q 3–5 minutes × 3.
- Atropine q 3–5 minutes × 3 if slow PEA rate.

Asystole

- Identify/treat underlying causes.
- Consider a transcutaneous pacemaker.
- Epinephrine q 3–5 minutes × 3.
- Atropine q 3–5 minutes × 3.

Bradycardia

- Atropine q 3–5 minutes × 3 prn.
- Transcutaneous pacemaker (also if 2° or 3° **AV block**).
- Dopamine drip.
- Epinephrine drip.
- Isoproterenol drip.

Unstable Tachycardia

- Synchronized cardioversion.

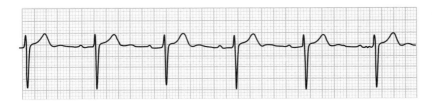

FIGURE 2.3-2. First-degree atrioventricular block.

(Reproduced, with permission, from Gomella LG, Haist SA. *Clinician's Pocket Reference*, 10th ed. New York: McGraw-Hill, 2004:394.)

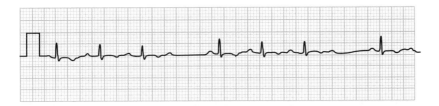

FIGURE 2.3-3. Second-degree atrioventricular block, Mobitz I/Wenckebach.

(Reproduced, with permission, from Gomella LG, Haist SA. *Clinician's Pocket Reference*, 10th ed. New York: McGraw-Hill, 2004:394.)

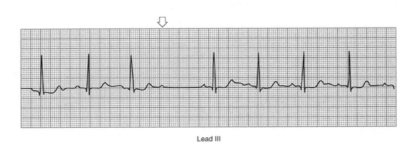

Lead III

FIGURE 2.3-4. Second-degree atrioventricular block, Mobitz II, non-Wenckebach.

(Reproduced, with permission, from Sondheimer HM, Boucek MM, Ivy DD, Lorts A, Schaffer MS, Wolfe RR. *Current Pediatric Diagnosis and Treatment*, 16th ed. Denver: McGraw-Hill/Appleton & Lange, 2002.)

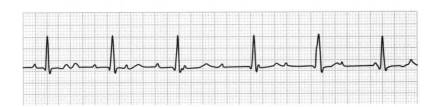

FIGURE 2.3-5. Third-degree atrioventricular block.

(Reproduced, with permission, from Gomella LG, Haist SA. *Clinician's Pocket Reference*, 10th ed. New York: McGraw-Hill, 2004:395.)

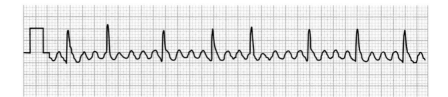

FIGURE 2.3-6. Atrial flutter.

(Reproduced, with permission, from Gomella LG, Haist SA. *Clinician's Pocket Reference*, 10th ed. New York: McGraw-Hill, 2004:391.)

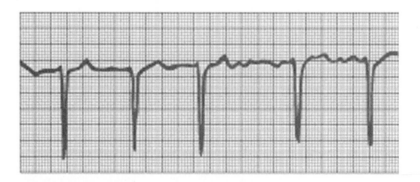

FIGURE 2.3-7. Atrial fibrillation.

(Reproduced, with permission, from Josephson ME, Zimetbaum P. *Harrison's Principles of Internal Medicine*, 15th ed. New York: McGraw-Hill, 2001.)

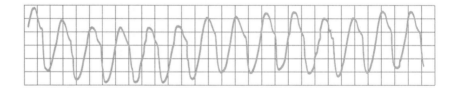

FIGURE 2.3-8. Ventricular tachycardia.

(Reproduced, with permission, from Katzung BG. *Basic & Clinical Pharmacology*, 8th ed. New York: McGraw-Hill, 2001:1016.)

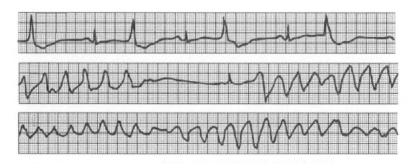

FIGURE 2.3-9. Torsades de pointes.

(Reproduced, with permission, from Josephson ME, Zimetbaum P. *Harrison's Principles of Internal Medicine*, 15th ed. New York: McGraw-Hill, 2001).

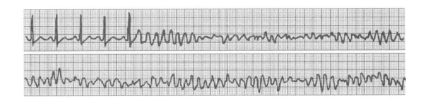

FIGURE 2.3-10. Ventricular fibrillation.

(Reproduced, with permission, from Josephson ME, Zimetbaum P. *Harrison's Principles of Internal Medicine*, 15th ed. New York: McGraw-Hill, 2001).

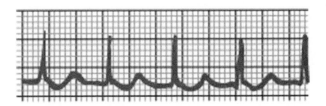

FIGURE 2.3-11. AV nodal reentrant tachycardia.

(Reproduced, with permission, from Harrison's Principles of Internal Medicine Online, www.AccessMedicine.com, © 2004 McGraw-Hill.)

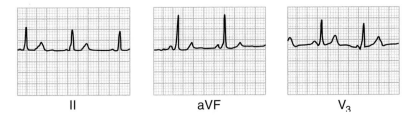

| II | aVF | V₃ |

FIGURE 2.3-12. Wolff-Parkinson-White syndrome (preexcitation).

(Reproduced, with permission, from Gomella LG, Haist SA. *Clinician's Pocket Reference*, 10th ed. New York: McGraw-Hill, 2004:402.)

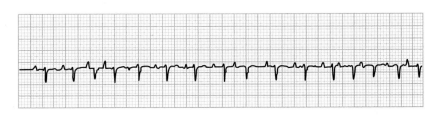

FIGURE 2.3-13. Multifocal atrial tachycardia.

(Reproduced, with permission, from Gomella LG, Haist SA. *Clinician's Pocket Reference*, 10th ed. New York: McGraw-Hill, 2004:390.)

Stable Supraventricular Tachycardia (SVT)

- Vagal stimulation.
- Adenosine 6 mg IV push.
- Adenosine 12 mg IV push.
- IV diltiazem if no CHF.
- Adenosine 12 mg IV push.

Stable Monomorphic VT

- Procainamide or sotalol.
- Amiodarone or lidocaine.
- If CHF, amiodarone or lidocaine followed by DC cardioversion.

Stable Wide-Complex Tachycardia

- If no CHF, treat with DC cardioversion, procainamide, or amiodarone.
- If CHF, treat with DC cardioversion or amiodarone.

▶ HEAT EMERGENCIES

Heat Exhaustion

- Extreme fatigue with **profuse sweating.** Also presents with nausea/vomiting and dull headache.
- Body temperature is **normal** or **slightly** ↑. Patients are tachypneic, tachycardic, and hypotensive.
- Treat with IV NS and a cool environment.

Heat Stroke

- A true emergency!
- ↑ **body temperature;** altered mental status. Hot, dry skin, often with no sweating; ataxia.
- Treat with rapid and **aggressive cooling.** Remove from the heat source and undress. Atomized tepid water spray; ice packs to the groin/axillae.

Heat stroke presents with altered mental status and ↑ temperature, often with no sweating.

▶ COLD EMERGENCIES

Frostbite

- **Superficial:** Skin is soft under a frozen surface. Large, clear, fluid-filled vesicles develop within 1–2 days. Nonviable structures demarcate and slough off, leaving new skin that is pink and hypersensitive.
- **Deep:** Skin is hard under a frozen surface. Nonviable structures demarcate and slough off.
- Rapid rewarming is key but should not be started until refreezing can be prevented. Circulating water heated to 40°C. Local wound care; tetanus prophylaxis.

Do not rewarm frostbite until refreezing can be prevented.

Hypothermia

- Core body temperature < 35°C (95°F).
- Causes include environmental exposure, hypoglycemia, CNS or hypothalamic dysfunction, hypothyroidism, **alcohol,** drugs (barbiturates, benzodiazepines, narcotics), skin disorders, and sepsis.
- Look for **Osborn/J waves** on ECG.
- Risk of dysrhythmias, especially **ventricular fibrillation** at core temperatures < 30°C.

TREATMENT

- ABCs, CPR, and stabilization.
- Rewarming:
  - Passive external rewarming (blanket).
  - Active external rewarming (hot water bottles, warming blanket).
  - Active core rewarming (warm humidified O_2; heated IV fluids; gastric, colonic, bladder, or peritoneal lavage; extracorporeal rewarming).
  - Hypothermic patients should not be pronounced dead **until** after they have been rewarmed to 35°C.
- Bretylium is the drug of choice for ventricular fibrillation.

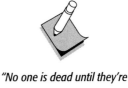

"No one is dead until they're warm and dead."

▶ BURNS

Determine if the victim is in an enclosed or an open space. Are there any toxic products of combustion? Any respiratory symptoms? Carbon monoxide poisoning?

EXAM

- Gauge the body surface area (BSA) involved. **Rule of 9's: 9%** BSA for head, each arm; **18%** BSA for back torso, front torso, each leg. In **children,** 9% BSA for each arm; 18% BSA for head, back torso, front torso; 14% BSA each leg.
- Determine the **depth of the burn** (see Table 2.3-4).

TREATMENT

- **Prehospital:**
  - IV fluid and high-flow O_2.
  - Remove the patient's clothes and cover with clean sheets or dressings.
  - Administer pain medications.
- **Hospital:**
  - **ABCs: Early airway control** is most important. Intubate if:
    - The patient is unconscious or obtunded.
    - The patient is in respiratory distress with facial burns, soot in the airway, singed nasal hairs, and carbonaceous sputum.

Table 2.3-4. Burn Classification

	TISSUE INVOLVEMENT	FINDINGS
First degree	Epidermis only.	Red and painful.
Second degree (superficial)	Epidermis and superficial dermis.	Red, wet, and painful with **blisters.**
Second degree (deep)	Epidermis and deep dermis.	White, dry, and tender.
Third degree	Epidermis and **entire dermis.**	Charred, pearly white, and **nontender.**
Fourth degree	Below the dermis to bone, muscle, and fascia.	

- **Fluid resuscitation** for patients with > 20% BSA second-degree burns:
    - Give 4 cc/kg per % total BSA (**Parkland formula**) over 24 hours—the first half over the first 8 hours and the second half over the next 16 hours.
    - Maintain a urine output of 1 cc/kg/hr.
  - Tetanus prophylaxis.
  - Pain control.
- **Disposition:**
  - **Minor burns:** Discharge with pain medications.
  - **Moderate burns** (partial thickness 15–25% BSA or full thickness < 10% BSA): Hospital admission.
  - **Major burns** (partial thickness > 25% BSA or full thickness > 10% BSA; burns to the face, hands, joints, feet, or perineum; electrical or circumferential burns): Refer to a burn center.

▶ ELECTRICAL INJURIES

Electrical current flows most easily through tissues of low resistance (nerves, blood vessels, mucous membranes, and muscles). The current pathway determines which organs are affected.

SYMPTOMS

- **Alternating current (household and commercial):**
  - Explosive exit wounds.
  - Effects are worse with AC than with DC current at the same voltage.
  - Ventricular fibrillation is common.
- **Direct current (industrial, batteries, lightning):**
  - Discrete exit wounds.
  - Asystole is common.

TREATMENT

- ABCs.
- IV fluids for severe burns.
- Pain medications.
- Treat burns.
- Treat **myoglobinuria** with IV fluids to maintain a urine output of 1.5–2.0 cc/kg/hr.
- Tetanus prophylaxis.
- Asymptomatic low-voltage (< 1000 V) burn victims can go home.

▶ TETANUS

Presents with trismus ("lockjaw"), glottal spasm, and convulsive spasms. High-risk patients include the elderly (due to inadequate immunization), IV drug abusers, and ulcer patients.

TREATMENT

- Benzodiazepine to control muscle spasms.
- Neuromuscular blockade if needed to control airway.
- **Metronidazole** is the antibiotic of choice.
- Tetanus immune globulin (TIG), tetanus and diphtheria toxoid adsorbed (Td) as indicated in Table 2.3-5.

Table 2.3-5. Tetanus Prophylaxis Schedule

HISTORY OF ADSORBED TETANUS TOXOID (DOSES)	NON-TETANUS-PRONE WOUNDS	TETANUS-PRONE WOUNDS[a]	
	TD	TD	TIG
Unknown or < 3 doses	✓	✓	✓
Three doses:			
Last dose > 5 years		✓	
Last dose > 10 years	✓	✓	

[a]Tetanus-prone wounds are those that are present > 6 hours; are nonlinear; are > 1 cm deep; and show signs of infection, devitalized tissue, and contamination.

▶ ANIMAL BITES

- If the bite is from a domestic animal and if the animal can be captured/secured and its behavior observed as normal for 10 days, no treatment is necessary.
- If the bite is from a domestic animal that exhibits abnormal behavior or becomes ill, the animal should be sacrificed and the head/brain tested for rabies via a direct immunofluorescent antibody study. If that study is ⊖, no treatment is necessary. If it is ⊕, immediate treatment is indicated.
- If the animal is wild, immediate treatment is indicated.
  - **Active immunization** with human diploid cell vaccine (HDCV).
  - **Passive immunization** with **human rabies immune globulin (HRIG)**.
- See Table 2.3-6 for a summary of bite types, associated infecting organisms, and treatment.

▶ EYE CONDITIONS

Corneal Abrasion

- Presents with **pain out of proportion to the exam** as well as with foreign-body sensation and photophobia.
- **Fluorescein staining** (cobalt blue light source via slit lamp or Wood's lamp) reveals an abraded area.
- Treat with topical broad-spectrum antibiotics (e.g., gentamicin, sulfacetamide, bacitracin), tetanus prophylaxis, and oral analgesics.

Viral Conjunctivitis

- Painful, itchy, red eye with watery discharge. **Frequently bilateral.** Often concomitant with cold symptoms (e.g., rhinorrhea, sore throat, cough).
- Look for diffuse conjunctival injection with normal vision and **preauricular lymphadenopathy.** Multiple superficial punctate corneal lesions are seen on fluorescein staining.
- Treat with topical antibiotics to prevent bacterial superinfection.

Bacterial Conjunctivitis

- Painful, red eye. **Usually unilateral.** Also presents with photophobia, gritty foreign-body sensation, and purulent exudate. Causative organisms in-

Table 2.3-6. Bite Types, Infecting Organisms, and Treatment

Bite Type	Likely Organisms	Treatment
Dog	α-hemolytic streptococcus, *S. aureus,* and *Pasteurella multocida.*	**Amoxicillin/clavulanate** or a first-generation cephalosporin. +/– tetanus and rabies prophylaxis.
Cat	**P. multocida** (high rate of infection).	**Amoxicillin/clavulanate** +/– tetanus.
Human	Polymicrobial. Viridans streptococci most frequent.	Second- or third-generation cephalosporins, dicloxacillin + penicillin, **amoxicillin/clavulanate,** or clarithromycin. +/– tetanus prophylaxis. +/– hepatitis B vaccine +/– hepatitis B immunoglobulin. +/– postexposure prophylaxis for HIV.

clude *Neisseria gonorrhoeae* and *Chlamydia trachomatis* in newborns and in sexually active adults.

- Diffuse conjunctival injection with normal visual acuity. See bacteria on Gram stain.
- Treat with topical **10% sulfacetamide** or aminoglycoside for *Staphylococcus* or *Streptococcus;* IV ceftriaxone and topical erythromycin or tetracycline for suspected *N. gonorrhoeae.* IV and topical erythromycin for *Chlamydia.* Warm compresses and frequent flushes.

Allergic Conjunctivitis

- Intensely pruritic, watery eyes. Most commonly affects males with a family history of **atopy.**
- Look for diffuse conjunctival injection with normal visual acuity. Lid edema; cobblestone papillae under the upper lid.
- Treat with topical antihistamine/vasoconstrictor preparations such as **naphazoline/pheniramine** or with mast cell stabilizers such as **cromolyn** or **olopatadine.** Cool compresses.

Chemical Conjunctivitis

Alkali burns do far more damage than acid burns.

- Caused by acid or alkali exposure.
- Determine pH from litmus paper. **Coagulation necrosis** is seen in acid burns, **liquefaction necrosis** in alkali burns.
- Copious irrigation with a Morgan's lens until pH is neutral. Tetanus prophylaxis.

Ruptured Globe

- Patients present with trauma and loss of vision.
- Look for vitreous humor leak → a teardrop-shaped pupil; marked ↓ in visual acuity.
- Do a CT scan. Often, diagnosis can be made only by clinical means.
- Manage with a rigid eye shield to prevent pressure on the globe. Immediate ophthalmologic consultation.

Endocrinology

"Honeymoon period": A remission phase that occurs in type 1 diabetics days after the initiation of insulin therapy. During this phase, which inevitably ends after a few months, patients often have ↓ insulin requirements.

Type 1 DM— the 3 P's

Polyuria
Polydipsia
Polyphagia

DM is classified into two types (see Table 2.4-1).

SYMPTOMS/EXAM

Patients present with the classic symptoms of Polyuria (including nocturia), Polydipsia, and Polyphagia **(the 3 P's)**. They can also have rapid or unexplained weight loss, blurry vision, or recurrent infections (e.g., candidiasis).

DIFFERENTIAL

Pancreatic disease (e.g., chronic pancreatitis), glucagonoma, Cushing's disease, iatrogenic factors (e.g., corticosteroids), gestational diabetes, diabetes insipidus (DI).

DIAGNOSIS

At least one of the following is required to make the diagnosis:

- A random plasma glucose concentration ≥ 200 mg/dL with classic symptoms of diabetes.
- A fasting plasma glucose ≥ 126 mg/dL on two separate occasions.
- Two-hour postprandial glucose ≥ 200 mg/dL after a 75-g oral glucose tolerance test (on two separate occasions).

Patients with a clinical picture suggestive of diabetes should be screened with a **fasting blood glucose.** Screening should also be conducted every three years if the patient:

Table 2.4-1.   Type 1 vs. Type 2 DM

	TYPE 1 (INSULIN-DEPENDENT DM)	TYPE 2 (NON-INSULIN-DEPENDENT DM)
Pathophysiology	Failure of the pancreas to secrete insulin as a result of autoimmune destruction of B cells.	Insulin resistance and inadequate insulin secretion by the pancreas to compensate.
Incidence	15%.	85%.
Age (exceptions are common)	< 30 years of age.	> 40 years of age.
Association with obesity	No.	Yes.
"Classic symptoms"	Common.	Sometimes.
Diabetic ketoacidosis (DKA)	Common.	Rare.
Genetic predisposition	Weak, polygenic.	Strong, polygenic.
Association with HLA system	Yes (HLA-DR3 and -DR4).	No.
Serum C-peptide	↓; Can be normal initially during the "honeymoon period."	↑; ↓ Late in the disease.

- Is > 45 years of age.
- Has a fasting glucose level of 110–126 mg/dL.
- Is obese.
- Is habitually physically inactive.
- Is of African-American, Hispanic, or Native American ethnicity.
- Has delivered a baby weighing > 9 lb.
- Has a family history of diabetes in a first-degree relative.
- Has a history of gestational diabetes, hypertension, dyslipidemia, or polycystic ovarian disease.

TREATMENT

- **Type 1 diabetics** should be started on insulin (see Table 2.4-2). The most popular regimen for insulin therapy is as follows:
    - **Estimated total daily insulin requirement (ETDIR):** 0.5 U/kg.
    - Divide the ETDIR as shown in Figure 2.4-1.
- **Type 2 diabetics** should be started on an oral antidiabetic medication (see Table 2.4-3).
    - Typical stepwise management includes metformin, a "glitazone," and a sulfonylurea (e.g., glyburide).
    - If the patient continues to have inadequate control on three oral antidiabetic drugs, glyburide should be replaced with NPH insulin at bedtime.

MAINTENANCE

- **Monitor blood glucose** (see Table 2.4-4).
    - **Type 1:**
        - Pre-breakfast glucose level reflects pre-dinner NPH dose.
        - Pre-lunch glucose level reflects for all pre-breakfast regular insulin dose.
        - Pre-dinner glucose level reflects for all pre-breakfast NPH dose.
        - Bedtime glucose level reflects for all pre-dinner regular insulin dose.
    - **Type 2:**
        - Check a fasting glucose level once a day.
- Check a **hemoglobin A_{1c} (HbA_{1c})** level every three months. Maintain $HbA_{1c} < 7$.
- Maintain a low-fat, reduced-carbohydrate diet. Refer to a dietitian.
- Manage **CAD risk factors**—hypertension, smoking, obesity, and hyperlipidemia.

HbA_{1c} is used to monitor the efficacy of and compliance with treatment, since it reflects glucose levels over the previous three months.

Table 2.4-2. Insulin Formulations

TYPE	TIME OF ONSET OF ACTION	PEAK EFFECT
Aspart	10–15 minutes	0.5–1.5 hours
Lispro	10–15 minutes	1–2 hours
Regular	45 minutes	2–5 hours
NPH	2–4 hours	6–10 hours
Glargine	4 hours	None (lasts 16–20 hours)

(Reproduced, with permission, from Le T et al. *First Aid for the USMLE Step 2,* 4th ed. New York: McGraw-Hill, 2004:124.)

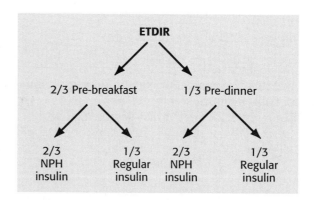

FIGURE 2.4-1. ETDIR dosing by meal and insulin type.

- Obtain a baseline ECG if the patient has heart disease or is > 35 years of age.
- Check eyes annually for retinopathy or cataracts. Also do an eye exam if the patient is planning a pregnancy.
- Screen for **thyroid disease** in newly diagnosed type 1 diabetics.
- Order an annual BUN/creatinine and UA for **microalbuminuria** to screen for diabetic nephropathy.
- Check the **feet** annually for neuropathy, ulcers, and peripheral vascular disease. Patients should inspect feet daily and wear comfortable shoes.
- Give an annual flu shot. Keep pneumococcal vaccination up to date.

COMPLICATIONS

Acute complications include DKA, hyperosmolar nonketotic coma, and hypoglycemia 2° to excessive drug treatment.

▶ DIABETIC KETOACIDOSIS (DKA)

Runaway catabolism due to lack of insulin action plus ↑ counterregulatory hormones → life-threatening metabolic acidosis. DKA may be the initial manifestation of type 1 DM.

SYMPTOMS/EXAM

Typically seen in **type 1 diabetics.** Patients are dehydrated and present with altered mental status, **"fruity" breath** (acetone), anorexia, nausea, vomiting,

Table 2.4-3. Oral Antidiabetic Medications

MEDICATION	MECHANISM OF ACTION	SIDE EFFECTS	CONTRAINDICATIONS
Metformin	↑ glucose uptake in peripheral tissue.	GI upset, lower extremity edema, weight gain.	Lactic acidosis, renal failure, CHF.
"Glitazone"	Same as above.	Hepatotoxicity, anemia.	Lactic acidosis.
Glyburide or glipizide	Promotes ↑ insulin secretion from the pancreas.	Hypoglycemia.	

Table 2.4-4. **Target Glucose Levels in Diabetics**

	NORMAL GLUCOSE LEVEL (MG/DL)	TARGET GLUCOSE LEVEL WITH DRUG TREATMENT (MG/DL)	ADJUST DOSAGE OF DRUG WHEN GLUCOSE LEVEL IS:
Preprandial glucose	< 110	80–120	< 80 or > 140
Bedtime glucose	< 120	100–140	< 100 or > 160

fatigue, abdominal pain, and Kussmaul respirations (**rapid, deep breathing**). DKA can be preceded by 1–2 days of polyuria and polydipsia.

DIAGNOSIS

- Hyperglycemia > 250 mg/dL.
- Acidosis with blood pH < 7.3 (anion gap metabolic acidosis).
- Serum bicarbonate < 15 mEq/L.
- Serum/urine $\oplus$ for ketones.

Establish the diagnosis by ordering a CBC, electrolytes, BUN/creatinine, glucose, ABG, and serum ketones. DKA is usually **precipitated by a stressor** that must be identified and treated. Do a CXR, blood culture, and UA/urine culture to look for infection. Look for MI with an ECG. Other precipitating factors include medication noncompliance, surgery, and trauma.

TREATMENT

Patients must be admitted to the ICU for fluid resuscitation (3–4 L in eight hours) with NS and IV insulin. Identify and treat the precipitating cause (e.g., antibiotics). Sodium, potassium, phosphate, and glucose (change NS fluids to D_5NS when glucose < 250 mg/L) must be monitored and repleted every two hours. Change IV insulin to an SQ insulin sliding scale once the anion gap normalizes.

▶ HYPERGLYCEMIC HYPEROSMOLAR NONKETOTIC STATE (HHNK)

Severe hyperglycemia in the absence of significant ketosis, with hyperosmolarity and dehydration.

SYMPTOMS/EXAM

Patients are typically **older type 2 diabetics.** They appear acutely ill and dehydrated with altered mental status.

DIAGNOSIS

Diagnostic criteria are as follows:

- Hyperglycemia > 600 mg/dL.
- Serum pH > 7.3.
- Serum bicarbonate > 15 mEq/L.
- Normal anion gap < 14 mEq/L.
- Serum osmolality > 310 mOsm/kg.

DKA is often triggered by infection, surgery, MI, or poor diabetic management.

HIGH-YIELD FACTS

ENDOCRINOLOGY

As with DKA, look for a stressor such as infection, MI, medication noncompliance, surgery, or trauma. Table 2.4-5 compares HHNK to DKA.

TREATMENT

ICU care and 4–6 L NS within the first eight hours. Identify the precipitating cause (e.g., antibiotics) and treat. Monitor and replete sodium, potassium, phosphate, and glucose every two hours. Give IV insulin only if glucose levels remain elevated after sufficient fluid resuscitation.

▶ DIABETIC NEPHROPATHY

- Usually asymptomatic, but can present with bilateral lower extremity edema (from nephrotic syndrome).
- Patients with microalbuminuria or proteinuria should be started on an ACEI to keep their BP < 120/80.
- End-stage nephropathy requires chronic hemodialysis or transplantation.
- Kimmelstiel-Wilson lesions (nodular glomerulosclerosis) may be seen on kidney biopsy.
- Look for **coexisting retinopathy**.

▶ FUNCTIONAL THYROID DISEASE

Classified as hyperthyroidism or hypothyroidism. **Myxedema coma** is a form of severe hypothyroidism characterized by altered mental status and hypothermia. **Thyroid storm** is a form of severe hyperthyroidism characterized by high fever, dehydration, tachycardia, coma, and high-output cardiac failure.

SYMPTOMS/EXAM

Table 2.4-6 lists the clinical characteristics of hypo- and hyperthyroidism.

Table 2.4-5. DKA vs. HHNK

	DKA	HHNK	LACTIC ACIDOSIS
Diabetic types	Type 1 > type 2	Older type 2	On metformin or critically ill
Hyperglycemia (mg/dL)	> 250	> 600	+/–
Blood pH	< 7.3	≥ 7.3	< 7.3
Serum bicarbonate (mEq/L)	< 15	> 15	< 15
Anion gap	↑↑	None	↑↑ (↑ lactate)
Ketosis	+++	+/–	+/–

Table 2.4-6.   **Clinical Presentation of Functional Thyroid Disease**

	HYPOTHYROIDISM	HYPERTHYROIDISM
General	Fatigue, lethargy.	Hyperactivity, nervousness, fatigue.
Temperature	Cold intolerance.	Heat intolerance.
GI	Constipation → ileus; weight gain despite poor appetite.	Diarrhea; weight loss despite good appetite.
Cardiac	Bradycardia, pericardial effusion, hyperlipidemia.	Tachycardia, atrial fibrillation, CHF; systolic hypertension, ↑ pulse pressure.
Neurologic	Delayed DTRs.	Fine resting tremor.
Menstruation	Heavy.	Irregular.
Dermatologic	Dry, coarse skin; thinning hair; thin, brittle nails; myxedema.	Warm, sweaty skin; fine, oily hair; nail separation from matrix.
Other	Arthralgias/myalgias.	**Osteoporosis,** proptosis.

DIFFERENTIAL

- **Hyperthyroidism:** Anxiety, malignancy, pheochromocytoma, pregnancy, mania, chronic alcoholism.
- **Hypothyroidism:** Depression, CHF, dementia, malnutrition, 1° amyloidosis, sick euthyroid syndrome, chronic fatigue.

DIAGNOSIS

- Order a TSH and free T_4 to distinguish hyperthyroidism from hypothyroidism.
- **Hyperthyroid patients (↓TSH):** Order a radioactive iodine uptake scan, thyroglobulin antibody, anti-thyroid peroxidase (TPO) antibody, and thyroid-stimulating immunoglobulin.
- **Hypothyroid patients (↓TSH):** Order a thyroglobulin antibody and anti-TPO antibody.
- Figure 2.4-2 and Table 2.4-7 outline the workup, differential, and treatment of functional thyroid disease.

Free T_4 is more accurate than total T_4 because it is not affected by changes in thyroxine-binding globulin (TBG).

TREATMENT

- **Symptomatic hyperthyroidism** is treated with **propranolol,** hydration, rest, and adequate nutrition. Cooling measures are required for severe hyperthermia. Mild cases of hyperthyroidism can then be treated with **propylthiouracil** or **methimazole.** More severe cases require radioactive ^{131}I thyroid ablation. **Thyroidectomy** is indicated for large goiters, pregnant patients, or obstruction of the trachea. Patients who have undergone radioactive ablation or thyroidectomy become hypothyroid and are treated with PO levothyroxine.
- **Hypothyroidism** is treated with **levothyroxine.** Patients with myxedema coma need IV levothyroxine and IV hydrocortisone. Mechanical ventilation and warming blankets are required for hypoventilation and hypothermia, respectively.

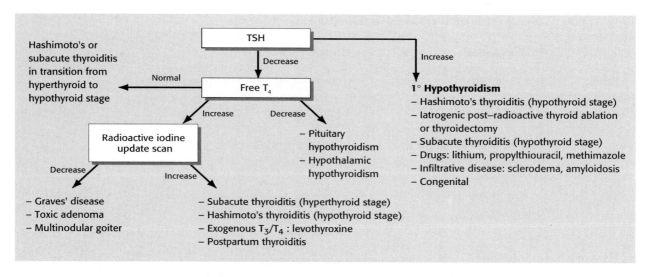

FIGURE 2.4-2. **Workup of Functional Thyroid Disease**

► **OSTEOPOROSIS**

A common metabolic bone disease characterized by osteopenia with normal bone mineralization. More common in inactive, **postmenopausal Caucasian women.**

SYMPTOMS/EXAM

Commonly asymptomatic. Patients may present with **hip fractures, vertebral compression fractures** (resulting in loss of height and progressive thoracic kyphosis), and/or distal radius fractures after minimal trauma.

DIFFERENTIAL

Osteomalacia (inadequate bone mineralization), hyperparathyroidism, multiple myeloma, metastatic carcinoma (pathologic fracture).

DIAGNOSIS

- All patients > 65 years of age as well as those 40–60 years of age with at least one risk factors for osteoporotic fractures after menopause should be screened with a dual-energy x-ray absorptiometry (DEXA) scan of the spine and hip.
- Take the lowest **T-score** between the hip and the spine:
  - **Osteopenia:** T-score −1 to −2.5.
  - **Osteoporosis:** T-score ≤ 2.5.
- Rule out **2° causes,** including smoking, alcoholism, renal failure, hyperthyroidism, multiple myeloma, heparin, and chronic steroid use.

TREATMENT

Avoid hormone replacement therapy because of the risk of cardiovascular mortality and breast cancer.

Treat when a T-score is < −2 or when a T-score is < −1.5 in a patient with risk factors for osteoporotic fractures. Drugs of choice, in order of efficacy, include **bisphosphonates** (alendronate, etidronate), selective estrogen receptor modulators (raloxifene), and intranasal calcitonin. Eliminate or treat 2° causes. Add weight-bearing exercise and calcium and vitamin D supplementation. A DEXA scan should be repeated 1–2 years after initiation of drug therapy. If the T-score is found to have worsened, combination therapy (e.g., a selective estrogen receptor modulator [SERM] and a bisphosphonate) should be tried.

Table 2.4-7. **Differential and Treatment of Thyroid Diseases**

	GRAVES' DISEASE	SUBACUTE THYROIDITIS	HASHIMOTO'S THYROIDITIS
Etiology	Antibody directed at TSH receptor.	Viral (possibly mumps or coxsackievirus).	Autoimmune disorder.
History/exam	Hyperthyroidism. More prevalent in females. Diffuse, painless goiter. Proptosis, lid lag, diplopia, conjunctival injection. Pretibial myxedema.	Hyperthyroidism → hypothyroidism. Tender thyroid. Malaise, upper respiratory tract symptoms, fever early on.	Hyperthyroidism → hypothyroidism. Painless thyroid enlargement.
Tests	↓ radioactive iodine uptake scan. ⊕ thyroglobulin antibody. ⊕ thyroid-stimulating immunoglobulin.	↑ radioactive iodine uptake scan. ⊕ thyroglobulin antibody.	↑ radioactive iodine uptake scan. ⊕ thyroglobulin antibody. ⊕ anti-TPO antibody.
Treatment specific to disease	Ophthalmopathy may require surgical decompression, steroids, or low-dose orbital radiation.	NSAIDs for pain control; add steroids for severe pain.	

▶ **CUSHING'S SYNDROME**

Results from hypercortisolism. **Cushing's disease** is Cushing's syndrome caused by hypersecretion of ACTH from a pituitary adenoma.

SYMPTOMS/EXAM

Look for truncal obesity with moon facies and a **"buffalo hump."** Psychiatric disturbances, hypertension, impotence, oligomenorrhea, growth retardation, hirsutism (excessive hair growth, acne), easy bruisability, and purple striae can also be seen.

DIFFERENTIAL

Chronic alcoholism, depression, DM, chronic steroid use, adrenogenital syndrome.

DIAGNOSIS

Elevated 24-hour urine cortisol is diagnostic for Cushing's syndrome. Low DHEA is seen only with exogenous steroids. Check A.M. serum ACTH.

- **If A.M. serum < 5 pg/mL:** Exogenous steroids or obtain an adrenal CT or MRI to look for adrenal adenoma or carcinoma (unilateral) or adrenal hyperplasia (bilateral).
- **If A.M. serum > 5 pg/mL:** High-dose dexamethasone suppression test.
  - **Suppressed cortisol response:** Cushing's disease (e.g., ACTH-secreting pituitary adenoma). Confirm with a pituitary MRI.

- **Nonsuppressed cortisol response:** Ectopic ACTH-producing tumor such as carcinoid tumors and small cell lung cancer. Can be seen on octreotide scan and/or MRI/CT chest. If ⊖, do a pituitary MRI.

TREATMENT

- **Ectopic secreting ACTH tumor:** Surgical resection of the tumor.
- **Adrenal carcinoma, adenoma, or hyperplasia:** Adrenalectomy.
- **ACTH-secreting pituitary adenoma:** Transsphenoidal resection or radiation treatment.
- **Exogenous steroids:** Minimize use.

▶ ADRENAL INSUFFICIENCY

Adrenocortical hypofunction can stem from adrenal failure (1° adrenal insufficiency, also known as **Addison's disease**) or from ↓ ACTH production from the pituitary (2° adrenal insufficiency).

- **Causes of 1° adrenal insufficiency:** Autoimmune (idiopathic), metastatic tumor, hemorrhagic infarction (from coagulopathy or septicemia), adrenalectomy, granulomatous disease (TB, sarcoid).
- **Causes of 2° adrenal insufficiency:** Withdrawal of exogenous steroids, hypothalamic or pituitary pathology (tumor, infarct, trauma, infection, iatrogenic). **AdD**ison's disease is due to **A**drenocortical **D**eficiency.

SYMPTOMS/EXAM

Symptoms include weakness, anorexia, weight loss, nausea, vomiting, postural hypotension, diarrhea, abdominal pain, myalgias, and arthralgias. Infection, surgery, or other stressors can trigger an **addisonian crisis** with symptomatic adrenal insufficiency, confusion, and vasodilatory shock.

DIAGNOSIS

An A.M. serum cortisol < 5 μg/dL or < 20 μg/dL after ACTH simulation test, is diagnostic. Nonspecific findings include hyponatremia, hyperkalemia, and eosinophilia. Check A.M. serum ACTH to distinguish 1° from 2° adrenal insufficiency (see Table 2.4-8).

TREATMENT

Treat with glucocorticoids and mineralocorticoids. **Hydrocortisone** is the drug of choice. Add **fludrocortisone** for orthostatic hypotension, hyponatremia, or hyperkalemia. Glucocorticoid doses should be ↑ in times of illness, trauma, or surgery. Patients in **adrenal crisis** need immediate fluid resuscitation and IV hydrocortisone.

Table 2.4-8. 1° vs. 2° Adrenal Insufficiency

	ADDISON'S DISEASE	2° ADRENAL INSUFFICIENCY
ACTH	↑	↓
Cortisol after ACTH challenge	↓	↑

(Reproduced, with permission, from Le T et al. *First Aid for the USMLE Step 2,* 4th ed. New York: McGraw-Hill, 2004:121.)

AdDison's disease is due to

Adrenocortical
Deficiency

Hyperpigmentation, dehydration, and salt craving are specific to 1° adrenal insufficiency.

Ethics and Statistics

Be familiar with the following principles:

- **Autonomy:** Governing of oneself according to one's own system of morals and beliefs.
- **Beneficence:** The state of doing or producing good.
- **Nonmaleficence:** The state of not doing harm or evil.
- **Truth telling:** Remembering to tell the facts as they are to patients.
- **Proportionality:** Ensuring that a medical treatment or plan is commensurate with the illness and with the goals of treatment.
- **Distributive justice:** Distribution of the same level of goods or services to each person.

Informed Consent

Involves discussions with patients about their diagnosis, their prognosis, the proposed treatment, the risks and benefits of that treatment, and alternatives. Only with such information can a patient reach a decision. **Do not hide a diagnosis from a patient.** However, respect your patients' wishes if they tell you to share only certain things with them.

Use of Restraints

Psychiatric patients can be held against their will only if they are a danger to themselves or others (in accordance with the principle of beneficence). The use of restraints can be considered if a patient is at risk of doing harm to self or others, but such use must be evaluated on at least a daily basis.

Rights of Minors

Patients < 18 years of age do not require parental consent:

- If they are emancipated (i.e., financially independent, married, raising children, living on their own, or serving in the armed forces).
- Parental consent is also not needed for contraception or for the treatment of pregnancy, STDs, or psychiatric illness.
- In general, for the Step 3 test, the governing principle should be to let minors make their own decisions.

The determination of competency is made by the courts. In the case of incompetency, if there is no prior assigned guardian or next of kin, a court-appointed guardian should be arranged.

Health Care Power of Attorney (HCPOA)

HCPOA refers to an individual whom patients have previously chosen to represent them and to express their wishes in the event that they themselves are no longer able to do so.

Surrogate/Proxy

If no person has been formally designated to represent the patient, the responsibility to do so falls to relatives according to a hierarchy that may vary from state to state (typically, a spouse is at the top of this hierarchy). Relevant language varies from state to state as well; depending on which state you are in, the terms *proxy, surrogate,* or *HCPOA* may mean either a formally designated individual or a de facto spokesperson.

Do Not Resuscitate (DNR) Orders

Physicians should inquire about and follow DNR orders during each hospitalization. Similarly, if a family informs you that a patient would not want to be on a ventilator and this decision is congruent with your medical decision, respect the wishes of the family.

▶ CONFIDENTIALITY

The confidentiality of patient information is critical. The rules and guidelines outlined in the Health Insurance Portability and Accountability Act (HIPAA) work to preserve the privacy and confidentiality of patient information as well as that of the patient-doctor relationship.

When to Violate Confidentiality

In a situation in which a physician learns about a threat to an individual's life or well-being, violating confidentiality is permissible. Similarly, information about child abuse must be reported.

Reportable Conditions

Include syphilis, gonorrhea, chlamydia, TB, mumps, measles, rubella, smallpox, and other infections that may vary by state.

▶ END-OF-LIFE CARE

Mentally competent adults in the end stages of a terminal illness have the right to obtain medical treatment that is intended to preserve human dignity in dying. There is no legal difference between withholding and withdrawing care.

The best means of reaching an agreement with the patient and family regarding end-of-life care is to continue to talk about the patient's condition and to resolve decision-making conflicts. Ultimately, this is the same task that the ethics consult will try to do for you and the patient.

The Principle of "Double Effect"

A given action can have more than one consequence, one of which may be intended and the other not. If the intended consequence is legitimate and proportionate, then an unintended but unavoidable bad consequence may be acceptable. For example, it is acceptable for a dying patient to receive medical care that is intended to relieve suffering but that will have the unintended consequence of shortening life (e.g., opiates given for air hunger that also suppress respiratory drive).

The Elisabeth Kübler-Ross psychological stages at the end of life are denial, anger, bargaining, depression, and acceptance.

Advance Directives

These are oral or written statements regarding what patients would want in the event that they require intensive resuscitative efforts. Such conversations or documents should guide what happens to patients in the event that they become incompetent. Oral statements are ethically binding but are not legally binding in all states. Well-informed, competent adults have the right to refuse treatment even if it means that doing so would lead to death.

Pain in Terminally Ill Patients

Terminally ill patients are often inadequately treated for pain. Therefore, do not be afraid to prescribe as much narcotic medication as is needed to relieve patients' pain and suffering. Do not worry about addiction in this setting. Two-thirds of patients in their last three days of life stated that they felt moderate to severe pain.

Persistent Vegetative State (PVS)

Defined as a state in which the brain stem is intact and the patient has sleep-wake cycles, but there is no consciousness and no ability to interact with the environment.

Euthanasia

Currently, the act of physician-assisted suicide (euthanasia) is illegal in all states except Oregon.

Withdrawal of Care

Withdrawal of care is appropriate when all parties are in agreement. However, if the medical team feels that it is futile to continue the care, it may also be appropriate to withdraw care. If the patient's representatives and the doctors have made clear decisions regarding how long they may continue a trial of therapy, it may be easier to withhold care that is not going to change the outcome.

Quality of Life

Refers to the extent to which patients' lives are affected by their current physical, emotional, and social well-being or by treatment. This principle is subjective and must be evaluated from the perspective of the patient.

Palliation

An attempt to manage symptoms and to bolster psychosocial as well as physical care in a manner that preserves dignity and makes the patient and family as comfortable as possible in a difficult time. Involves an interdisciplinary collaboration focusing on patient-defined goals of care.

Sensitivity

The probability that a person with a certain disease will have a positive test result. Because the goal of a screening test is to identify everyone with a given disease, high sensitivity is desirable in such a test.

Specificity

The probability that a person without the disease will have a negative test result. High specificity is desirable for a confirmatory test.

Positive Predictive Value (PPV)

The probability that a person with a positive test result has the disease (true positives/all those who tested positive; see Table 2.5-1). If a disease has a higher prevalence, then the PPV is higher. Conversely, in a population with a low disease prevalence, most positive tests will be false positives.

Negative Predictive Value (NPV)

The probability that a person with a negative test result is disease free (see Table 2.5-1). A test has a higher NPV value when a disease has a lower prevalence.

Relative Risk (RR)

Seen with cohort (prospective) studies. Compares the chance of a given disease in the group exposed to the particular risk factor with the chance of disease in those not exposed to the risk factor (see Table 2.5-2).

Odds Ratio (OR)

Part of case-control (retrospective) studies. Describes the odds of exposure to a given risk factor in individuals with the disease compared to those without the disease (see Table 2.5-2). In rare diseases, the OR approximates the RR.

Incidence

The number of new cases of disease/total population.

Prevalence

The number of existing cases of disease/total population.

| **PID** = **P**ositive **I**n **D**isease. |

| **NIH** = **N**egative **I**n **H**ealth. |

HIGH-YIELD FACTS

ETHICS AND STATISTICS

Table 2.5-1. **Determination of PPV and NPV**

	DISEASE PRESENT	**NO DISEASE**	
Positive test	a	b	PPV = a/(a + b)
Negative test	c	d	NPV = d/(c + d)
	Sensitivity = a/(a + c)	Specificity = d/(b + d)	

Table 2.5-2. Determination of RR and OR

	DISEASE DEVELOPS	NO DISEASE	
Exposure	a	b	RR = [a/(a + b)]/[c/(c + d)]
No exposure	c	d	OR = ad/bc

Note the large difference that can occur between absolute and relative risk reduction. RRR has the potential to look deceptively large, so watch out for drug advertising that touts RRR rather than ARR.

If a 95% CI crosses or includes 1, the results are not significant. So if an RR is 1.9 but the 95% CI is 1.0–4.6, the RR is not significant.

Absolute Risk Reduction (ARR)

A useful statistical tool in randomized controlled trials. Numerically, ARR = the absolute adverse event rate in placebo – the absolute adverse event rate for the treated patients. It takes into account the background rate of the disease.

Relative Risk Reduction (RRR)

In randomized controlled trials, the fractional reduction in the risk of the measured outcome when a group of patients is treated. Numerically, RRR = (the event rate in untreated patients – the event rate in treated patients)/the event rate in untreated patients.

Number Needed to Treat (NNT)

Expresses the number of patients that would need to be treated to prevent one event. NNT = 1/ARR. *Example:* A randomized control trial shows that treatment with a medication reduces the risk of heart attack from 7% to 4%. The ARR is 7% – 4% = 3%. The NNT is 1/0.03 = 33. The RRR is (0.07 – 0.04)/0.07 = 0.42 (i.e., 42%).

Statistical Significance/*p*-Value

The *p*-value expresses the chance that an observed outcome is the product of random chance. A *p*-value of < 0.05 means that the observed outcome has a < 5% chance that it was a random occurrence. A *p*-value of < 0.05 is accepted as the cutoff for a genuine difference in outcome.

Confidence Interval (CI)

Like the *p*-value, the CI expresses the certainty that the observation is real or is a product of random chance. Used with ORs and RR, the 95% CI says the observed risk or odds have a 95% chance of being within the interval. Thus, in Figure 2.5-1, the relative risk of cancer with smoking is 2.0 with a 95% CI of 1.3–3.5—meaning that the **observed** RR of cancer was 2.0, and that there is a 95% certainty that the **actual** RR of cancer from smoking falls somewhere between 1.3 and 3.5.

▶ **STUDY DESIGN**

Cohort Study

Takes a large population and divides it into groups on the basis of exposure status to a risk factor being studied. The population is then observed over time to see what outcomes occur. Can be prospective or retrospective; gives RR if prospective. Not good for rare conditions.

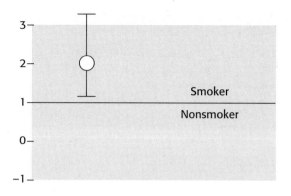

FIGURE 2.5-1. **Relative risk of cancer.**

Case-Control Study

A group of people with a given disease and an otherwise similar group of people without the disease are retrospectively compared for exposure to risk factors. Good for rare disease; can see the correlation of multiple exposures. Comparison is expressed as OR. Always retrospective.

Randomized Control Trial

A study in which people are randomly assigned to a treatment group or a placebo group. The placebo group and the treatment group are then compared to determine if the treatment made a difference.

Gastroenterology

► ESOPHAGEAL DYSPHAGIA

Obstruction of passage of food or liquid through the esophagus.

SYMPTOMS/EXAM

Patients note difficulty swallowing or say that food sticks or hangs up. Distinguish from **odynophagia,** which is pain with swallowing that is typically caused by *Candida,* CMV, or HSV infections in immunocompromised patients (HIV or chemotherapy).

DIAGNOSIS

Workup includes barium swallow and/or EGD.

- If difficulty is with **solids alone,** consider:
    - **Lower esophageal ring:** Intermittent symptoms or sudden obstruction with a food bolus (**"steakhouse syndrome"**). The ring is located at the gastroesophageal junction.
    - **Plummer-Vinson syndrome:** Cervical esophageal web and iron deficiency anemia. Associated with esophageal cancer.
    - **Peptic stricture:** Progressive symptoms with long-standing heartburn.
    - **Carcinoma:** Progressive symptoms in an older person.
- If difficulty is with both **solids and liquids,** consider:
    - **Esophageal spasm:** Intermittent symptoms with chest pain. Triggered by acid, stress, and hot and cold liquids. Presents with **"corkscrew esophagus"** on barium swallow.
    - **Achalasia:** Progressive symptoms that worsen at night with no heartburn (see Figure 2.6-1). Presents with **"bird beak"** on barium swallow. Characterized by the **AAA** syndrome: **A**lacrima, **A**drenal insufficiency, and **A**chalasia.
    - **Scleroderma:** Progressive symptoms with heartburn and Raynaud's phenomenon (**CREST** syndrome: **C**alcinosis cutis, **R**aynaud's phenomenon, **E**sophageal dysmotility, **S**clerodactyly, and **T**elangiectasia).

► GASTROESOPHAGEAL REFLUX DISEASE (GERD)

Risk factors include hiatal hernia, obesity, collagen vascular disease, alcohol, caffeine, nicotine, chocolate, fatty foods, and pregnancy.

SYMPTOMS/EXAM

- Uncomfortable hot and burning sensation beneath the sternum.
- Usually worsens after meals and with reclining and tight clothes.

DIAGNOSIS

Barium swallow, endoscopy, esophageal biopsy, ambulatory pH monitoring (pH < 4 for > 4.5% of a 24-hour period).

TREATMENT

- **Lifestyle modifications:** Elevate the head of the bed; promote weight loss; avoid bedtime snacks, trigger foods, cigarettes, and NSAIDs.
- **Drugs:** Antacids, prokinetics, H_2 blockers, proton pump inhibitors (PPIs).
- **Other:**
    - If the disease is refractory to medical therapy, consider evaluation for Nissen fundoplication or hiatal hernia repair.

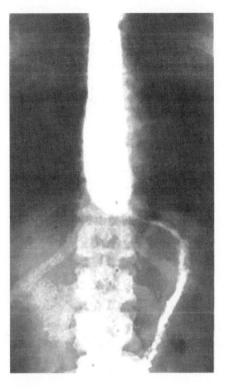

FIGURE 2.6-1. Achalasia of the esophagus.

Moderately advanced achalasia. Note the dilated body of the esophagus and the smoothly tapered lower portion. (Reproduced, with permission, from Way LW, Doherty GM [eds]. *Current Surgical Diagnosis & Treatment*, 11th ed. New York: McGraw-Hill, 2003:478.)

- Consider endoscopy to screen for Barrett's, especially in patients requiring continual medical therapy.

▶ PEPTIC ULCER DISEASE (PUD)

The most common sites are the **stomach** and **duodenum**. *H. pylori* infection and **NSAIDs/aspirin** are major causes. Rarely from Zollinger-Ellison syndrome, HSV infection, CMV, and cocaine use.

SYMPTOMS/EXAM

- **Epigastric** abdominal pain described as **"gnawing"** or **"aching"** that comes in waves. May also present with dyspepsia and upper GI bleed.
  - **Duodenal ulcers** are relieved by food, and the pain comes on a few hours **postprandially.**
  - **Stomach ulcers** are worsened by food and are characterized by **pain with eating.**
- **Red flags:** With diarrhea, weight loss, and gastric pH = 1, think of the rare causes (Zollinger-Ellison syndrome, systemic mastocytosis, hyperparathyroidism, small bowel resection).

DIAGNOSIS

- **Detect the ulcer: Endoscopy** with rapid urease testing; biopsy any gastric ulcers.

- Look for *H. pylori* infection:
  - **Urease testing** of biopsy sample.
  - **Serum antibody:** Easy to obtain, but a ⊕ antibody may not necessarily mean active infection. Remains ⊕ even after treatment.
  - **Urea breath test:** Good for detecting active infection, but the patient must be off PPIs, antibiotics, or bismuth for several weeks.
  - Fecal antigen test for *H. pylori*.

TREATMENT

- **Discontinue aspirin/NSAIDs;** stop smoking.
- PPIs to control symptoms and ↓ acid secretion.
- For *H. pylori* infection, initiate multidrug therapy. Can use two of the following three drugs—**amoxicillin 1 g TID, clarithromycin 500mg BID,** or **metronidazole 500 mg BID**—plus a PPI (**omeprazole, lansoprazole**).

▶ INFLAMMATORY BOWEL DISEASE (IBD)

Two distinct chronic inflammatory diseases consisting of **Crohn's** and **ulcerative colitis.** Clusters in families; twice as common among **Jews** and four times more common in **Caucasians** than in other ethnicities.

Crohn's Disease

- **Transmural inflammation** anywhere from the mouth to the anus (**skip lesions**).
- Most commonly affects the **terminal ileum,** small bowel, and colon. Presents with **linear ulcerations** with areas of normal mucosa and with **fissures** and **cobblestoning.**
- ↑ incidence in Caucasians, especially Jews.
- Bimodal with peaks in the 20s and 50s–70s.

SYMPTOMS/EXAM

- **GI symptoms: Colicky RLQ pain,** diarrhea (mucus-containing, non-bloody stools), weight loss, anorexia, low-grade fever, **perirectal abscess/fistula,** periodic joint pain, fecal incontinence with small amounts of stool.
- **Other symptoms:** Erythema nodosum, pyoderma gangrenosum (see Figure 2.6-2), iritis and episcleritis, gallstones, kidney stones, arthritis.
- Patients are thin and pale with temporal wasting and RLQ tenderness/fullness; many present with perianal fistula.

DIAGNOSIS

- **Labs:** CBC, iron, folate, B_{12}, ESR, LFTs, stool WBC, RBC, and O&P.
  - **Anemia:** Look for normocytic anemia of chronic disease or anemias from malabsorption of iron, B_{12}, or folate.
  - ↑ ESR.
  - O&P is ⊖, but fecal leukocytes and occult blood may be ⊕.
  - Expect normal LFTs.
- **Skip lesions** are seen on colonoscopy; **"cobblestoning"** is seen on barium enema. Biopsy shows noncaseating granuloma with mononuclear cell infiltrate. Stricture formation and a pseudodiverticulum may be seen on imaging (see Figure 2.6-3).

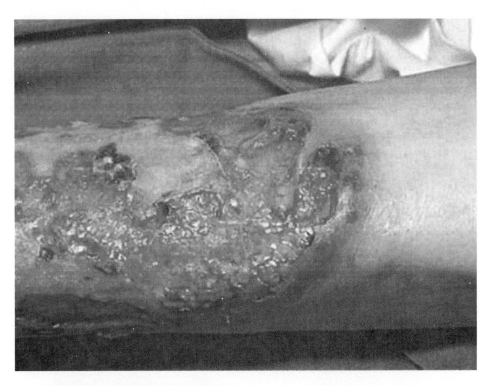

FIGURE 2.6-2. Pyoderma gangrenosum.

(Reproduced, with permission, from Bondi EE, Jegasothy BV, Lazarus GS [eds]. *Dermatology: Diagnosis & Therapy*. Stamford, CT: Appleton & Lange, 1991.)

TREATMENT

- **Mild cases:** 5-aminosalicylic acid **(5-ASA)** compounds.
- **Moderate cases:** Oral corticosteroids +/– azathioprine, 6-mercaptopurine (6-MP), or methotrexate.
- **Refractory disease:** IV steroids +/– cyclosporine, +/– anti-TNF antibody. Place the patient on bowel rest, TPN, and antibiotics. Serial imaging to rule out perforation, megacolon, or abscess formation. In some cases, stricturoplasty +/– resection may be needed.

Ulcerative Colitis

Usually occurs in **young females** (mid-30s). Commonly seen in **Caucasians,** especially **Ashkenazi Jews.** Can lead to **toxic megacolon.**

SYMPTOMS/EXAM

- **Cramping** abdominal pain, **urgency, bloody diarrhea,** weight loss, fatigue.
- Low-grade fever, tachycardia, orthostatic hypotension, heme-⊕ stools, mild tenderness in the lower abdomen.

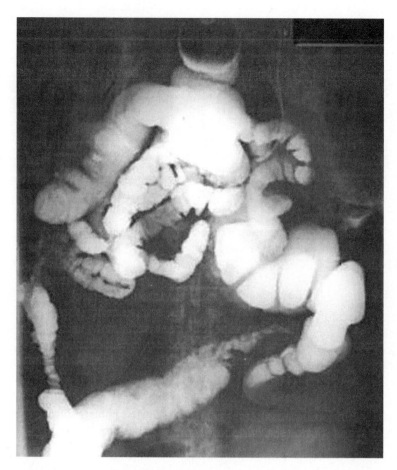

FIGURE 2.6-3. **Crohn's disease of the colon.**

The rectum and sigmoid colon appear normal. The descending colon is narrowed and has an irregular contour with areas of ulceration. In the midtransverse colon, there is a second area of involvement that shows ulcerations, abrupt narrowing, and irregularity consistent with a thickened colon wall. (Adapted, with permission, from Kenneth McQuaid Current Medical Diagnosis and Treatment Online, GI Diseases of the Colon and Rectum. www.AccessMedicine. com, © 2004 McGraw-Hill.)

DIAGNOSIS

- **Labs: Normocytic, normochromic anemia;** low albumin; ⊕ **p-ANCA;** ⊖ stool **cultures.**
- Colonoscopy shows **friable mucosa** with ulcerations and erosions, along with inflammation that is continuous from the anus up. Barium enema shows **lead-pipe colon** and loss of haustra (see Figure 2.6-4). Biopsy reveals crypt abscess and microulcerations but no granuloma.

TREATMENT

- **Mild cases: 5-ASA** compounds.
- **Moderate cases:** Oral corticosteroids +/– azathioprine, 6-MP, or methotrexate.
- **Refractory disease:** IV steroids +/– cyclosporine, +/– anti-TNF antibody. Place the patient on bowel rest, TPN, and antibiotics. Serial imaging to rule out perforation, megacolon, or abscess formation. In some cases resection may be needed, especially if complications ensue or the patient fails medical therapy.

- **Follow-up:** Surveillance colonoscopy 8–10 years after diagnosis and annually thereafter.
- Some patients may elect to get a **prophylactic colectomy** given that the incidence of colon cancer is 1% per year after 10 years of disease.

▶ IRRITABLE BOWEL SYNDROME (IBS)

A GI disorder characterized by abdominal pain and episodes of either diarrhea or constipation with or without bloating. Theories for its etiology include altered gut motor function, autonomic nervous system (**ANS**) **abnormality**, and **psychological factors**.

SYMPTOMS/EXAM

- **Abdominal pain** with incomplete relief by defecation; **intermittent diarrhea and constipation;** a feeling of incomplete rectal evacuation; urgency, passage of mucus, and bloating.
- Abdominal pain that is poorly localized, migratory, and variable in nature.

DIAGNOSIS

A **diagnosis of exclusion.** Basic labs to exclude other causes include CBC,

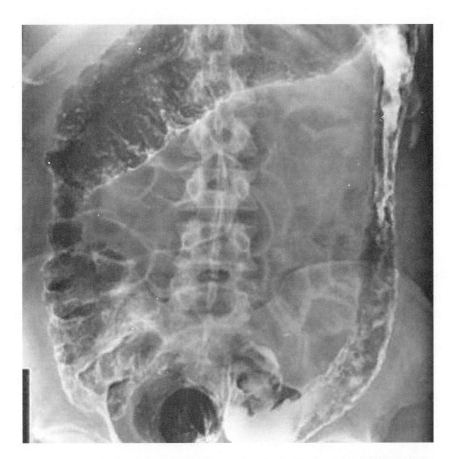

FIGURE 2.6-4. Barium enema showing acute colonic dilation in ulcerative colitis.

Note dilation of the transverse colon, the multiple irregular densities in the lumen that represent pseudopolyps, and the loss of haustral markings. (Reproduced, with permission, from Way LW [ed]. *Current Surgical Diagnosis & Treatment*, 10th ed. Stamford, CT: Appleton & Lange, 1994.)

Pain unrelated to defecation or pain induced with activity, menstruation, or urination is unlikely to be IBS.

BMP, calcium, TSH, and stool O&P. Also rule out chronic constipation or diarrhea. After everything else is ruled out, consider diagnosing on the basis of the history and physical exam. Also aiding in diagnosis are the **Manning criteria:**

- Relief of pain with bowel movement.
- More frequent stools with onset of pain.
- Visible abdominal distention.
- Mucus per rectum; feeling of incomplete rectal emptying.

TREATMENT

- **High-fiber diet** (20–30 g/day), **exercise,** and adequate fluid intake.
- **TCAs** are often used even in the absence of depression, especially in cases of chronic pain.
- **If constipation predominates:** Use bulking agents (psyllium, lactulose) or enemas. Tegaserod, a 5-HT4 receptor agonist, can also be used.
- **If diarrhea predominates:** Loperamide or cholestyramine; avoid laxatives and bulking agents.
- **If bloating predominates:** Simethicone, charcoal, or *Lactobacillus* may be used.
- **Postprandial symptoms:** Treat with anticholinergic agents, dicyclomine, or hyoscyamine.

▶ DIARRHEA

Described as watery consistency with an ↑ frequency of bowel movements. Stool weight is > 30 g. Small bowel pathology will → voluminous watery diarrhea; large bowel pathology will → more frequent but smaller-volume output. Distinguish acute diarrhea from chronic:

- **Acute diarrhea:** Defined as < 2 weeks in duration; usually infectious.
- **Chronic diarrhea:** Defined as lasting > 4 weeks.

SYMPTOMS/EXAM

The most important goal is to assess the degree of fluid loss/dehydration and nutritional depletion. If bloating predominates, it is suggestive of malabsorption. If fever is present, think of infectious causes. If guaiac ⊕, consider inflammatory processes or enteroinvasive organisms. Etiologies can be further distinguished as follows:

- **Infectious:** The **number one cause of acute diarrhea.** Characterized by vomiting, pain, fever, and chills. If stools are bloody, think of enteroinvasive organisms. To diagnose, check stool leukocytes, Gram stain, culture, and O&P. Treat severe disease with ciprofloxacin or metronidazole for *Clostridium difficile.*
- **Osmotic:** Lactose intolerance; ingestion of magnesium, sorbitol, or mannitol. ↑ stool osmotic gap. Bloating and gas are prominent with malabsorption. Treat by stopping the offending agent.
- **Secretory:** Caused by ↑ fat content in the diet or by viruses or toxins. Normal stool osmotic gap; no change in the diarrhea with fasting. Treatment is mainly supportive.
- **Exudative:** Mucosal inflammation, enteritis, TB, colon cancer, IBD. ↑ ESR and C-reactive protein (CRP). Characterized by tenesmus, often

small volume, and frequent diarrhea. Diagnose by colonoscopy. Treatment varies depending on the etiology.

- **Rapid transit:** Associated with laxative abuse or bowel surgery with large-portion resections. Treatment is supportive; where applicable, stop laxative use.

DIAGNOSIS

- **Evaluation of acute diarrhea:** In the presence of high fever, bloody diarrhea, or duration > 4–5 days, obtain fecal leukocytes and bacterial cultures and test for *C. difficile* toxin for inpatients; obtain an O&P for AIDS patients and for those under suspicion for *Giardia*. If symptoms start within six hours of ingestion, think of a preformed toxin such as *S. aureus* or *Bacillus cereus*. If symptoms start after 12 hours, the etiology is more likely to be bacterial or viral, especially if those symptoms are accompanied by vomiting.
- **Evaluation of chronic diarrhea:** Consider malabsorption syndromes, lactose intolerance, previous bowel surgery, medications, systemic disease, and IBD. Tests to consider include fecal leukocytes, occult blood, flex sigmoidoscopy with biopsy, an upper GI series, and a barium enema.
- **Calculate the osmotic gap:** 290 − 2 (stool Na + stool K). A normal gap is < 50.
  - **Normal gap:** If the patient is of normal weight, consider IBS and factitious causes. If weight is ↑, consider secretory or laxative abuse.
  - **↑ Gap:** Normal stool fat points to lactose intolerance or sorbitol, lactulose, or laxative abuse. ↑ stool fat is associated with malabsorption, pancreatic insufficiency, and bacterial overgrowth.

Common bugs in acute diarrhea:

- *Bacterial:* E. coli, Shigella, Salmonella, Campylobacter jejuni, Vibrio parahaemolyticus, Yersinia.
- *Viral: Rotavirus, Norwalk virus.*
- *Parasitic:* Giardia, Cryptosporidium, Entamoeba histolytica.

TREATMENT

Treat according to the etiology as indicated above. General treatment guidelines are as follows:

- If acute, give oral or IV fluids, electrolyte repletion, and loperamide or bismuth salicylate.
- Avoid antimotility agents in the presence of high fever, bloody diarrhea, or systemic toxicity.

▶ ACUTE PANCREATITIS

Gallstones and **alcohol** account for 70–80% of cases. Other causes include **obstruction** (pancreatic or ampullary tumors, pancreas divisum), **metabolic** factors (hyperlipidemia, hypercalcemia), abdominal **trauma**, endoscopic retrograde cholangiopancreatography (**ERCP**), **infection** (mumps, CMV, clonorchiasis, ascariasis), and **drugs** (thiazide, azathioprine, pentamidine, sulfonamide). Can lead to **pseudocyst**, peripancreatic **effusions**, infected **necrosis** or **abscess**, **ARDS**, and **hypotension**.

SYMPTOMS

Presents with abdominal pain, typically in the **midepigastric** region, that **radiates to the back** and is accompanied by nausea, vomiting, fever, and pain that is relieved by sitting forward. If chronic, may present with **steatorrhea** (foul-smelling, loose, bulky, greasy stool), weight loss, and mild fever.

EXAM

- **Midepigastric tenderness,** ↓ bowel sounds, jaundice, fever.
- **Cullen's sign** (periumbilical ecchymoses) and **Grey Turner's sign** (flank ecchymoses) reflect retroperitoneal hemorrhage.

DIAGNOSIS

- Typically, both **amylase and lipase** will be ↑; however, amylase may be normal, especially if the disease is due to hyperlipidemia. **Lipase** has the **greatest specificity.**
- **Abdominal CT** is especially useful in detecting complications of pancreatitis. In **chronic pancreatitis, calcification** may be seen.
- If patients are female and > 60 years of age, or if patients abstain from alcohol or use it only moderately, gallstone is a more likely diagnosis.

TREATMENT

- **Acute:**
  - **Supportive** (NPO, IV fluids, pain management).
  - If **gallstone pancreatitis,** perform an ERCP with papillotomy if the common bile duct is obstructed or if there is evidence of cholangitis. If the gallstone has passed, perform a cholecystectomy once the patient is sufficiently stable for surgery.
  - **Prophylactic antibiotics:** Imipenem monotherapy or fluoroquinolone + metronidazole. Used in the setting of severe pancreatitis.
- **Chronic:** Treat the malabsorption with pancreatic enzyme replacement and vitamin B_{12}. Treat any diabetes that develops.

> **Causes of acute pancreatitis— GET SMASH'D**
>
> **G**allstones
> **E**thanol
> **T**rauma
> **S**teroids
> **M**umps
> **A**utoimmune
> **S**corpion bites
> **H**yperlipidemia
> **D**rugs

▶ APPROACH TO LIVER FUNCTION TESTS

The algorithm in Figure 2.6-5 outlines a general approach toward the interpretation of LFTs.

▶ VIRAL HEPATITIS

May be acute and self-limited or may be chronic and symptomatic. May not be detected until years after initial infection.

SYMPTOMS/EXAM

- In **acute** cases, patients present with anorexia, **nausea,** vomiting, malaise, and fever. Often **asymptomatic.**
- Exam is often normal. An enlarged and tender liver, dark urine, and jaundice may be seen.

DIFFERENTIAL

- **High level of transaminase elevation (> 10–20 times upper limit of normal):** Infection (acute viral), ischemia ("shock liver"), or toxins.
- **Moderate level of transaminase elevation:** Chronic viral, autoimmune, or nonalcoholic fatty liver disease (NAFLD). Also consider mononucleosis, CMV, 2° syphilis, drug-induced illness, and autoimmune disease.

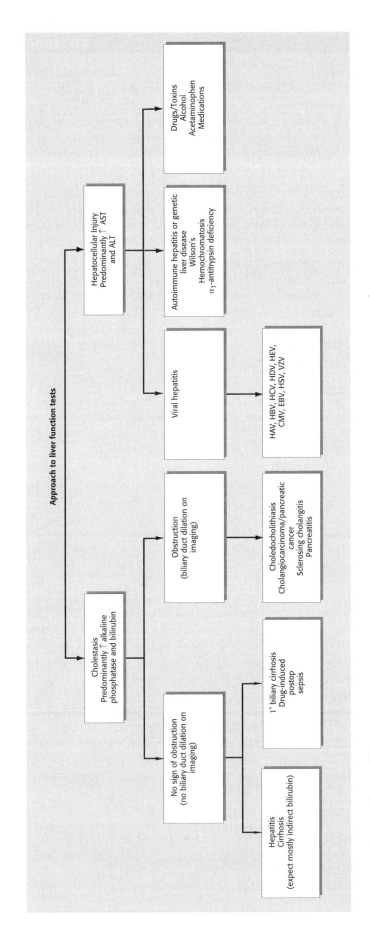

Approach to liver function tests

Cholestasis
Predominantly ↑ alkaline
phosphatase and bilirubin

Hepatocellular Injury
Predominantly ↑ AST
and ALT

No sign of obstruction
(no biliary duct dilation on
imaging)

Obstruction
(biliary duct dilation on
imaging)

Viral hepatitis

Autoimmune hepatitis or genetic
liver disease
Wilson's
Hemochromatosis
α₁-antitrypsin deficiency

Drugs/Toxins
Alcohol
Acetaminophen
Medications

Hepatitis
Cirrhosis
(expect mostly indirect bilirubin)

1° biliary cirrhosis
Drug-induced
postop
sepsis

Choledocholithiasis
Cholangiocarcinoma/pancreatic
cancer
Sclerosing cholangitis
Pancreatitis

HAV, HBV, HCV, HDV, HEV,
CMV, EBV, HSV, VZV

FIGURE 2.6-5. Abnormal liver tests

There is an ↑ (25–40%) risk of cirrhosis and hepatocellular carcinoma with chronic hepatitis B.

DIAGNOSIS

Diagnose on the basis of the following:

- The presence of hepatitis based on clinical presentation as well as on ↑ transaminases.
- Serology and/or PCR testing confirming a specific virus (see Table 2.6-1).
- Biopsy showing hepatocellular necrosis (rarely indicated).
- May do an RUQ ultrasound to see if the liver is enlarged in acute hepatitis (vs. cirrhotic nodular liver in the advanced disease state).

TREATMENT

Treat according to subtype as outlined in Table 2.6-1. Additional guidelines are as follows:

- Rest during the acute phase.
- Avoid hepatotoxic agents; avoid morphine.
- Although most symptoms resolve in 3–16 weeks, LFTs may remain ↑ for much longer.

► ACETAMINOPHEN TOXICITY

SYMPTOMS/EXAM

Within 2–4 hours of acute overdose, patients present with nausea, vomiting, diaphoresis, and pallor. Within 24–48 hours, hepatotoxicity is manifested by RUQ tenderness, hepatomegaly, and ↑ transaminases.

TREATMENT

- Begin N-acetylcysteine administration up to 36 hours after ingestion if the acetaminophen level is above the "no-risk zone" or if the time of ingestion is unknown and ↓ levels are seen (see Figure 2.6-6).
- Administer a 140-mg/kg loading dose followed by 70 mg/kg q4h × 17 additional doses.

► HEREDITARY HEMOCHROMATOSIS (HHC)

- An **autosomal-recessive** disorder of **iron overload.** Usually affects **middle-aged men** at a rate of 1 in 300. Presents with **hepatitis, bronzing** of the skin, **diabetes mellitus, arthritis,** and heart failure.
- Diagnosis is made with ↑ iron saturation (> 60% in men and > 50% in women) and in the presence of the **HFE gene mutation.**
- Treat with **phlebotomy** and **deferoxamine** to ↓ the iron burden. Genetic counseling is useful to assess the likelihood of transmission.

► WILSON'S DISEASE

- An **autosomal-recessive** disorder of **copper overload.** Examination reveals **Kayser-Fleischer rings** and **neuropsychiatric** disorders.
- Labs reveal ↑ urinary copper, ↓ serum **ceruloplasmin,** and ↑ hepatic copper content.
- Treatment is via **chelation** with penicillamine and trientine.

SUBTYPE	TRANSMISSION	CLINICAL/LAB FINDINGS	TREATMENT	OTHER COMMENTS
Hepatitis A virus (HAV)	Transmitted via **contaminated food, water,** milk, and shellfish. Known day care center outbreaks. Fecal-oral transmission; associated with a 30-day incubation period; virus is shed in stool up to two weeks before onset of symptoms.	⊕ IgM antibody to HAV (acute infection). ⊕ IgG antibody to HAV (past exposure). Chronic infection does not occur.	Supportive; usually resolves with no sequelae.	Give immunoglobulin to close contacts.
Hepatitis B virus (HBV)	Transmitted through infected blood, through sexual contact, or perinatally. Incubation is six weeks to six months. HDV can coinfect with HBV. Percutaneous transmission >> sexual.	Surface antigen (HBsAg) indicates active infection (see Figure 2.6-6). High prevalence in homosexuals and IV drug users; < 1% of cases are fulminant. Adult-acquired infection usually does not become chronic.	Interferon, lamivudine, and other nucleotide/ nucleoside analogs. (Goal is to reduce viral load and improve liver histology; cure is uncommon.)	Vaccinate patients with chronic HBV against HAV. Associated with arthritis, glomerulonephritis, and **polyarteritis nodosa.**
Hepatitis C virus (HCV)	Transmitted through blood transfusion or **IV drug use** as well as through intranasal cocaine use or body piercing. Incubation 6–7 weeks.	Illness is often mild or asymptomatic; characterized by waxing and waning aminotransferases. HCV antibody is not protective. Antibody appears six weeks to nine months after infection; diagnose acute infection with PCR. Most infections become chronic.	Interferon + ribavirin combination therapy.	Vaccinate patients with HCV against HAV and HBV. Cryoglobulinemia, membranoproliferative glomerulonephritis.
Hepatitis E (HEV)	Fecal-oral transmission.	Will test ⊕ on serology for HEV.	Supportive.	Self-limited. Endemic to India, Afghanistan, Mexico, and Algeria. Carries a **10–20% mortality rate in pregnant women.**

HIGH-YIELD FACTS

GASTROENTEROLOGY

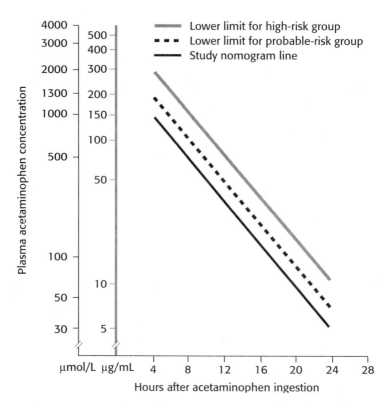

FIGURE 2.6-6. **Estimation of the severity of acetaminophen ingestion.**

(Adapted, with permission, from Christopher Linden and Michael Burns. Harrison's Online. Poisoning and Drug Overdose. www.AccessMedicine.com)

► α₁-ANTITRYPSIN DEFICIENCY

- Usually affects the **liver** (cirrhosis) and the **lung** (emphysema).
- Diagnosed by the absence of α_1-antitrypsin globulin on serum protein electrophoresis (SPEP).
- Treatment is via **liver transplantation** and α_1-antitrypsin replacement for the lung.

► AUTOIMMUNE HEPATITIS

- Primarily affects **young women;** usually suspected when transaminases are ↑.
- Hypergammaglobulinemia is seen on SPEP; autoantibodies are sometimes seen (antinuclear antibody [**ANA**], antismooth muscle antibody [**ASMA**], and liver-kidney microsomal antibody [**LKMA**]). Ultimately, a **liver biopsy** is needed to confirm the diagnosis.
- Treat with **corticosteroids and azathioprine.** A significant number of patients relapse when off therapy and thus require long-term treatment.

► GALLSTONE DISEASE

In the United States, most likely due to **cholesterol stones.** In trauma patients, burn patients, or those on TPN, acute cholecystitis may occur in the absence of stones (**acalculous cholecystitis**).

- Most patients with gallstones are **asymptomatic** (80%).
- **Biliary colic:** Characterized by **episodic RUQ** or epigastric pain that may radiate to the right shoulder; usually **postprandial** and accompanied by vomiting. **Nocturnal** pain awakening the patient is common. Associated with **fatty food** intolerance.
- **Cholangitis:** Fever and persistent RUQ pain suggest cholangitis.
    - **Charcot's triad:** RUQ pain, jaundice, and fever/chills.
    - **Reynold's pentad:** Charcot's triad plus shock and altered mental status may be seen in suppurative cholangitis.
- Look for RUQ tenderness and **Murphy's sign** (inspiratory arrest during deep palpation of the RUQ). Look for jaundice as a sign of common bile duct obstruction.

DIAGNOSIS

- Leukocytosis, ↑ amylase, ↑ LFTs.
- **Ultrasound** is 85–90% sensitive for gallstones and cholecystitis (**echogenic focus that casts a shadow;** pericholecystic fluid = acute cholecystitis). A thickened gallbladder wall and biliary sludge are less specific findings.
- Magnetic resonance cholangiopancreatography (MRCP) is 85% sensitive for bile duct obstruction by stones.
- If ultrasound is equivocal and suspicion is high for the diagnosis of acute cholecystitis, proceed to a **HIDA** scan.

TREATMENT

- **Acute cholecystitis:**
    - IV antibiotics, IV fluids, electrolyte repletion.
    - Early cholecystectomy within 72 hours with an intraoperative cholangiogram to look for common bile duct stones. If the patient is a high-risk surgical candidate, may wait for elective surgery if the clinical condition allows.
    - If the patient is not a candidate for surgery, consider percutaneous biliary drain.
- **Cholangitis:**
    - **ICU** admission, hydration, pressors if needed, **IV antibiotics.**
    - **Endoscopic sphincterotomy** may be needed. Other emergency options are percutaneous hepatic drainage and operative decompression. Once the acute presentation is managed, **ERCP** or percutaneous transhepatic cholangiography will be necessary to locate the obstruction, remove it, and place a stent or do a sphincterotomy.

Symptoms of ascending cholangitis:

RUQ pain

Fever

Jaundice

Risk factors for acute cholecystitis— the 5 F's

Female
Fertile
Fat
Forties
Fifties

HIGH-YIELD FACTS

GASTROENTEROLOGY

▶ 1° BILIARY CIRRHOSIS

Autoimmune destruction of intrahepatic bile ducts. Usually occurs with other autoimmune diseases. More commonly occurs in **women** and is **familial.**

SYMPTOMS/EXAM

Fatigue, **pruritus,** fat **malabsorption.**

DIAGNOSIS

Suggested by markedly ↑ alkaline phosphatase, ↑ bilirubin, and **antimitochondrial antibody (AMA).** Confirmed by biopsy.

TREATMENT

Ursodeoxycholic acid, fat-soluble vitamins, cholestyramine for pruritus, and transplantation. None of these measures is disease modifying.

▶ 1° SCLEROSING CHOLANGITIS

- **Idiopathic** intra- and extrahepatic fibrosis of bile ducts. Affects **men** 20–50 years of age; associated with **IBD.**
- Can present with **RUQ pain** and pruritus but is often **asymptomatic.**
- Look for ↑ bilirubin and alkaline phosphatase; ⊕ **ASMA**; ⊕ **p-ANCA**; and multiple areas of beaded bile duct strictures on ERCP.
- Treat with ursodeoxycholic acid, cholestyramine, fat-soluble vitamins, stenting of the strictures, and ultimately liver transplantation.

▶ UPPER GI BLEED

Bleeding in the section of the GI tract extending from the upper esophagus to the duodenum at the **ligament of Treitz.** Mostly due to **PUD, gastritis,** or **varices** (see Figure 2.6-7).

SYMPTOMS

May present with **dizziness,** lightheadedness, weakness, and nausea. Patients may also report vomiting of blood or dark brown contents (**hematemesis**—vomiting of fresh blood, clots, or coffee-ground material) or passing black stool (**melena**—dark, tarry stools composed of degraded blood from the upper GI tract).

EXAM

Associated with pallor, **abdominal pain,** and peritonitis; rectal exam reveals blood. Patients show signs of **cirrhosis** (telangiectasia, spider angiomata, gynecomastia, testicular atrophy, palmar erythema, caput medusae). **Vital signs** reveal **tachycardia** at 10% volume loss, orthostatic **hypotension** at 20% blood loss, and **shock** at 30% loss.

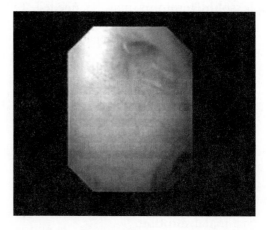

FIGURE 2.6-7. Duodenal ulcer with oozing.

(Adapted, with permission, from Kenneth McQuaid. Current Medical Diagnosis and Treatment Online. GI Diseases of the stomach and duodenum PUD. www.AccessMedicine.com, © 2004 McGraw-Hill.)

DIAGNOSIS

- Assess the severity of the bleed; start with the **ABCs.**
- Check **hematocrit** (may be normal in acute blood loss), **platelet count, BUN/creatinine** ($\uparrow$ ratio reflects volume depletion), PT/PTT, and LFTs.
- NG tube placement and lavage to assess the activity and severity of the bleed (if clear, could be an intermittent bleed or from the duodenum).
- If perforation is suspected, obtain upright and abdominal x-rays.
- Endoscopy (can be both diagnostic and therapeutic in some cases).

TREATMENT

- Start with the **ABCs.** Use at least **two large-bore** peripheral IV catheters. **Transfusion** and intravascular volume replacement.
- Consult GI and surgery if bleeding does not stop or if difficulty is encountered with resuscitation 2° to a brisk bleed.
- Treat a **variceal bleed** with **octreotide,** endoscopic **sclerotherapy,** or **band ligation.** Balloon tamponade if very severe; then embolization or transjugular intrahepatic portosystemic shunt (**TIPS**) if endoscopic therapy fails.
  - For variceal bleed prevention, treat with **nonselective β-blockers** (e.g., propranolol), obliterative endoscopic therapy, **shunting,** and liver transplantation if the patient is a candidate.
  - For **PUD,** use **PPIs, endoscopic** epinephrine injection, thermal contact, and laser therapy. Institute *H. pylori* eradication.
  - **Mallory-Weiss tears** usually stop bleeding **spontaneously.**
  - Treat **esophagitis/gastritis** with PPIs or H$_2$ antagonists. Avoid aspirin and NSAIDs.

► LOWER GI BLEED

- Bleeding that is distal to the ligament of Treitz. Presents with **hematochezia** (fresh blood or clot per rectum).
- Diarrhea, tenesmus, bright red blood per rectum, or maroon-colored stools.
- As with upper GI bleeds, check vital signs to assess the severity of the bleed. Obtain orthostatics. Perform a rectal exam for hemorrhoids, fissures, or a mass.

DIAGNOSIS

- First, **rule out upper GI bleed.**
- Bleeding usually **stops spontaneously.** However, colonoscopy should be performed; in the majority of cases, the diagnosis can be made at the time of visualization.
- If the bleed continues, a bleeding scan (**^{99}Tc-tagged RBC scan**) can be done to detect bleeding if > 1.0 mL/min.
- If unstable, **arteriography** or **exploratory laparotomy** may be done.

Think diverticulosis with painless lower GI bleeding.

TREATMENT

- Although bleeding generally stops spontaneously, resuscitative efforts should be initiated, as with upper GI bleeds, until the source is found and the bleeding stops.
- With diverticular disease, bleeding usually stops spontaneously, but **epinephrine injection,** catheter-directed **vasopressin,** or **embolization** can be used. In some cases, surgery may be needed.

▶ ASCITES

- **Portal hypertension (serum-ascites albumin gradient [SAAG] ≥ 1.1; see below):** Cirrhosis, heart failure, Budd-Chiari syndrome (hepatic vein thrombosis).
- **Not portal hypertension (SAAG < 1.1):** Peritonitis (e.g., TB), cancer, pancreatitis, trauma, nephrotic syndrome.

DIAGNOSIS

- **Ultrasound** and **paracentesis:** Check cell count, differential, albumin, and bacterial cultures +/− acid-fast stain and +/− cytology.
- If a patient with cirrhosis and established ascites presents with worsening ascites, fever, and abdominal pain, think of **spontaneous bacterial peritonitis (SBP).**

Diagnose SBP with ⊕ cultures or peritoneal fluid neutrophil count > 250.

TREATMENT

- **Portal hypertension:**
    - **Sodium restriction** to < 2 g/day.
    - **Diuretics:** Furosemide and spironolactone in combination.
    - Large-volume paracentesis for painful distention.
    - TIPS can be used in refractory cases, but this ↑ the rate of encephalopathy.
    - Ultimately, liver transplant if the patient is a candidate.
- **Not portal hypertension:** Treat the underlying disorder. Therapeutic paracentesis can also be performed.
- Treat SBP with a **third-generation cephalosporin** (first-line therapy) or fluoroquinolone. Often recurs.

▶ CELIAC SPRUE

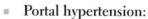

Usually affects people of **Northern European** ancestry. Often **familial;** thought to be an **autoimmune disease** triggered by an environmental agent. Associated with arthritis and an ↑ risk of GI malignancies (lymphoma), and **dermatitis herpetiformis** (see Figure 2.6-8).

SYMPTOMS/EXAM

Celiac sprue → **malabsorption** with **chronic diarrhea.** Patients complain of **steatorrhea** and **weight loss.**

DIAGNOSIS

- Histology reveals **loss of villi.**
- **Antibodies: Antigliadin** or **antiendomysial antibody** or **anti-tissue transglutaminase** (highly specific and sensitive).
- A gluten-free trial improves symptoms and the histology of the small bowel.

TREATMENT

Gluten-free diet. Gluten is found in most grains in the Western world—e.g., wheat, barley, additives, and many prepared foods.

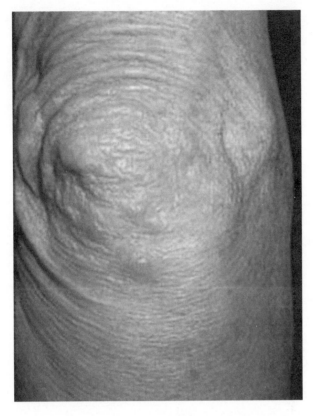

FIGURE 2.6-8. Dermatitis herpetiformis presenting as pruritic papulovesicles.

(Courtesy of J. Reeves; adapted with permission, from Timothy G. Berger. Current Medical Diagnosis and Treatment Online, www.AccessMedicine.com, © 2004 McGraw-Hill.)

Hematology

Anemias are classified by the size of the **MCV** (microcytic, normocytic, or macrocytic).

DIAGNOSIS

- Initially, order a CBC, MCV, blood smear, reticulocyte count, iron studies (ferritin, serum iron, TIBC), serum folate, TSH, serum B_{12}, hemolysis labs (LDH, unconjugated bilirubin, haptoglobin, Coombs' test), DIC panel (D-dimer, fibrinogen, blood smear).
- Look for a bleeding source. Consider cross and typing some RBCs if the patient is actively bleeding.
- Look for **pancytopenia.** Causes include SLE, congenital causes, toxins, drugs, infection, myelodysplasia, malignancy, radiation, and vitamin B_{12}/folate deficiency.

TREATMENT

Severe anemia initially requires fluid resuscitation and RBC transfusion. Transfuse to keep serum hemoglobin > 9 mg/dL, or > 8 g/dL for CAD patients. Identify the cause of the anemia and treat the underlying disorder.

Microcytic Anemia

Anemia with an MCV < 80 fL.

SYMPTOMS/EXAM

Iron-deficient patients may have **pica.** Ask about melena and blood in the stools, and check for stool occult blood. For females, ask about for heavy menstrual periods.

DIAGNOSIS

Examine iron studies, blood smear, and CBC to identify the cause of the microcytic anemia (see Table 2.7-1). Suspect **colorectal cancer** in elderly patients with microcytic anemia, and refer these patients for a colonoscopy.

TREATMENT

If iron-deficiency anemia is the cause, identify the site of blood loss and initiate oral iron supplementation. **Epogen** should be administered to patients with anemia of chronic disease. Patients with thalassemia should be treated with transfusions when necessary.

Macrocytic Anemia

Anemia with an MCV > 100 fL.

DIAGNOSIS

Emphasis should be placed on serum B_{12} level, serum folate level, and blood smear to look for megaloblastic anemia.

- **Hemolysis:** ↑ reticulocyte count, ↑ LDH, ↑ unconjugated bilirubin, ↓ haptoglobin.

Causes of microcytic anemia—TICS

Thalassemia
Iron deficiency
Chronic disease
Sideroblastic anemia

Serum ferritin, a measure of iron stores, is the most useful test with which to diagnose iron-deficiency anemia but is falsely ↑ by infection and inflammation.

Table 2.7-1. **Causes of Microcytic Anemia**

	SERUM FERRITIN (μg/L)	SERUM IRON	IRON-BINDING CAPACITY	OTHER TESTS TO EXAMINE	FURTHER COMMENTS
Iron-deficiency anemia	Low	Low	High		Etiology: malabsorption, chronic blood loss, malnutrition.
Thalassemia	Normal to high	Normal to high	Normal to high	If MCV/RBC < 13, order hemoglobin electrophoresis to confirm the diagnosis.	Characterized by reduced or absent production of one or more globin chains in the hemoglobin.
Anemia of chronic disease (late)	Normal to high	Slightly low	Normal to low		Etiology: chronic inflammation, infection, malignancy.
Sideroblastic	High	Low	Normal	Smear shows normal and dimorphic RBCs. Bone marrow biopsy is required for diagnosis.	Etiology: chronic alcohol use, drugs (antituberculosis, chloramphenicol), lead poisoning.

- **Megaloblastic anemia:** Hypersegmented neutrophils (see Figure 2.7-1). Causes include B_{12} or **folate** deficiency and **drugs** (e.g., azathioprine, AZT, hydroxyurea, chemotherapeutic agents).
- Other causes include **liver disease, alcohol abuse,** and **myelodysplasia.**

TREATMENT

- Treat B_{12} deficiency with monthly B_{12} shots; treat folate deficiency with oral replacement.
- Discontinue any medications that could be contributing to megaloblastic anemia; minimize alcohol use.

Normocytic Normochromic Anemia

Anemia with an MCV of 80–100 fL.

SYMPTOMS/EXAM

Look for evidence of acute bleeding on history and exam. Patients with hemolytic anemia may present with jaundice from unconjugated hyperbilirubinemia as well as with dark urine.

DIAGNOSIS

The initial workup should focus on reticulocyte count, creatinine, hemolysis labs, and blood smear (see Figure 2.7-1).

- ↓ reticulocyte count: **Anemia of chronic disease** or **chronic renal failure (CRF).**

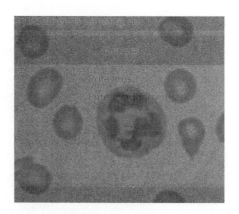

FIGURE 2.7-1.   Hypersegmented neutrophil.

(Courtesy of Dr. Peter McPhedran, Yale University.)

- ↑ reticulocyte count with normal hemolysis labs: Hemorrhage.
- ↑ reticulocyte count, ↑ LDH, ↑ unconjugated bilirubin, ↓ haptoglobin: **hemolysis.** Causes include the following:
  - **Microangiopathic hemolytic anemia:** Schistocytes or helmet cells on blood smear (see Table 2.7-2).
  - **Hereditary spherocytosis:** Spherocytes and ⊖ Coombs' test.
  - **Autoimmune hemolytic anemia:** Spherocytes with ⊕ Coombs' test.
  - **Sickle cell anemia.**

TREATMENT

Patients who are hemorrhaging need to be resuscitated with fluids and RBC transfusions. The cause of the bleeding must be identified and treated. Anemia from CRF can be treated with Epogen and iron.

Microangiopathic Hemolytic Anemia

A group of disorders in which a coagulopathy is associated with **thrombocytopenia** and **hemolysis** (schistocytes and helmet cells on blood smear). Distinguished as follows (see also Table 2.7-2):

- **DIC:** Overwhelming systemic activation of the coagulation system stimulated by serious illness. Treat the underlying condition; transfuse platelets, cryoprecipitate.
- **HUS:** Triad of hemolytic anemia, thrombocytopenia, and ARF causes include viral illness or *E. coli* O157:H7. Treat with dialysis for ARF.
- **TTP: Pentad** of HUS triad + fever and neurologic signs causes include HIV, pregnancy, or OCP use. Treat with plasmapheresis, steroids, ASA, or splenectomy.

Sickle Cell Anemia

An autosomal-recessive disease resulting from the substitution of valine for glutamic acid at the sixth position in the globin chain.

SYMPTOMS/EXAM

Sickle cell patients often have a ⊕ family history. They may also have a history of gallstones and poorly healing ulcers. Exam could be significant for jaundice, splenomegaly (usually during childhood), or CHF.

Table 2.7-2. **Differential of Microangiopathic Hemolytic Anemia**

	PLATELETS	PT/PTT	D-DIMER	OTHER FINDINGS
Thrombotic thromboytopenic purpura/hemolytic-uremic syndrome (TTP/HUS)	↓↓↓	–	–	Acute renal failure (ARF)
DIC	↓↓	↑	↑↑	↑ fibrin split products, ↓ fibrinogen
Mechanical valve	–	–	–	Heart murmur
Severe vasculitis, severe hypertension, HELLP	↓	–	–	

> **Causes of DIC—MOIST**
>
> **M**alignancy
> **O**bstetric complications
> **I**nfection
> **S**hock
> **T**rauma

DIAGNOSIS

Hemoglobin electrophoresis is the definitive diagnostic test.

TREATMENT

All patients should be vaccinated for *Streptococcus pneumoniae, Haemophilus influenzae,* and hepatitis B. Tranfusion for severe anemia. Patients should be put on folic acid. Instruct patients to avoid dehydration, hypoxia, intense exercise, and high altitudes.

COMPLICATIONS

- **Pain crisis:**
    - Sickled cells cause occlusion of arterioles → tissue infarction.
    - Characterized by pain in the back, limbs, and ribs.
    - Precipitated by dehydration, acidosis, infection, fever, or hypoxia.
    - Treat with hydration, analgesia, and supplemental O_2.
- **Aplastic crisis:** Sudden ↓ in hemoglobin and reticulocyte count caused by parvovirus B19. Support with transfusions.
- **Acute chest crisis:**
    - Sickled cells cause occlusion of pulmonary blood supply → lung infarctions.
    - **Clinical findings:** Fever, chest pain, cough, wheezing, tachypnea, and new pulmonary infiltrate on CXR.
    - Treat with O_2, analgesia, and antibiotics (second-generation cephalosporin with erythromycin).
- **Lungs:** Pulmonary infarcts that can cause pulmonary hypertension.
- **Heart:** Sickle cell cardiomyopathy → heart failure.
- **GI:** Cholecystitis, splenic infarcts.
- **Renal failure:** Sickling of cells can cause infarcts leading to ARF.
- **Genital:** Priapism, impotence in males.
- **Infections:** Patients are predisposed to *Streptococcus pneumoniae, Haemophilus influenzae, Neisseria meningitidis,* and gram-negative bacterial infections.
- **Bones:** Avascular necrosis, *Salmonella* osteomyelitis.
- **Pregnancy:** Patients are at ↑ risk of spontaneous abortions.

Sickle cell pain crises are precipitated by infection, dehydration, and hypoxia.

HIGH-YIELD FACTS

HEMATOLOGY

A group of disorders resulting from ↓ synthesis of α- or β-globin protein subunits.

- **α-thalassemia:** Most common in **Asians** and African-Americans. If **all four** α alleles are affected, the baby is stillborn with **hydrops fetalis** or dies shortly after birth. **HbH** disease with **three** affected alleles → **chronic hemolytic microcytic anemia** and **splenomegaly.** Carriers of one or two affected alleles are usually asymptomatic.
- **β-thalassemia:** Most common in people of **Mediterranean** origin, Asians, and African-Americans. **Thalassemia major** (homozygote, no β-globin production) presents in the first year of life as the fraction of HbF declines. Manifestations include growth retardation, **bony deformities,** hepatosplenomegaly, and jaundice. β-thalassemia minor (heterozygote): is less severe.

TREATMENT

Treatment includes **transfusions,** splenectomy, folic acid, and bone marrow transplant. SQ **deferoxamine** ↑ urinary excretion of iron and ↓ iron toxicity, the most serious complication of which is cardiac toxicity.

- Classically affects males ≥ 60 years old. The most common cause of erythrocytosis is **chronic hypoxia** 2° to lung disease rather than 1° PCV.
- Patients present with malaise, fever, pruritus (especially after a warm shower), and signs of vascular sludging—**stroke,** angina, MI, claudication, hepatic vein thrombosis, headache, and blurred vision. Exam may reveal **plethora,** large retinal veins on funduscopy, and **splenomegaly.**
- Labs show ↑ **hematocrit** (≥ 50%), ↑ RBC mass, and ↓ **erythropoietin** level (↑ in chronic hypoxia-induced polycythemia). Basophilia suggests proliferative myelopoiesis. Bone marrow biopsy shows hypercellular marrow.
- Treatment includes **serial phlebotomy** until hematocrit < 45 and **daily ASA** +/– anagrelide to ↓ platelets. Hydroxyurea for difficult-to-treat PCV. PCV is associated with an ↑ **risk of conversion** to CML, myelofibrosis, or AML.
- Table 2.7-3 outlines the laboratory features of PCV as well as those of other myeloprdiferative disorders.

Disorders in coagulation or platelets that predispose patients to bleed (see Table 2.7-4).

DIAGNOSIS

Initial tests to order include PT/PTT, CBC, platelet count, and DIC panel (D-dimer, fibrinogen, blood smear). Use these laboratory data to determine if the cause of the bleeding is 2° to a coagulopathy or platelet problem.

- Think **thrombocytopenia** when the platelet count is < 90,000 cells/μL (see the section on platelet problems).
- Think **coagulopathy** if the PT or PTT time is ↑ (see the section on coagulopathies).

Table 2.7-3. Laboratory Features of Myeloproliferative Disorders

	WBC COUNT	HEMATOCRIT	PLATELET COUNT	RBC MORPHOLOGY
CML	↑↑	Normal	Normal or ↑	Normal
Myelofibrosis	Normal or ↓ or ↑	Normal or ↓	↓ or normal or ↑	Abnormal
PCV	Normal or ↑	↑	Normal or ↑	Normal
Essential thrombocytosis	Normal or ↑	Normal	↑↑	Normal

(Reproduced, with permission, from Tierney LM et al. *Current Medical Diagnosis and Treatment: 2004.* New York: McGraw-Hill, 2004:481.)

- If platelet count and PT/PTT are normal, check bleeding time and thrombin time. An ↑ bleeding time suggests a **platelet dysfunction** (see the section on platelet problems). An ↑ thrombin time suggests a **defect in the cross-linking of fibrin.**

> **P**etechiae = **P**latelet deficiency.
> **C**avity/joint bleeding = **C**lotting factor deficiency.

TREATMENT

Patients who are hemodynamically unstable need immediate resuscitation with IV fluids. The source of hemorrhage should be identified and stopped. Blood transfusions should be given to maintain a hemoglobin > 8 g/dL. Fresh frozen plasma (FFP) should be given to normalize PTT and PT. Platelets should be given if the platelet count is < 50,000 cells/μL.

▶ PLATELET PROBLEMS

Disorders associated with a ↓ in the number of platelets (thrombocytopenia) or a ↓ in the function of platelets that predisposes patients to bleed. Look for petechiae and easy bruising. In addition to DIC, TTP, and HUS, other platelet problems include the following:

Table 2.7-4. Coagulopathy vs. Platelet Problems

	PLATELET PROBLEM	COAGULOPATHY
Amount of bleeding after surface cuts	Excessive, prolonged.	Normal to slightly prolonged.
Onset of bleeding after injury	Immediate bleeding.	Delayed bleeding after surgery or trauma. Spontaneous bleeding into joints or hematomas.
Clinical presentation	Superficial and mucosal bleeding (GI tract, gingival, nasal). Petechiae, ecchymosis.	Deep and excessive bleeding into joints, muscles, GI tract, and GU tract.

- **Idiopathic thrombocytopenic purpura (ITP):** Severe thrombocytopenia. A diagnosis of exclusion. ⊖ DIC panel; ⊕ **platelet-associated IgG** antibodies. **Prednisone** and splenectomy if the patient is unresponsive to steroids.
- **Heparin-induced thrombocytopenia:** Thrombocytopenia occurring 4–14 days after starting heparin. Stop heparin immediately and start an alternative anticoagulant such as lepirudin, argatroban, or danaparoid sodium (**not** warfarin).
- **Platelet dysfunction:** Normal platelet count.
    - **Acquired:** Severe liver disease, severe renal disease, DIC, aspirin use, multiple myeloma.
    - **Inherited:** Includes von Willebrand's disease, Bernard-Soulier syndrome, Glanzmann's thrombasthenia, and storage pool disease.
    - **Treatment:** Desmopressin. OCPs for menorrhagia. FFP or cryoprecipitates for major bleeding. No ASA.

▶ COAGULOPATHIES

Conditions in which a defective clotting cascade predisposes patients to bleeding. Ask about medications that predispose to bleeding (e.g., warfarin, enoxaparin [Lovenox], heparin); note factors that predispose to **vitamin K** deficiency (malnutrition, antibiotic use, alcoholism). A history of recurrent spontaneous bleeding suggests a factor deficiency. Look for evidence of liver disease on exam.

DIAGNOSIS

Order liver enzymes. Defects in the clotting cascade can be classified into four categories:

- ↑ **PT and normal PTT:** The differential diagnosis includes early DIC, liver disease, warfarin use, and vitamin K deficiency. If these causes are eliminated, order a factor VII level to see if it is deficient.
- ↑ **PT and** ↑ **PTT:** The differential diagnosis includes severe DIC, severe liver disease, warfarin overdose, severe vitamin K deficiency, and heparin use. If these causes are eliminated, order a factor II, V, and X level to see if they are deficient.
- ↑ **PTT and normal PT:** Usually caused by heparin therapy. If the patient is not on heparin, order a **50:50 mixing study.**
    - If the **PTT normalizes** with 50:50 mixing, determine factor VIII (hemophilia A), IX (hemophilia B), and XI levels to look for a deficiency.
    - If the **PTT does not normalize** with 50:50 mixing, test for the presence of a factor VII inhibitor and antiphospholipid syndrome (order a lupus anticoagulant and anticardiolipin antibody). Patients with antiphospholipid syndrome are predisposed to thrombosis, not to bleeding. The ↑ PTT is artifactual.
- ↑ **TT:** Indicates a disorder that involves a defect in the cross-linking of fibrin.

TREATMENT

Coagulopathic patients who are actively bleeding need **FFP** to normalize their PT and PTT levels. Heparin and warfarin must be stopped. If vitamin K deficiency is suspected, it is reasonable to empirically give a patient 10 mg of oral vitamin K for three days to see if the PT normalizes. Patients with hemophilia A or B require **factor VIII** (cryoprecipitate) or **factor IX** replacement, respectively. Patients with antiphospholipid syndrome and a history of thrombosis require anticoagulation with warfarin.

A group of conditions that predispose patients to blood clotting. Suspect a hypercoagulable state in the presence of the following:

- Thrombosis (DVTs, pulmonary emboli, and CVAs) at an early age.
- A **family history** of hypercoagulable state.
- Thrombosis at an unusual site (cerebral or mesenteric vein, upper extremities).
- **Recurrent** thromboses.
- Multiple **miscarriages.**

DIAGNOSIS

The major causes of a hypercoagulable state are listed in Table 2.7-5. Patients with a first venous thrombosis event before age 50, a history of recurrent thombotic episodes, or thrombotic event with a first-degree relative with a thromboembolic event before age 50 need to be screened two weeks after completion of anticoagulation for 1° causes of hypercoagulability—activated protein C resistance, prothrombin mutation, antiphospholipid antibody, plasma homocysteine, antithrombin deficiency, protein C deficiency, and protein S deficiency.

TREATMENT

Acute thrombosis must be treated with at least six months of anticoagulation with warfarin. Indications for lifelong warfarin use include > 2 spontaneous thromboses, antithrombin deficiency, antiphospholipid syndrome, spontaneous life-threatening thrombosis, and thrombosis in an unusual site (e.g., the mesenteric or cerebral vein). Patients with a history of hypercoagulable state who become pregnant need to be treated with low-molecular-weight heparin.

COMPLICATIONS

The complications of hypercoagulable state are listed in Table 2.7-6.

Factor V Leiden is the most common inherited hypercoagulable disorder.

Table 2.7-5. **Causes of Hypercoagulable States**

INHERITED	ACQUIRED
Factor V Leiden mutation	Prolonged bed rest or immobilization
Protein C or S deficiency	MI
Antithrombin III deficiency	Tissue damage (surgery, fracture)
Homocystinemia	DIC
Fibrinolysis defects	Hyperlipidemia
	Vasculitis
	Multiple myeloma
	Lupus anticoagulant (antiphospholipid syndrome)
	Nephrotic syndrome
	Smoking
	Cancer
	Warfarin (on initiation of therapy)
	OCPs
	Pregnancy

(Reprinted, with permission, from Le T et al. *First Aid for the USMLE Step 2,* 4th ed. New York: McGraw-Hill, 2003:202.)

Table 2.7-6. **Transfusion Complications**

	CLINICAL	TESTS	MANAGEMENT
Major/minor hemolytic reaction	Chills, fever, SOB, nausea, chest/flank pain, hypotension, flushing. Complications: ARF (from hemoglobinuria), DIC.	⊕ Coombs' test, agglutination of RBC on smear, low haptoglobin (best test). UA for hemoglobinuria (⊕ urine dip for hematuria in setting of few RBCs on microscopy).	Stop transfusion. Maintain BP and urine output with IV fluids; give patient furosemide (Lasix) if urine output < 100 cc/hr. Type and cross RBCs just transfused.
Delayed hemolysis	Onset 4–14 days post-transfusion. Jaundice, anemia, hemoglobinuria, fever.	↑ LDH, unconjugated hyper-bilirubinemia, ↓ haptoglobin.	Type and screen blood before future transfusions. Acetaminophen for fever.
Febrile, nonhemolytic reaction	Onset within two hours post-transfusion. Fever, rigors, nausea, vomiting, chills.	Rule out biochemical evidence of hemolysis.	Leukocytes reduce any future packed RBC transfusions. Avoid transfusion when febrile.
Anaphylaxis	↑ risk in patients with congenital IgA deficiency. Sudden onset, flushing, hypertension followed by hypotension, edema, respiratory distress, shock, wheezing, chest pain.	None.	IV epinephrine. Use saline-washed packed RBCs in future RBC transfusions.
Urticaria	Rash, pruritus.		Stop transfusion; monitor for anaphylaxis. Give diphenhydramine (Benadryl) and antihistamines. Resume transfusion at slower rate when symptoms resolve.
Acute lung injury (TRALI)	Occurs 1–6 hours post-transfusion. Like ARDS of lung. Acute respiratory distress, cyanosis, fever; gone in 24 hours. Differential: fluid overload.	CXR shows bilateral pulmonary infiltrates without CHF.	Ventilation (O_2, intubation), diuretics, steroids.
Bacterial infection	More likely with platelets. Fever, hypotension, onset within four hours.	Culture remaining blood product.	Antibiotics.

SECTION II

Oncology

Leukemias are the most common cancer in children.

Lymphade-nopathy and splenomegaly are common in ALL but rare in AML.

Recombinant human hematopoietic growth factors (G-CSF or GM-CSF) are used to treat granulocytopenia in acute leukemia.

Most patients have B-cell ALL, which has a poorer prognosis than T-cell variants.

Administer allopurinol to patients with acute leukemia before initiating chemotherapy.

- Characterized as malignant proliferations of hematopoietic cells.
- Categorization is based on cellular origin (promyeloid, myeloid, lymphoid) and on the level of differentiation of neoplastic cells.
- **Acute leukemias** are proliferations of minimally differentiated blast cells.
- **Chronic leukemias** are proliferations of more mature, differentiated cells.

Acute Lymphocytic Leukemia (ALL)

Most common in children; occurs in whites more often than blacks.

SYMPTOMS/EXAM

- Often a **viral-like prodrome** of fever, sore throat, and lethargy begins weeks before the diagnosis of ALL.
- Children may present with limpness, refusing to walk, with **bone pain,** easy bruising, and **fever.**
- Exam may reveal pallor, widespread **petechiae/purpura,** adenopathy, **hepatosplenomegaly,** multiple ecchymoses, and bleeding.

DIFFERENTIAL

Aplastic anemia, **mononucleosis** or other viral infection, rheumatic disease, ITP, TTP, other neoplasms.

DIAGNOSIS

Leukocyte count may be ↑ or ↓. Look for ↓↓ platelets and ↑ **LDH and uric acid.**

- Obtain a CXR, LP, and CT scan to rule out mediastinal involvement and brain metastasis.
- **Bone marrow biopsy** is necessary for diagnosis and is superior to blood for cytogenetic studies (CALLA ⊕, TdT ⊕).

TREATMENT

There is a **good prognosis** with **chemotherapy;** nearly all children achieve complete remission, and 80% achieve long-term leukemia-free survival. For adults, these numbers are 80% and 30%, respectively. Phases of treatment include:

- **Remission induction therapy:** Usually a cocktail of vincristine + prednisone + daunorubicin.
- **Consolidation therapy:** High-dose methotrexate started within a month of complete remission.
- **Remission maintenance therapy:** Daily methotrexate, 6-mercaptopurine (6-MP) or both.

Acute Myelogenous Leukemia (AML)

Although AML is the most common acute leukemia in the **perinatal period,** most cases occur in adults; the incidence ↑ with each decade of life.

SYMPTOMS/EXAM

Adults present with **fatigue, easy bruising, dyspnea due to anemia,** fever, leukemia cutis (small, raised, painless skin lesions), CNS symptoms, and a

HIGH-YIELD FACTS

ONCOLOGY

history of **frequent infections.** AML may present with **DIC, gingival hyperplasia,** or CNS involvement. Exam will show fever, lethargy, bleeding, **petechiae/purpura,** and hepatosplenomegaly.

DIAGNOSIS

- In addition to ↑ myelocytic cell lines, there is ↓ **leukocyte alkaline phosphatase (LAP). Hyperuricemia is often seen from** ↑ **cell turnover. Auer rods** and **myeloperoxidase staining** may be present and are diagnostic for AML.
- Leukemoid reactions due to infection, stress, chronic inflammation, and certain neoplasms can cause WBC counts of 40,000–100,000 cells/μL but lack the cytogenetic changes and ↓ LAP seen with AML and CML.

TREATMENT

- Cytosine arabinoside + daunorubicin or idarubicin.
- **All-*trans*-retinoic acid** is used for induction and maintenance therapy for the promyelocytic form (AML M3).
- Prognosis depends on subtype, but generally 70–80% of adults < 60 years of age achieve complete remission.
- Allogeneic or autologous **bone marrow transplantation (BMT)** with high-dose chemotherapy +/– total body irradiation is considered for patients with poor prognostic factors for long-term disease-free survival and those < 60 years of age.

Chronic Lymphocytic Leukemia (CLL)

Malignant cells resemble mature lymphocytes. The typical patient is **> 65 years of age.** CLL is a slowly progressive disease, and median survival is approximately 6–8 years. **Anemia** and **thrombocytopenia** are associated with ↓ survival.

SYMPTOMS/EXAM

Lymphadenopathy, fatigue, and hepatosplenomegaly may be present on exam. This is usually an **indolent disease,** and many patients are diagnosed by incidental lymphocytosis.

DIAGNOSIS

Isolated lymphocytosis on CBC with a normal hematocrit and platelet count. Bone marrow will be infiltrated with lymphocytes. Aberrant **CD5+** expression is characteristic, and **smudge cells** may be present on peripheral smear.

TREATMENT

Most patients are **managed supportively.** Fludarabine may be used to ameliorate fatigue, lymphadenopathy, anemia, or thrombocytopenia. **Splenectomy + steroids** are used to treat associated autoimmune hemolytic anemia and immune thrombocytopenia.

Chronic Myelogenous Leukemia (CML)

An overproduction of myeloid cells, CML is often stable for several years (chronic phase) until it transforms into an acute leukemia **(blast crisis),**

AML is associated with exposure to smoking, benzene, radiation, and chemotherapeutic agents.

Auer rods are diagnostic for AML.

CLL may be complicated by autoimmune hemolytic anemia and may transform to intermediate- or high-grade lymphoma (Richter's transformation).

which is fatal within a few months. CML is associated with prior radiation exposure and most commonly affects people 40–60 years of age.

SYMPTOMS/EXAM

Typically, CML is diagnosed on a routine CBC that demonstrates **leukocytosis** with myeloid precursors. Patients may have mild, nonspecific symptoms (**fatigue, fever, malaise,** ↓ exercise tolerance, weight loss, night sweats). **Blast crisis** presents as fever, bone pain, weight loss, and ↑ **splenomegaly.**

DIAGNOSIS

The presence of the Philadelphia chromosome is not only diagnostic for CML but also the causative genetic event.

Peripheral smear reveals ↑↑ WBC count (median of 150,000 cells/μL at the time of diagnosis) and prominent myeloid cells with basophilia. Also seen are ↓ **LAP** and ↑↑ B_{12} levels. Confirm diagnosis by detection of the **t(9;22) Philadelphia chromosome *bcr-abl* gene** by karyotyping, PCR, or fluorescent in situ hybridization (FISH) analysis of the blood or bone marrow aspirate.

TREATMENT

Hydroxyurea and SQ **interferon-α** can suppress the malignant clone, normalize blood counts, and delay the onset of blast crisis. However, all patients eventually progress to terminal blast crisis.

- **Imatinib mesylate (Gleevec)** specifically targets and inhibits *bcr-abl* tyrosine kinase and eliminates CML clone → rapid hematologic and cytogenetic remission.
- **Allogeneic BMT,** if performed while the patient is in the **chronic phase** (within one year of diagnosis), may result in long-term survival in CML. Best results are achieved in patients < 40 years of age. Can be complicated by graft-versus-host disease.

> ▶ **LYMPHOMAS**

Lymphomas are made up of a single clone of lymphocytes. Approximately 90% of lymphomas are derived from B cells, 9% from T cells, and 1% from monocytes or natural killer (NK) cells.

Hodgkin's Lymphoma

SYMPTOMS/EXAM

EBV is a common cause of aggressive lymphoma in patients with congenital or acquired immune deficiencies.

Usually presents with cervical lymphadenopathy and spreads in a predictable manner along lymph nodes. The spleen is the most commonly involved intraabdominal site. If the patient presents late, he or she may complain of *B symptoms*—**10% weight loss in six months, night sweats requiring change of clothes, and fever > 38.5°C.** These indicate bulky disease and a poorer prognosis.

DIAGNOSIS

Reed-Sternberg cell = Hodgkin's lymphoma.

Usually made on biopsy of an enlarged lymph node. Staging is based on the anatomic-based **Ann Arbor system.** Staging workup involves determining the Ann Arbor stage and the presence of prognostic factors. Chest and abdominal/pelvic CT as well as bilateral bone marrow biopsies and aspirates are routine.

TREATMENT

Chemotherapy consisting of doxorubicin, bleomycin, vinblastine, and dacarbazine (**ABVD cocktail**), with or without radiation of the involved field, is the current treatment of choice. This is capable of effecting long-term survival in 40–50% of patients, and salvage high-dose therapy with stem cell transplantation can achieve long-term survival in 20–25% of those not cured with initial therapy.

Non-Hodgkin's Lymphoma (NHL)

- Classified as low, intermediate, or high grade based on histologic type.
- Diagnosis is similar to that of other lymphomas.
- The addition of **rituximab** (monoclonal anti-CD20) to chemotherapy appears to result in a significantly improved response rate and overall survival.
- The treatment of **high-grade NHL** may be complicated by **tumor lysis syndrome** → hyperkalemia, hyperphosphatemia, hyperuricemia, and hypocalcemia.

NHL is spread hematogenously.

▶ MULTIPLE MYELOMA

A malignancy of **plasma cells** seen in **older adults** within bone marrow, often with unbalanced, excessive production of immunoglobulin heavy/light chains.

SYMPTOMS/EXAM

Symptoms include **back pain** (presenting symptom in 80% of patients), **hypercalcemic symptoms** ("stones, bones, abdominal moans, and psychiatric overtones"), **pathologic fractures,** fatigue, and frequent infections (2° to dysregulation of antibody production). Exam may reveal pallor, fever, bone tenderness, and lethargy.

DIFFERENTIAL

Monoclonal gammopathy of undetermined significance (MGUS), Waldenström's macroglobulinemia (plasma cell proliferation in which **IgM** is produced), 1° amyloidosis, metastatic carcinoma, lymphoma, hyperparathyroidism.

DIAGNOSIS

Critical tests to evaluate for the presence of multiple myeloma are **serum and urine protein electrophoresis** (monoclonal immunoglobulin, most commonly **IgG**), **bone marrow** aspirate to enumerate plasma cells, and **full-body skeletal survey** (x-rays showing **punched-out osteolytic lesions** of the skull and long bones).

Plain radiographs of the axial skeleton, including skull, vertebral bodies, ribs, and pelvis, will show the characteristic lytic lesions of multiple myeloma. Bone scans are not helpful, since they show blastic activity.

TREATMENT

Therapy is aimed at reducing tumor burden, relieving symptoms, and preventing complications.

- **Melphalan** is effective at reducing tumor burden; **thalidomide** is also used but can produce quality-of-life-altering somnolence at effective doses. **High-dose chemo and stem cell transplantation** are used for patients < 60 years of age and in advanced stages of disease.
- **Hypercalcemia:** Treat with hydration, glucocorticoids, and natriuresis.
- **Bone pain/destruction:** Bisphosphonates.
- **Renal failure:** Prevent with hydration to help excrete light-chain immunoglobulins.

- **Infections:** Vaccinate against preventable infections; diagnose early and treat aggressively.
- **Fractures:** Local radiation.
- **Anemia:** Erythropoietin.

▶ CNS MALIGNANCIES

1° brain tumors make up < 2% of all tumors diagnosed. Meningioma, glioma, vestibular schwannoma, pituitary adenoma, and 1° CNS lymphoma are the most common CNS tumors in adults.

Meningioma

- The **most common** tumor of the brain; **usually benign.**
- Most are small, asymptomatic, and discovered incidentally. When symptoms are present, they usually consist of **progressive headache** or **focal neurologic deficit** reflecting the location of the tumor.
- CT of the head typically demonstrates a partially **calcified, homogeneously enhancing extra-axial mass adherent to the dura.**
- Surgical resection for large or symptomatic tumors; observation with serial scans for small or asymptomatic ones.

Glial Tumors

- Include astrocytomas, oligodendrogliomas, mixed gliomas, and ependymomas.
- Headache is the most common symptom; it may be generalized or unilateral, often **awakens** the patient from sleep and induces **vomiting,** and is **worse with Valsalva maneuver.**
- Tumors appear as a **diffusely infiltrating area** of low attenuation on CT or as an ↑ T2 signal on MRI.
- **Glioblastoma multiforme** is usually a **unifocal and centrally necrotic** enhancing lesion with surrounding edema and mass effect.
- **Biopsy** is required for definitive diagnosis.
- **Surgical resection** followed by **external-beam radiation** is used for high-grade tumors. Chemotherapy is reserved for high-grade gliomas in patients < 60 years of age with good performance status.

▶ BREAST CANCER

The most common cancer and the second most common cause of cancer death in women (after lung cancer) in the United States. Risk factors include th following:

- Female gender.
- Older age.
- Breast cancer in first-degree relatives.
- Prior history of breast cancer.
- History of atypical ductal or lobular hyperplasia.
- Early menarche, early menopause, or late first full-term pregnancy (before age 35).
- HRT > 5 years.

SYMPTOMS/EXAM

Most masses are discovered by the patient. They often present as a **hard, irregular, immobile, painless breast lump,** possibly with nipple discharge. **Skin changes** (dimpling, erythema, ulceration) and **axillary adenopathy** indicate more advanced disease. The most common location is the **upper outer quadrant.** Metastatic sites include **lymph nodes, bones, brain, lung,** and **liver.**

DIFFERENTIAL

Mammary dysplasia, fibroadenoma, mastitis, fat necrosis.

DIAGNOSIS

Diagnosis is suggested by a palpable mass or **mammographic abnormalities** (e.g., microcalcifications, hyperdense regions).

- A ⊖ mammogram should be followed by **ultrasound, MRI,** tissue collection by **FNA** (of a palpable lump), **stereotactic** core biopsy (of a nonpalpable lesion), or **excisional** biopsy until convincing evidence for absence of cancer is gathered.
- The specimen should be tested for prognostic factors such as estrogen/progesterone receptors (**ER⊕/PR⊕**), and **HER-2.**

Special forms of breast cancer include the following:

- **Inflammatory breast cancer:** A highly aggressive, rapidly growing cancer; invades lymphatics and causes skin inflammation. Poor prognosis.
- **Paget's disease:** Ductal carcinoma in situ (DCIS) of the nipple with itching, burning, and nipple erosion (may be mistaken for infection). Associated with a focus of invasive carcinoma.

TREATMENT

Breast-preserving therapy for most women involves tumor excision and radiation therapy. About 25% of women are better served by **mastectomy,** especially if complete excision cannot be achieved or radiation is contraindicated. Adjuvant treatment includes **endocrine** and **chemotherapy.**

- **Intraductal carcinoma (DCIS** or pure ductal carcinoma in situ) warrants only local therapy (either mastectomy or wide excision + radiation therapy).
- **Endocrine** therapy is beneficial only for patients with **ER⊕ or PR⊕ tumors;** tamoxifen has become the standard of care for both premenopausal and postmenopausal women.
- **Adjuvant chemotherapy** (two or more agents such as 5-FU, methotrexate, doxorubicin, cyclophosphamide, or epirubicin for 3–6 months) is usually given for tumors > 2 cm or those with axillary lymph node involvement.

► LUNG CANCER

Carcinoma of the lung is the **leading cause of cancer death.** The major risk factor is **tobacco** use. Other risk factors include radon and asbestos exposure.

- **Adenocarcinoma:** The most common lung cancer; **peripheral** location.
- **Bronchoalveolar type of adenocarcinoma:** Associated with multiple nodules, bilateral lung infiltrates, and metastases late in the course.

BRCA-1 and BRCA-2 mutations are seen in < 5% of breast cancer patients. Test women who have "genetic" risk–i.e., a strong premenopausal family history of breast/ovarian cancer.

The sensitivity of mammography for breast cancer is 75–80%. Never stop with a negative mammogram!

⊕ estrogen/ progesterone receptor status is a good prognostic indicator in breast cancer.

Breast-preserving therapy results in survival rates equivalent to those of mastectomy.

DCIS increases the risk for a new breast cancer.

- Squamous cell carcinoma: Presents **centrally**.
- Large cell/neuroendocrine carcinomas: Least common.
- Small cell lung cancer (SCLC): Highly related to **cigarette exposure**. Usually **centrally** located and always presumed to be **disseminated** at the time of diagnosis. **Chemotherapy** is the treatment of choice.

SYMPTOMS/EXAM

Some patients have an asymptomatic lesion discovered incidentally on either x-ray or chest CT. Most patients, however, develop signs that herald a problem—e.g., **cough, hemoptysis, weight loss,** or **postobstructive pneumonia. Less frequently, patients may present late with complications of large tumor burden:**

- **Pancoast's syndrome:** Shoulder pain, Horner's syndrome, lower brachial plexopathy.
- **Superior vena cava syndrome:** Swelling of the face and arm, most often on the right side.
- **Hoarseness:** Vocal cord paralysis from entrapment of the recurrent laryngeal nerve, more often on the left.
- **Hypercalcemia:** Most often seen with squamous cell carcinoma.
- **Trousseau's syndrome:** Hypercoagulable state seen with adenocarcinoma.
- **Hyponatremia/SIADH:** Small cell carcinoma.

DIFFERENTIAL

TB/other granulomatous diseases, fungal disease (aspergillus, histoplasmosis), lung abscess, metastasis, benign tumor (bronchial adenoma), hamartoma.

DIAGNOSIS

- **Chest CT** is usually the initial imaging modality. Nodules that double in size in one year are usually malignant.
- **Centrally** located cancers can be diagnosed by **bronchoscopy** or **sputum cytology.**
- **Staging** includes chest and abdominal CT, bone scan, and CT (or MRI) of the head.

TREATMENT

Non–small cell lung cancer (NSCLC) is **potentially curable with resection of localized disease but is only modestly responsive to chemotherapy.** Patients are classified into one of three clinical groups at the time of diagnosis:

- **Stages I and II:** Early-stage disease = candidacy for surgical resection.
- **Locally or regionally advanced disease** (supraclavicular or mediastinal lymphadenopathy or chest wall/pleura/pericardium invasion): chemotherapy and radiation combination; surgery is not indicated.
- **Distant metastases:** The goal of any chemo or radiation is **palliation only.**
- **SCLC: Chemotherapy** is the treatment of choice.

▶ **GI MALIGNANCIES**

Pancreatic Cancer

Diets rich in vegetables and fruits ↓ risk of pancreatic cancer.

Typically seen in patients > 50 years of age. **Ductal adenocarcinoma** accounts for 90% of 1° tumors; > 50% arise in the head of the pancreas. Risk factors include smoking, chronic pancreatitis, and diabetes mellitus (DM).

Symptoms are usually vague and nonspecific. The most common symptoms are **nausea, anorexia, lumbar back pain, new-onset DM, venous thromboembolism,** and **painless obstructive jaundice** (associated with adenocarcinoma in the **head** of the pancreas).

DIAGNOSIS

↑ bilirubin; aminotransferases; normocytic, normochromic anemia; frequent elevation of **CA 19-9**. **Ultrasound** is useful as an initial diagnostic test. Abdominal/pelvic CT can evaluate the extent of disease; **thin-section helical CT** through the pancreas can determine if the mass is resectable. **Endoscopic ultrasonography** yields excellent anatomic detail and is useful to confirm if the tumor is resectable.

TREATMENT

- **Pancreaticoduodenectomy** (Whipple procedure) for patients with resectable tumors. Postoperative mortality rates depend on the experience of the surgeon and treatment center.
- **Chemotherapy** or **radiation** is used for **palliative care** in patients with advanced or unresectable disease.

Hepatocellular Carcinoma (Hepatoma)

Risk factors include viral hepatitis (HBV, HCV), alcoholic cirrhosis, hemochromatosis, and α_1-antitrypsin deficiency.

SYMPTOMS/EXAM

Patients may present with abdominal discomfort and laboratory abnormalities (↑ aminotransferases, bilirubin, coagulopathy) warranting abdominal imaging.

TREATMENT

Surgical resection and liver transplantation can provide long-term survival. Alternatives for unresectable tumors include percutaneous alcohol injections, arterial chemoembolization, and radiofrequency ablation.

Colorectal Cancer

Incidence is similar among men and women until age 50, after which the incidence is higher in men. Most cases occur after age 50. Table 2.8-1 discusses risk factors.

SYMPTOMS/EXAM

Symptoms depend on the site of the 1° tumor and may include change in bowel habits, melena or bright red blood per rectum, weight loss, fatigue, vomiting, and abdominal discomfort.

Painless jaundice? Think cancer involving the head of the pancreas.

HIGH-YIELD FACTS

ONCOLOGY

Table 2.8-1. Risk Factors for Colorectal Cancer

FACTOR	COMMENTS
Age > 50 years	
Personal history	Colorectal cancer Adenomatous polyps IBD Ovarian, uterine, or breast cancer
Family history of colorectal cancer or adenomatous polyps	In one first-degree relative < 60 years or two first-degree relatives of any age
Family history of hereditary colorectal cancer syndromes	Familial adenomatous polyposis (FAP) Hereditary nonpolyposis colorectal cancer (HNPCC) Hamartomatous polyposis syndromes

DIAGNOSIS

Physical exam should include DRE and fecal occult blood testing. Iron-deficiency anemia or ↑ transaminases may be seen. CXR, abdominal and pelvic CT or MRI, **CEA level** (> 5 ng/mL is associated with poorer prognosis), and colonoscopy.

TREATMENT

- Treatment decisions are influenced by tumor stage at diagnosis. 1° surgical resection involves resection of the bowel segment with adjacent mesentery and regional lymph nodes.
- Stage I patients have an excellent prognosis with **surgery** alone (90% survival at five years).
- **Adjuvant chemotherapy** is warranted for patients at stage III and above.

▶ GU MALIGNANCIES

Bladder Carcinoma

The most common malignant tumor of the urinary tract. Most cases are **transitional cell carcinoma**. Risk factors include **smoking**, aniline dyes, and chronic bladder infections (e.g., **schistosomiasis**)

SYMPTOMS/EXAM

Gross hematuria is the most common presenting symptom. Other urinary symptoms, such as frequency, urgency, and dysuria, can also occur. Most patients are asymptomatic during early stages.

DIAGNOSIS

- **UA** is the most basic evaluation and often shows hematuria (macro- or microscopic); cytology (first morning specimen is best) may show dysplastic cells.
- **IVP** can examine the upper urinary tracts as well as defects in bladder filling.
- **Cystoscopy with biopsy is diagnostic.**

TREATMENT

Treatment depends on the extent of spread beyond the bladder mucosa.

- **Carcinoma in situ (CIS):** Intravesicular chemotherapy.
- **Invasive cancers without metastases:** Aggressive surgery, radiotherapy, or both.
- **Patients with distant metastases:** Chemotherapy alone.

Prostate Carcinoma

SYMPTOMS/EXAM

Many patients are asymptomatic and incidentally diagnosed either by DRE or by **PSA** level done for screening purposes. Symptoms may include **urinary urgency/frequency/hesitancy** and, in late or aggressive disease, anemia, hematuria, or other symptoms from local invasion or metastasis.

DIAGNOSIS

- Based on DRE, PSA level, and ultrasound-guided needle biopsy of the prostate with 6–12 biopsy specimens.
- **Gleason score** is still the best predictor of tumor biology. It sums the scores of the two most dysplastic biopsy samples on a scale of 1–5 (well differentiated to poorly differentiated). A Gleason score of 2–4 has the most favorable prognosis; 5–6 is intermediate, and ≥ 7 is worse.

TREATMENT

Treatment choice is based on the aggressiveness of the tumor and the patient's risk of dying from the disease.

- **Watchful waiting** may be the best approach for elderly patients with low Gleason scores.
- **Radical prostatectomy** and **radiation therapy** (e.g., brachytherapy or external beam) are associated with an ↑ risk of incontinence and/or impotence.
- Treat metastatic disease with **androgen ablation** (e.g., GnRH agonists, orchiectomy, flutamide) and chemotherapy.

PSA may be used to follow patients post-treatment for disease recurrence.

Testicular Carcinoma

The most common solid malignant tumor in men 20–35 years of age. Highly treatable and often curable. Risk factors include **cryptorchid testis** and Klinefelter's syndrome.

SYMPTOMS/EXAM

The initial finding is usually a **unilateral scrotal mass,** which may be painless. Other presentations include testicular discomfort or swelling suggestive of orchitis or epididymitis.

DIAGNOSIS

- Serum levels of α-fetoprotein (**AFP**) and β-hCG should be measured. Definitive diagnosis is made by radical inguinal orchiectomy.
- Staging (TNM is widely used) evaluation should include serum LDH, AFP, β-hCG, and CT of the chest/abdomen and pelvis.

Rising AFP and β-hCG levels postoperatively indicate recurrence or persistent tumor.

TREATMENT

All patients undergo **radical inguinal orchiectomy** with initial ligation of the spermatic cord.

Ovarian Carcinoma

More than 90% are adenocarcinomas. Risk factors include age, infertility drugs, and familial cancer syndromes (e.g., BRCA-1, BRCA-2). Risk is ↓ with sustained use of OCPs, having children, breast-feeding, bilateral tubal ligation, and TAH-BSO.

SYMPTOMS/EXAM

Usually **asymptomatic** until the disease has reached an advanced stage. Patients may have abdominal pain, bloating, pelvic pressure, urinary frequency, early satiety, constipation, vaginal bleeding, and systemic symptoms (fatigue, malaise, weight loss). Exam findings may include a palpable **solid, fixed, nodular pelvic mass; ascites; and pleural effusion.**

DIFFERENTIAL

Uterine leiomyomas, ectopic pregnancy, pelvic kidney, retroperitoneal fibrosis/tumor, colorectal cancer, PID, ovarian cyst, metastasis (e.g., Krukenberg tumor), endometriosis.

TREATMENT

- Evaluate an adnexal mass with **pelvic ultrasound** and possibly CT or MRI; serum **CA-125**, CXR.
- Staging is surgical and includes **TAH-BSO, omentectomy, and tumor debulking.**

Cervical Carcinoma

Despite the **screening Pap smear**, cervical cancer remains the third most common gynecologic malignancy. Risk factors include **HPV infection, tobacco use,** early onset of sexual activity, multiple sexual partners, immunocompromised status (e.g., HIV), and STDs.

Infection with HPV types 16, 18, and 31 ↑ risk of cervical cancer.

DIAGNOSIS

- Patients are usually asymptomatic and diagnosed on a routine **Pap smear.** Otherwise, patients may present with meno- and/or metrorrhagia, **postcoital bleeding,** pelvic pain, and vaginal discharge.
- **Colposcopy** and biopsy usually follow the abnormal Pap smear.
- Cancers are categorized as **invasive cervical carcinoma** (depth > 3 mm, width > 7 mm) or **cervical intraepithelial neoplasia (CIN).**

TREATMENT

- **CIN I (mild dysplasia or low-grade squamous intraepithelial lesion [LGSIL]):** Most regress spontaneously. Reliable patients can be **observed** (Pap smears and colposcopy every three months for one year).
- **CIN II/III:** Treat with **cryosurgery,** laser, or **loop electrocautery excision procedure (LEEP).**
- **Invasive cancer:** Early stages may be treated with **radical hysterectomy and lymph node dissection.** All stages can be treated with **radiation and chemotherapy** or less radical surgeries. Use radiation +/– chemotherapy with bulky tumors or advanced disease to improve survival.

Cervical cancer is a preventable disease with a screening test (Pap smear) and a good prognosis if diagnosed early.

Melanoma

An aggressive malignancy of melanocytes. The **leading cause of death** from skin diseases. Risk factors include **sun exposure,** fair skin, family history, large number of nevi, and the presence of dysplastic nevi (see Table 2.8-2).

SYMPTOMS/EXAM

Melanoma is usually **asymptomatic** until late in the disease process. Patients may present with pruritus and mild discomfort. **A pigmented skin lesion that has recently changed in size or appearance should raise concern.** Lesions are characterized by the **ABCDs** of melanoma (see mnemonic) and may occur **anywhere** on the body. They are most commonly found **on the trunk for men** and on the **legs for women.**

DIAGNOSIS

Skin biopsy shows **melanocytes with marked cellular atypia** and melanocytic invasion into the dermis.

TREATMENT

Surgical excision is the treatment of choice. **The thickness of the melanoma (depth of invasion)** is the most important prognostic factor. Depending on depth, lymph node dissection may be necessary. Systemic **chemotherapy** is used for metastatic disease.

> **The ABCDs of melanoma:**
>
> **A**symmetric shape
> **B**orders irregular
> **C**olor variegated
> **D**iameter > 6 mm

Basal Cell Carcinoma

The **most common skin cancer;** associated with excessive sun exposure. Lesions take many forms, including nodular, ulcerative, pigmented, and superficial.

SYMPTOMS/EXAM

Exam reveals a **pearly-colored papule** of variable size. The external surface is frequently covered with fine **telangiectasias** and appears **translucent.** Lesions may be anywhere on the body but are most commonly on **sun-exposed** areas. Large ulcers are described as **"rodent ulcers."**

HIGH-YIELD FACTS

ONCOLOGY

Table 2.8-2.   **Types of Malignant Melanoma**

	SUPERFICIAL SPREADING	NODULAR	ACRAL-LENTIGINOUS	LENTIGO MALIGNA
Appearance	Dark brown, irregular borders, asymmetric.	Uniform, dark, "blueberry-like" nodule.	Marked variegation of brown/black macule.	Flat, brown/black with "stain-like" appearance.
Distribution	Back, legs.	Any area; grows rapidly.	Palms, soles, mucous membranes.	Sun-exposed areas.
Epidemiology	Comprise 70% of all melanomas.	50s, M = F.	M > F, African-Americans and Asians.	60s, fair-skinned.

DIAGNOSIS

Skin biopsy shows characteristic basophilic **palisading cells with retraction.**

TREATMENT

Therapy depends on the size and location of the tumor, the histologic type, the history of prior treatment, the underlying health of the patient, and cosmetic considerations. Options include curettage, surgical excision, cryosurgery, and radiation.

Squamous Cell Carcinoma

Risk factors include exposure to **sun** or ionizing radiation, **actinic keratosis,** immunosuppression, arsenic, and industrial carcinogens.

SYMPTOMS/EXAM

Usually slowly evolving and **asymptomatic;** occasionally, bleeding or pain may develop. Exam reveals small, red, **exophytic nodules** with varying degrees of scaling or crusting. Lesions are commonly found in **sun-exposed areas.**

Prevent all types of skin cancers with UVA/UVB sunscreens.

DIAGNOSIS

Biopsy shows irregular masses of anaplastic epidermal cells proliferating down to the dermis.

TREATMENT

- **Surgical excision** is necessary for larger lesions and for those involving the periorbital, periauricular, perilabial, genital, and perigenital areas.
- **Mohs' micrographic surgery** may be performed for recurrent lesions and on areas of the face that are difficult to reconstruct.
- **Radiation** may be necessary in cases in which surgery is not a viable option.

SECTION II

Infectious Disease

> ## ENCEPHALITIS

- Usually involves the brain parenchyma. HSV is the leading cause (see Table 2.9-1).
- Patients may have nonspecific complaints initially consistent with a viral prodrome (e.g., **fever,** malaise, body aches) and then go on to develop headaches, photophobia, seizures, focal neurologic deficits (weakness, cranial nerve/sensory deficits), and meningeal signs.

Herpes Simplex Virus (HSV) Encephalitis

- The majority of cases are due to HSV-1 reactivation.
- Think of HSV when patients present with **bizarre behavior,** speech disorders, gustatory or olfactory hallucinations, or acute hearing impairment.
- Key CSF studies—**HSV polymerase chain reaction (PCR) tests and HSV culture.** MRI will show a characteristic pattern in the temporal lobes, usually bilaterally.
- Empiric treatment with IV acyclovir for 14–21 days.

West Nile Encephalitis

- Suspect in anyone with an acute febrile illness presenting in late spring, summer, or early autumn.
- Patients have fever +/− maculopapular rash. Look for acute flaccid paralysis suggestive of Guillain-Barré syndrome.
- CSF findings resemble **viral meningitis.** Test serum or CSF by ELISA for IgM antibody to West Nile virus.
- Treatment is supportive (fluids, etc.).

> ## BACTERIAL MENINGITIS

Common causative organisms vary with age group (see Table 2.9-2).

SYMPTOMS/EXAM

- Typical symptoms include fever, malaise, headaches, photophobia, and neck stiffness. Patients may also complain of nausea and vomiting.
- Be sure to look for fever, nuchal rigidity, and Kernig or Brudzinski signs. Funduscopic exam may reveal papilledema, indicating ↑ ICP.

TABLE 2.9-1. **Common Causes of Viral Encephalitis by Time of Year**

TIME OF YEAR	VIRAL ENCEPHALITIS
Summer/fall	West Nile virus
Winter/spring	VZV
	Measles
	Mumps
Year round	HSV-1
	HIV

Table 2.9-2. Common Causes of Bacterial Meningitis by Age

PREDISPOSING FACTORS	TYPICAL BACTERIAL PATHOGEN
Neonates (0–4 weeks)	**Group B strep, *E. coli*, *Listeria***
Infants (1–23 months)	***Streptococcus pneumoniae***, *Neisseria meningitidis*, *H. influenzae*
Age 2–50 years	***S. pneumoniae*, *N. meningitidis***
Elderly (> 50 years)	*S. pneumoniae*, *N. meningitidis*, ***L. monocytogenes***

DIAGNOSIS

Obtain an LP in any patient suspected of having meningitis. When clinical features suggest possible intracranial mass or ↑ ICP, obtain a head CT. See Table 2.9-3 for common CSF findings in meningitis.

TREATMENT

Begin empiric therapy immediately in anyone suspected of having bacterial meningitis. Even a short delay ↑ mortality. Consider the patient's **risk factors,** and then choose an antibiotic regimen that will cover the most likely organisms (see Table 2.9-4).

Treat suspected meningitis immediately; don't wait for the LP results! You can always tailor therapy later.

▶ UPPER RESPIRATORY TRACT INFECTIONS

Acute Sinusitis

- Defined as inflammation of the mucosal lining of the paranasal sinuses lasting > 4 weeks. The most common organisms include *S. pneumoniae*, *H. influenzae*, and *Moraxella catarrhalis*. Other causes may be anaerobes and rhinoviruses.
- Look for patients with acute onset of **fever, headache, face pain, or swelling.** Most cases have cough and purulent postnasal discharge. Patients are typically febrile and may have tenderness over the affected sinus.
- Diagnosis based on clinical findings. Imaging such as x-ray or CT may help (air-fluid level, inflammation of tissues).
- Empiric therapy consists of a 10-day course of TMP-SMX or amoxicillin +/– clavulanate.

Table 2.9-3. Common CSF Findings in Meningitis

CSF PARAMETER	BACTERIAL	VIRAL	TB	CRYPTO
Opening pressure (mmH$_2$O)	200–500	< 250	180–300	> 200
Cell type	PMNs	Lymphocytes	Lymphocytes	Lymphocytes
Glucose (mg/dL)	Low	Normal	Low to normal	Low
Protein (mg/dL)	High	Normal	Normal to high	High

Table 2.9-4. **Antibiotic Regimens for Bacterial Meningitis**

PATHOGEN	THERAPY OF CHOICE
S. pneumoniae	Vancomycin + third-generation cephalosporin +/– dexamethasone
N. meningitidis	Ampicillin or third-generation cephalosporin
L. monocytogenes	Ampicillin **(not cephalosporins)**
Streptococcus agalactiae	Ampicillin
H. influenzae type b	Third-generation cephalosporin

Chronic Sinusitis

- Defined as sinus symptoms lasting > 4 weeks.
- Sinus CT with bone windows is imaging modality of choice.

TREATMENT

- Amoxicillin +/– clavulanate for 21 days. Consider anaerobic coverage (clindamycin).
- Nasal steroid sprays are beneficial.
- Refractory cases require endoscopic surgery.

Otitis Media

- Causative agents are similar to those for acute sinusitis.
- Typical features include **fever,** unilateral **ear pain,** dizziness, or vertigo. There may be hearing loss. Children may be irritable or tug at their ears.
- The tympanic membrane is typically erythematous, without a normal light reflex, and may be bulging. Look for perforation of the tympanic membrane, with pus in the ear canal.
- First-line treatment is with amoxicillin or TMP-SMX for 10 days. Patients who do not respond to antibiotic therapy and develop hearing loss should have tympanostomy tubes placed.

Otitis Externa

- Predisposing factors include **swimming,** eczema, hearing aid use, and mechanical trauma (cotton swab insertion). In most patients, the causative organism is S. *aureus*. Think *Pseudomonas* in diabetics.
- Patients will have a painful ear along with foul-smelling drainage. The **external ear canal** will be swollen and erythematous. There may be pus. Patients will have tenderness upon **movement of the pinna** or tragus.
- Remove any foreign material from the ear canal and start a topical antibiotic (typically **ofloxacin**) with **steroids.**

Pharyngitis

- Typically due to **viral causes** such as rhinovirus or adenovirus. **Group A strep** occurs in up to 25% of cases. Untreated group A strep can lead to acute pyogenic complications and **rheumatic fever.**

- Symptoms include sore throat and fever +/– cough. Look for tonsillar exudates and tender anterior cervical adenopathy.

DIAGNOSIS

- Think about **infectious mononucleosis** in patients with lymphadenopathy and malaise.
- In **adults** with pharyngitis, always consider **HIV infection and acute retroviral syndrome.**
- In **children,** think about **epiglottitis** (febrile patients with complaints of severe sore throat/dysphagia and minimal findings on exam).
- Check a rapid antigen test (good sensitivity and specificity) as well as a throat swab for culture.

TREATMENT

Treat group A strep infections with penicillin G. Use a macrolide if penicillin allergy. Chronic carriers (i.e., $\oplus$ throat culture, asymptomatic) should be treated with clindamycin for eradication.

▶ PNEUMONIA

Community-Acquired Pneumonia (CAP)

Pneumonia still ranks as the sixth leading cause of death overall and is the leading cause of death from infection. Etiologies are as follows:

- Typical pathogens:
    - *S. pneumoniae*
    - *H. influenzae*
    - *S. aureus* (in setting of influenza virus)

- Atypical pathogens:
    - *Mycoplasma*
    - *Chlamydia*
    - *Moraxella*

SYMPTOMS/EXAM

Think of pneumonia in any patient with acute onset of fever, **chills, productive cough,** and **pleuritic chest pain. Atypical organisms** present with low-grade fevers, nonproductive cough, and myalgias ("walking pneumonia"). Look for evidence of consolidation (dullness to percussion, crackles, bronchial breath sounds) on lung exam.

DIAGNOSIS

- There should be radiographic evidence of an infiltrate in all immunocompetent patients and recovery of a pathogenic organism from blood, sputum, or pleural fluid.
- **Urine *Legionella* antigen** should be sent in patients with risk factors.
- Don't forget to check an ABG in patients who appear in distress to determine their acid-base status.

Think of Legionella *infection in a smoker with pneumonia, diarrhea, and elevated LDH.*

Sputum sample should have < 10 epithelial cells.

TREATMENT

Decide whether the patient needs to be hospitalized based on clinical risk factors. Admit patients who are > 50 years of age, with chronic underlying disease (e.g., COPD, CHF, cancer), unstable vitals, or high fever. Initiate empiric antibiotic therapy based on the patient's risk factors (e.g., community-dwelling and healthy, diabetic). Think about **methicillin-resistant S. aureus (MRSA)** with a history of colonization or if the patient has been in the hospital (see Table 2.9-5).

Ventilator-Associated Pneumonia (VAP)

- Typical agents in this setting include methicillin-sensitive S. *aureus*, MRSA, *Pseudomonas*, *Legionella*, *Acinetobacter*, and other gram-negative rods.
- *Candida* is rarely a pathogen.

TREATMENT

Remember to always obtain sputum cultures **before starting or changing antibiotics.** Tailor your empiric therapy **as soon as** culture data become available. Treatment should be for 7–10 days.

Pneumocystis carinii Pneumonia (PCP)

- Can be present in HIV-⊕ patients (CD4 < 200) as well as anyone on immunosuppressive therapies.

Table 2.9-5. Empiric Antibiotic Treatment Strategies for CAP

PATIENT PROFILE	INCLUDE COVERAGE FOR:	EMPIRIC ANTIBIOTIC CHOICE
Community-dwelling outpatients	S. pneumoniae H. influenzae Atypicals	Azithromycin PO
Patients with comorbidities (age > 60, DM, EtOH use, COPD)	S. pneumoniae Klebsiella Legionella	Fluoroquinolone or azithromycin PO
Inpatient (severe or multilobar pneumonia)	As above	Ceftriaxone IV + azithromycin IV
Nursing home–acquired CAP	Gram-negative rods Pseudomonas MRSA	Ceftriaxone IV + azithromycin IV +/– vancomycin
Patients with cystic fibrosis	Pseudomonas	Ceftazidime IV + levofloxacin IV + aminoglycoside
Aspiration	Anaerobes Gram-negative rods S. aureus	Ceftriaxone IV + azithromycin IV + clindamycin IV

- Fever, nonproductive cough, dyspnea on minimal exertion that resolves quickly on rest.
- Patients may have findings consistent with atypical pneumonia, or very few physical exam findings. Look for pneumothorax.

DIAGNOSIS

- CXR ranges from **normal** to bilateral interstitial or alveolar infiltrates. The classic appearance is of "ground-glass" infiltrates.
- Other findings include ↑ LDH.
- Do silver stain of sputum or bronchoalveolar lavage to look for PCP.

TREATMENT

First-line therapy is with IV TMP-SMX. Alternatives include inhaled pentamidine. Use **concomitant prednisone** if PaO_2 is < **70 mmHg** or if the patient has an A-a gradient of > 35 mmHg on room air.

▶ TUBERCULOSIS (TB)

- 1° **TB** usually involves the middle or lower lung zones and is associated with hilar adenopathy (Gohn complex).
- **Latent TB (LTB)** represents reactivation and typically involves the upper lungs and cavitation.
- Extrapulmonary TB is usually associated with HIV-⊕ persons and may involve any organ.
- Screening for LTB in **high-risk groups**—immigrants from endemic areas, HIV-⊕ persons, homeless persons, health care workers, IV drug users, and patients with chronic medical conditions (COPD, chronic renal failure, DM, post-transplant, cancer).
- BCG vaccination status should be disregarded in interpreting test results (see Table 2.9-6).

TREATMENT

- The most commonly used regimen includes four drugs described by the mnemonic **RIPE**—**R**ifampin, **I**soniazid (INH), **P**yrazinamide, and **E**thambutol daily for eight weeks, followed by INH and rifampin for an additional 16 weeks.
- Treatment of latent TB requires nine months of INH.
- Patients coinfected with TB and HIV should be treated with **rifabutin** instead of rifampin, since the latter can interact with anti-HIV meds.

Give vitamin B_6 to prevent INH-associated neuropathy.

Table 2.9-6. **PPD Interpretation**

POPULATION	⊕ TB SKIN TEST
Low risk of disease	≥ 15 mm
Patients with exposure risk (health care workers, immigrants, diabetics)	≥ 10 mm
HIV-⊕, immunocompromised, recent contact with TB, CXR c/w previous TB infection	≥ 5 mm

- Some 3–7% of central venous catheters become infected, with **femoral sites** having the highest risk, followed by internal jugular; subclavian catheters have the lowest rate of infections.
- Look for redness/induration +/− drainage at site of insertion as well as fevers, alteration in mental status.
- Draw two sets of blood cultures from peripheral sites; if the catheter is tunneled, obtain cultures through it. Treatment should be geared toward the causative organism. Empiric therapy should include coverage for MRSA.
- If peripheral blood cultures are ⊕ and/or the patient is febrile, remove the catheter as soon as possible.

► GENITOURINARY TRACT INFECTIONS

Uncomplicated Cystitis

- Some 10% of U.S. women have at least one uncomplicated UTI each year. The most common pathogen is *E. coli.*
- The most frequent complaints are those of dysuria, urgency, or frequency of urination.
- Think about urethritis/cervicitis in sexually active patients. Renal stones may also present with colicky pain and dysuria.
- Check the UA for the presence of bacteria, WBCs, leukocyte esterase, and nitrite.
- Give a three-day course of either TMP-SMX or fluoroquinolone. Cultures are not necessary. Seven-day courses are recommended for diabetics, women > 65 years, patients with symptoms > 7 days, and men.

Pyelonephritis

- Similar findings as in UTI, except more ill/acute appearing. Be sure to check for **CVA tenderness.** Also look for signs of bacteremia: fever, tachycardia, and hypotension.
- Urine specimens usually demonstrate significant bacteriuria, pyuria, and occasional WBC casts. Urine culture should be sent on all patients. **Always obtain blood cultures on admission—15–20% of cases will be bacteremic.**
- Begin ampicillin and gentamicin or a fluoroquinolone IV. If no clinical response, look for an **intrarenal abscess** or foreign bodies such as **renal calculi** with CT or ultrasound.

Prostatitis

- Presenting symptoms include spiking fevers, chills, dysuria, cloudy urine, and even obstructive symptoms if prostate swelling is significant. In patients with chronic infection, low back pain or perineal or testicular discomfort might be present.
- On gentle prostate DRE, the gland is exquisitely tender. Obtain urine cultures before and after a prostatic massage to look for gram-negative rods.
- Treat with TMP-SMX or fluoroquinolone for 14 days. In those with chronic prostatitis, treatment should be extended to a month with a fluoroquinolone or three months with TMP-SMX.

Syphilis

Caused by *Treponema pallidum*. Transmissible during early disease (1° and 2° syphilis) with exposure to open lesions (they're loaded with spirochetes!).

SYMPTOMS

- **1° syphilis:** Develops within several weeks of exposure; involves one or more painless, indurated, superficial ulcerations (chancre).
- **2° syphilis:** After resolution of chancre, patients may develop malaise, anorexia, headache, **diffuse lymphadenopathy,** or rash (involves mucosal surfaces, palms, and soles).
- **3° syphilis:** Includes cardiovascular, neurologic, and gummatous disease (e.g., general paresis, tabes dorsalis, aortitis, meningovascular syphilis).

EXAM

Findings depend on the stage of syphilis—the painless chancre for 1°, maculopapular rash or diffuse lymphadenopathy for 2°, and multiple neurologic and/or cardiovascular signs for 3° as mentioned above.

DIAGNOSIS

- **1°:** Do a nontreponemal serologic test (RPR or VDRL). Darkfield microscopy of the lesion's exudate will show the spirochetes. Direct antigen tests (MHA-TP or FTA-ABS) are used for confirmation.
- **2°:** Presence of clinical illness and ⊕ serologic tests.
- **3°:** Perform an LP when neurologic or ophthalmic signs and symptoms are present, in treatment failure, or with a VDRL of 1:32 or greater. Correlate with cardiovascular, neurologic, and systemic symptoms.

TREATMENT

- **1°/2°:** Penicillin G 2.4 million units in a single IM dose; alternatives include doxycycline or erythromycin for 14 days. If disease duration has been > 1 year, give three doses of penicillin G IM a week apart.
- **Neurosyphilis:** Penicillin G IV for 14 days.

Patients with HIV or syphilis longer than a year should always undergo LP.

Genital Herpes

- Painful grouped vesicles in the anogenital region. Caused by human herpes simplex virus, usually type 2.
- Frequently associated symptoms include tender inguinal lymphadenopathy, fever, myalgias, headaches, and aseptic meningitis. Those are usually more pronounced during the initial episode and less frequent with recurrences.
- Diagnosis can be confirmed by viral culture of the vesicle fluid.
- Use acyclovir for 7–10 days in 1° infections. Treatment should begin within a week of symptoms. For severe recurrences, repeat treatment with either acyclovir or valacyclovir for five days may be indicated. Daily suppressive therapy for frequent recurrences can be used.

Counsel patients regarding safe sex practices. HSV transmission can occur even in the absence of visible vesicles.

Chancroid

- Painful, nonindurated genital ulcer accompanied by bilateral inguinal lymphadenopathy that may suppurate. The edges of the ulcer are usually undermined.
- Caused by *Haemophilus ducreyi.* Rare outside tropical regions.

- Culture for *H. ducreyi* either from the ulcer or from lymph node aspirate.
- Ceftriaxone IM one dose or azithromycin 1 g PO once.

Cervicitis/Urethritis

- Chlamydial and gonococcal infections often present as cervicitis or urethritis.
- Dysuria, dyspareunia, and mucopurulent vaginal discharge are frequent complaints in women. In men, dysuria and purulent penile discharge predominate.
- A $\oplus$ endocervical or urethral culture or urine PCR for chlamydia/gonorrhea is diagnostic.
- Always treat for both infections simultaneously and treat sexual partners.
- **Chlamydia**—single PO dose of **azithromycin. Gonorrhea**—single PO dose of ofloxacin or ciprofloxacin or a single IM dose of ceftriaxone.

Pelvic Inflammatory Disease (PID)

- Upper genital tract infection in women; usually a complication of chlamydia/gonorrhea infection.
- Presents with pelvic pain, dyspareunia, vaginal discharge, fever, and menstrual irregularities and with lower abdominal tenderness, adnexal tenderness, and cervical motion tenderness (CMT).
- A finding of > 10 WBC/low-power field on Gram stain and endocervical smear is consistent with a diagnosis of PID.
- Treat with **second-generation cephalosporin** IV + IV doxycycline.

IUDs greatly ↑ the risk of PID and should be removed in a woman diagnosed with an STD.

Acute HIV Infection

- Occurs in 50–90% of cases.
- Incubation period is usually 2–6 weeks.
- Acute symptoms last 1–4 weeks, with an average of two weeks.
- Need for hospitalization averages 17% of cases.

SYMPTOMS/EXAM

Patients will have a typical viral prodrome (e.g., malaise, low-grade fever) followed by development of adenopathy. Unusual presentations include Bell's palsy, peripheral neuropathy, radiculopathy, cognitive impairment, and psychosis.

DIAGNOSIS

- HIV serology (ELISA) detects antibody to HIV. Becomes $\oplus$ 4–10 weeks after exposure with > 95% seroconversion at six months. Send confirmatory Western blot in patients with a $\oplus$ ELISA screen.
- For patients with suspected acute retroviral syndrome, check a viral load, since the ELISA may not have had time to turn $\oplus$.

TREATMENT

Begin highly active antiretroviral therapy (HAART) in any of the following situations:

- Symptomatic (any CD4 or viral load).
- Asymptomatic with CD4 < 200 and any viral load.
- Pregnant women.

Regimens should include three drugs, preferably from different categories (see Table 2.9-7).

Malaria Prophylaxis

Mefloquine is active against all plasmodial species, including chrloroquine-resistant *Plasmodium falciparum*. Given weekly.

- Currently 1° choice for malarial chemoprophylaxis.
- Potential for neuropsychiatric side effects; caution should be exercised in prescribing to people with recent or active depression, psychosis, schizophrenia, or anxiety disorders.
- Other effects include sinus bradycardia and QT-interval prolongation; avoid in patients on β-blockers or with known conduction disorders.

Traveler's Diarrhea (TD)

- Roughly 40–60% of people traveling to developing countries develop TD (see Table 2.9-8).
- Patients have watery, unformed stools with nausea, vomiting, or abdominal cramping or pain and fever. Stools may be bloody.

DIAGNOSIS

Since the disease is self-limited (48–72 hours), studies are usually not warranted and treatment is symptomatic. Stool culture should be considered in those with blood in the stool, fever, and symptoms of colitis. Viral studies should be considered if symptoms persist for 10–14 days. Stool examination for *Giardia* should be done in patients with predominantly upper GI symptoms—nausea, bloating, gas, and persistent nonbloody diarrhea.

Table 2.9-7. Prophylaxis in HIV

DISEASE	INDICATION	TREATMENT
PCP	CD4 < 200 or previous PCP or thrush.	TMP-SMX, dapsone, or atavaquone.
Mycobacterium avium-intracellulare (MAI)	CD4 < 50.	Azithromycin weekly.
Toxoplasma gondii	CD4 < 100 and Toxo IgG ⊕.	TMP-SMX or dapsone + leucovorin + pyrimethamine.
TB	Recent contact or PPD > 5 mm.	INH for nine months.
Pneumococcal pneumonia	All HIV-⊕.	Vaccine every five years.
Influenza	All HIV-⊕.	Yearly vaccine.
Hepatitis B	Surface antigen/core antibody ⊕.	Hepatitis B vaccine.

Table 2.9-8. Common Pathogens Causing TD

BACTERIA	VIRUSES	PARASITES
ETEC (enterotoxic *E. coli*)	Rotavirus	*Giardia*
Campylobacter	Enteric adenovirus	*Cryptosporidium*
Salmonella		*Cyclospora*
Shigella		Microsporidia
Vibrio		*Isospora belli*
Yersinia		*Entamoeba histolytica*

TREATMENT

Fluid replacement should be initiated in all cases; oral rehydration in children with cholera. Antibiotics are indicated for moderate to severe cases. **Quinolones** or **TMP-SMX** are first choices. Antimotility agents should not be used.

NEUTROPENIC FEVER

Defined as a single temperature of > 38.3°C (101.3°F), or a sustained temperature > 38°C (100.4°F) for > 1 hour in a neutropenic patient (ANC = PMNs + bands < 500).

EXAM

Elderly patients or those on corticosteroids might not be able to mount a fever that meets the diagnostic criteria for neutropenic fever.

- Examination of the skin should be conducted for signs of erythema, rash, cellulitis, ulcers, or line infection.
- All indwelling lines should be carefully examined for subtle signs of infection; erythema, tenderness, fluctuance, or exudate may be the only evidence of a serious "tunnel" infection.
- Avoid DRE unless perirectal abscess is suspected.

DIAGNOSIS

CBC with differential, complete metabolic panel, amylase, lipase, CXR; cultures of urine, blood, sputum, and stool should be sent. LP is warranted only if CNS symptoms are present.

TREATMENT

- Use a **third- or fourth-generation cephalosporin** IV or carbapenem IV.
- Consider vancomycin in patients with a history of MRSA infections, hypotension, persistent fever on empiric therapy, or skin or catheter site infections.
- Think about fungal infections (especially *Candida* and *Aspergillus*) in patients with 5–7 days of persistent fever, and begin amphotericin B or fluconazole.

SECTION II

Musculoskeletal

Joint aspiration aids in the preliminary diagnosis of arthritis by helping distinguish inflammatory from noninflammatory disease as well as infectious and hemorrhagic processes (see Table 2.10-1).

A multisystem chronic inflammatory disease that is 2° to ANA complex formation and deposition. Patients may experience acute flare-ups of their symptoms. SLE is generally 1° but sometimes occurs 2° to drug use (hydralazine, penicillamine, and procainamide). 2° SLE is reversible.

SYMPTOMS/EXAM

Patients tend to be young African-American females. Findings by organ system are as follows:

- **Constitutional:** Fatigue, weight loss, fever.
- **Arthritis:** Usually migratory and asymmetric; involves the hands.
- **Skin: Malar rash** (butterfly rash over the cheeks and nose), **discoid rash** (scaling papules that can leave residual scarring), alopecia, painless **oral ulcers,** Raynaud's phenomenon, **photosensitive rash.**
- **Renal failure.**
- **Pulmonary: Pleuritis,** pleural effusion, interstitial lung disease, pulmonary hypertension.
- **Cardiovascular: Pericarditis,** pericardial effusion.
- **CNS:** Seizures, neuropathies, headache.
- **Psychological:** Anxiety, depression, psychosis.
- **Hematologic:** Thrombocytopenia, hemolytic anemia, leukopenia.
- **GI: Peritonitis.**

Table 2.10-1. Interpretation of Joint Aspiration

	NORMAL	NONINFLAMMATORY	INFLAMMATORY	INFECTIOUS	HEMORRHAGIC
Color	Clear	Xanthochromic	Yellow	Opaque	Bloody
Viscosity	High	High	Low	Low	Variable
WBCs/mm^3	< 200	200–3000	3000–50,000	> 50,000	Variable
% PMNs	< 25	< 25	> 50	> 75	Variable
Crystals	None	None	May be present	None	None
Differential	None	Osteoarthritis, SLE, trauma, aseptic necrosis, scleroderma, Charcot's joint	Gout, pseudogout, rheumatoid arthritis, SLE, TB, scleroderma, ankylosing spondylitis, psoriatic arthritis	Bacterial, TB	Coagulopathy, trauma

DIAGNOSIS

- The diagnostic criteria for SLE are summarized in the mnemonic **DOPAMINE RASH.** The diagnosis is made in patients with at least four of the 11 criteria outlined.
- ANA is highly sensitive but nonspecific, whereas anti-dsDNA and anti-Sm antibodies are highly specific.
- Obtain anticardiolipin antibody and lupus anticoagulant to screens for antiphospholipid antibody syndrome in patients with SLE.
- Active SLE flare-ups: ↓ C3 and C4 but ↑ CRP and ESR.

TREATMENT

Arthritis and mild serositis are treated with NSAIDs. Hydroxychloroquine is used for rashes and for arthritis that is unresponsive to NSAIDs. Steroids and immunosuppressants are used in the presence of significant organ involvement. Patients undergoing active SLE flare-ups are treated with steroids, which are tapered when remission is induced. Patients with antiphospholipid antibody syndrome need lifelong anticoagulation with warfarin.

COMPLICATIONS

SLE patients who become pregnant have a higher incidence of spontaneous abortion. Neonates can get congenital complete heart block. Patients can also have antiphospholipid antibody syndrome, which predisposes them to arterial and venous thrombosis.

▶ RHEUMATOID ARTHRITIS (RA)

A chronic, symmetrical, and erosive synovitis.

SYMPTOMS/EXAM

Insidious onset of a symmetrical arthritis. **Nonspecific** complaints include fever, fatigue, anorexia, and weight loss. Affected joints are swollen and tender. Other findings include joint deformities (see Figure 2.10-1), atlantoaxial joint subluxation, carpal tunnel syndrome, and Baker's cyst rupture. **Extra-articular features** include neuropathy, episcleritis, Sjögren's syndrome (dry eyes and mouth), pulmonary fibrosis, hepatosplenomegaly, Hashimoto's thyroiditis, pleuritis, lung nodules, pericarditis, and myocarditis.

DIAGNOSIS

Diagnosed in the presence of four or more of the following criteria for six weeks:

- Morning stiffness (> 1 hour).
- Arthritis of three or more joint areas (most commonly the PIP, MCP, wrist, elbow, knee, or ankle).
- Arthritis of the hand joints (MCP, PIP, or wrists).
- Symmetric arthritis.
- Rheumatoid nodules.
- ⊕ serum RF.
- X-ray changes.

Think antiphospholipid syndrome in a woman with recurrent spontaneous abortion or premature delivery.

SLE criteria— DOPAMINE RASH

Discoid rash
Oral ulcers
Photosensitive rash
Arthritis
Malar rash
Immunologic criteria (⊕ anti-dsDNA or ⊕ anti-Sm)
NEurologic or psychiatric symptoms
Renal disease
ANA ⊕
Serositis (pleural, peritoneal, or pericardial)
Hematologic disorders (thrombocytopenia, anemia, or leukopenia)

Typical RA hands:

- *MCP and PIP involvement*
- *Sparing of the DIP joint*
- *Ulnar deviation*
- *Symmetric*
- *Swan-neck deformities*

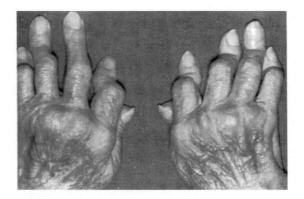

FIGURE 2.10-1. Rheumatoid arthritis.

The swan-neck deformities of the digits and severe involvement of the PIP joints are characteristic. (Reproduced, with permission, from Chandrasoma P. *Concise Pathology*, 3rd ed. Stamford, CT: Appleton & Lange, 1998:978.)

Methotrexate for RA is contraindicated in pregnant patients and in those with HIV, liver disease, renal failure, or bone marrow suppression.

RF is nonspecific but is ⊕ in 75% of RA cases. Joint aspiration is inflammatory (see Table 2.10-1). Look for periarticular osteoporosis with erosions around the affected MCP and PIP joints on x-rays (see Figure 2.10-1).

TREATMENT

Mild cases of RA are treated with NSAIDs. Add hydroxychloroquine if NSAIDs are inadequate. Moderate to severe cases are treated with NSAIDs and methotrexate. Give anti-TNF treatment (etanercept, infliximab, adalimumab) if methotrexate fails or is contraindicated. Gold and immunosuppressants are used in patients who fail methotrexate and etanercept therapy. Acute exacerbations of RA (i.e., patients who are febrile, toxic, or experiencing a rapid decline in function) are treated with a short course of prednisone. Other measures include weight loss, rest, and physiotherapy.

▶ GOUT

A metabolic condition resulting from the intra-articular deposition of monosodium urate crystals. Complications include nephrolithiasis and chronic urate nephropathy.

SYMPTOMS/EXAM

Typically presents in **middle-aged, obese men** (90%) from the Pacific Islands. Acute gout attacks often occur at night between periods of full remission. Patients present with severe pain, redness, and swelling in a single joint in a single lower extremity (typically the first MTP joint). Symptoms of pseudogout are less severe. Common precipitants of attacks include a high-purine diet (e.g., meats, alcohol), dehydration (2° to diuretic use), trauma, or tumor lysis syndrome. Patients with long-standing disease may develop **tophi** that lead to joint deformation.

DIAGNOSIS

Joint aspiration is inflammatory with needle-shaped, negatively birefringent (**yeLLow** when **paraLLel** to the condenser) crystals (see Figure 2.10-2 and Table 2.10-2). Radiographs are normal in early gout. Characteristic punched-

Monoarthritis? Think:

- *Gout*
- *Septic arthritis*
- *Lyme disease*
- *Traumas*

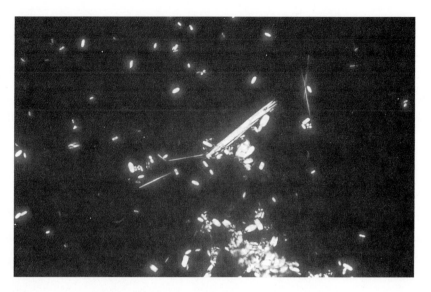

FIGURE 2.10-2. Gout crystals.

Needle-shaped, negatively birefringent crystals. (Reproduced, with permission, from Milikowski C. *Color Atlas of Basic Histopathology*, 1st ed. Stamford, CT: Appleton & Lange, 1997:546.)

out erosions with overhanging cortical bone ("rat bites") are seen in more advanced disease. Most patients have ↑ serum uric acid. A 24-hour urine collection for uric acid while patients are off hyperuricemia-inducing medications (diuretics, alchohol, cyclosporine) helps determine the etiology of hyperuricemia (see Table 2.10-3).

TREATMENT

For acute attacks, administer high-dose NSAIDs (e.g., indomethacin) or colchicine. Use steroids when first-line therapy fails. Once the acute attack resolves, patients need maintenance therapy to reduce serum uric acid levels to 5–6 mg/dL. Overproducers of uric acid are treated with allopurinol. Undersecreters of uric acid are treated with probenecid. Avoid precipitants of acute attacks and consume a low-purine diet (eggs, cheese, fruit, and vegetables).

Avoid allopurinol during acute gout attacks.

Table 2.10-2. Differential Diagnosis of Gout and Pseudogout

	GOUT CRYSTALS	PSEUDOGOUT CRYSTALS
Composition	Urate	Calcium pyrophosphate dihydrate
Shape	Needle-shaped	Rhomboid-shaped
Refringence	Negatively birefringent	Strongly positively birefringent
Red compensator	YeLLow when paraLLel	Blue when parallel
Response to colchicine	Good	Weak

Table 2.10-3. Causes of Hyperuricemia

	OVERPRODUCTION OF URIC ACID	UNDERSECRETION OF URIC ACID
24-hour urine collection for uric acid	> 800 mg/day	< 800 mg/day
Etiology	Idiopathic (1°), inherited enzyme defect, myeloproliferative disorders, lymphoproliferative disorders, tumor lysis syndrome, psoriasis	Chronic renal failure, aspirin, diuretics

► OSTEOARTHRITIS (OA)

A chronic, noninflammatory joint disease marked by degeneration of the articular cartilage, hypertrophy of the bone margins, and changes in the synovial membrane. OA can be 1° or 2° to trauma, any chronic arthritis, congenital joint disease, or a systemic metabolic disorder (hemochromatosis, Wilson's disease).

SYMPTOMS/EXAM

Insidious onset of joint pain without inflammatory signs (swelling, warmth, and redness). OA worsens with activity during the day and improves with rest. Crepitus is a common nonspecific finding. There are no systemic manifestations. 1° OA usually involves the following joints:

- **Hands: DIP,** PIP, and first carpometacarpal joint.
- **Feet:** First MTP joint.
- **Knees, hips.**
- **Spine:** C5, T9, and L3 are the most common spinal levels.

DIAGNOSIS

OA is diagnosed by an overall clinical impression based on the history and physical, radiographic findings (joint space narrowing, subchondral sclerosis, and osteophytes), and labs (which are normal).

TREATMENT

Acetaminophen or NSAIDs are used for mild symptoms. Intra-articular corticosteroid injections may be added if needed for further pain control. Joint replacement is used for severe OA in patients who fail medical management and have marked limitation of their daily activities. Nonpharmacologic interventions include weight loss, physiotherapy, and low-impact exercise.

► LOW BACK PAIN (LBP)

Table 2.10-4 outlines the common causes of LBP.

DIAGNOSIS

- Order a stat MRI if you suspect cauda equina syndrome. Assess the range of motion of the lower back. Localize the lower back tenderness to the spine or the paraspinal area.

Table 2.10-4. **Causes of Lower Back Pain**

	SYMPTOMS/EXAM	TESTS
Cauda equina syndrome	Bowel and bladder incontinence or retention, saddle anesthesia. **A medical emergency.**	Order a stat MRI if cauda equina is suspected.
Degenerative processes	Chronic and progressive. **Degeneration of disks** → localized pain that can also refer to adjacent spinal nerves (e.g., pain that radiates down the thigh). Severe disk disease can → **spinal stenosis** where LBP worsens with standing and walking but improves with sitting or stooping forward.	Order a lumbar spine x-ray to rule out other causes of LBP.
Neoplastic	1° or metastatic to bone. Suspect in elderly patients with weight loss or a history of cancer.	Tumor mass is seen on lumbar spine x-ray.
Traumatic	Acute onset of LBP temporally associated with a traumatic event. Local spinal tenderness 2° to a **fracture** or a **herniated disk** (pain worsens with cough; L4 or L5 nerve root compression). Perispinal tenderness indicates **myofascial strain.**	Fractures can be seen on lumbar spine x-ray. Myofascial strain and disk herniations cannot be seen.
Osteomyelitis	Fever, chills, or IV drug use.	Mass is seen on lumbar spine x-ray.
Ankylosing spondylitis	Young adult male with chronic LBP that is worse in the morning and with sacroiliitis and arthritis of the hip, knee, or shoulder. Acute anterior uveitis, restriction of chest wall expansion, dactylitis, Achilles tendonitis, plantar fasciitis. Reduced spinal mobility.	AP pelvic x-ray shows pseudowidening, erosions, and sclerosis of the sacroiliac joint. Lumbar spine x-ray shows "bamboo spine." HLA-B27 90% sensitive in Caucasians.
Referred	Can be 2° to disease from the aorta, kidneys, ureter, or pancreas.	Perform a thorough abdominal exam.

- Perform a neurologic exam to determine if the spinal nerves are affected (see Table 2.10-5).
- Suspect spinal cord involvement if the Babinski reflex is upgoing.
- A ⊕ **straight leg raise test** (a supine patient experiences leg, buttock, or back pain in the affected leg at < 60 degrees of elevation of the **affected** leg) is sensitive for spinal nerve irritation. A ⊕ **crossed straight leg raise test** (a supine patient experiences leg, buttock, or back pain in the affected leg at < 60 degrees of elevation of the **unaffected** leg) is specific for spinal nerve irritation.
- A **lumbar spine x-ray** is ordered for patients in whom osteomyelitis, cancer, fractures, or ankylosing spondylitis is suspected or for those who fail to improve after 2–4 weeks of conservative therapy. Consider screening patients for osteoporosis if fractures are seen on x-ray.

HIGH-YIELD FACTS

MUSCULOSKELETAL

Table 2.10-5. Spinal Nerve Damage and Associated Sensorimotor Deficits

SPINAL NERVE	MOTOR DEFICITS	SENSORY DEFICIT	REFLEXES
L3, L4	Problems rising from a chair and heel walking.	Over the anterior knee or the medial calf.	↓ knee jerk
L5	Problems heel walking, extending the big toe, or dorsiflexing the ankle.	Over the medial aspect of the foot.	
S1	Problems toe walking or plantar flexing the ankle.	Over the lateral aspect of the foot.	↓ ankle jerk

- An **MRI** should be ordered if the patient has neurologic deficits on exam where surgery is being considered.

TREATMENT

Patients with cauda equina syndrome, spinal stenosis, or spinal nerve involvement require surgical evaluation. Ankylosing spondylitis and degenerative LBP are treated with NSAIDs and physiotherapy. Avoid heavy lifting. Most LBP from disk herniation will improve within six weeks; otherwise, surgery should be considered.

▶ COMMON ORTHOPEDIC INJURIES

Tables 2.10-6 and 2.10-7 outline common adult and childhood orthopedic injuries.

▶ TEMPORAL ARTERITIS (GIANT CELL ARTERITIS)

Affects older women more often than men by a ratio of 2:1. Can cause **blindness** 2° to occlusion of the **central retinal artery** (a branch of the internal carotid artery). Half of patients also have polymyalgia rheumatica (see below).

SYMPTOMS/EXAM

A new headache associated with scalp pain (e.g., pain combing hair), **temporal tenderness, jaw claudication,** fever, and **monocular blindness** are classic. Temporal arteritis is also associated with weight loss, myalgias/arthralgias, and fever.

DIAGNOSIS

Obtain an **ESR** (often > 100), an ophthalmologic evaluation, and a **temporal artery biopsy.** Biopsy will reveal thrombosis, necrosis of the media, and lymphocytes, plasma cells, and giant cells.

TREATMENT

Treat immediately with **high-dose prednisone** (40–60 mg/day) for 1–2 months before tapering. Unless a biopsy is immediately available, do not delay treatment, as blindness is permanent. Continue to follow the eye exam for improvements or changes.

HIGH-YIELD FACTS

MUSCULOSKELETAL

Table 2.10-6. Common Adult Orthopedic Injuries

INJURY	MECHANICS	TREATMENT
Shoulder dislocation	Most commonly an anterior dislocation with the **axillary artery and nerve** at risk. Posterior dislocations are associated with seizures and electrocutions and can injure the **radial artery.** Patients with anterior injuries hold the arm in external rotation; those with posterior injuries hold the arm in internal rotation.	Closed reduction followed by a sling and swath. Recurrent dislocations may need surgical repair.
Hip dislocation	Most commonly a posterior dislocation via a posteriorly directed force **on an internally rotated, flexed,** adducted hip **("dashboard injury").** Anterior dislocations can injure the obturator nerve; posterior dislocations can injure the sciatic nerve and cause avascular necrosis (AVN).	Closed reduction followed by abduction pillow/bracing. Evaluate with CT scan after reduction.
Colles' fracture	**The most common wrist fracture.** Involves the distal radius and commonly results from a **fall onto an outstretched hand,** resulting in a dorsally displaced, dorsally angulated fracture. Commonly seen in the **elderly** (osteoporosis) and in children.	Closed reduction followed by application of long arm cast. May need open reduction if fracture is intra-articular.
Boxer's fracture	Fracture of the fifth metacarpal neck. Often results from forward trauma of a **closed fist** (e.g., punching a wall, an individual's jaw, or another fixed object).	Closed reduction and ulnar gutter splint; percutaneous pinning if fracture is excessively angulated. If skin is broken, assume infection by human oral pathogens **("fight bite")** and treat with surgical irrigation, debridement, and IV antibiotics to cover *Eikenella.*
Humerus fracture	Results from direct trauma and puts the **radial nerve** at risk (nerve travels in the spiral groove of the humerus). Signs of radial nerve palsy include **wrist drop** and loss of thumb abduction.	Hanging arm cast versus coaptation splint and sling. Functional bracing.
Hip fracture	**Most common in osteoporotic women** who sustain a fall. Patients present with a **shortened** and **externally rotated leg.** Displaced femoral neck fractures are associated with a high risk of AVN and fracture nonunion. Patients are at risk for subsequent DVTs.	Open reduction with internal fixation (ORIF) with parallel pinning of the femoral neck. Displaced fractures in elderly patients (> 80 years of age) may require a hip hemiarthroplasty. **Anticoagulation** is necessary for DVT prevention.
Achilles tendon rupture	Most commonly seen in unfit men who are participating in sports and hear a sudden **"pop" like a rifle shot.** Exam shows **limited plantar flexion** and a **positive Thompson test** (pressure on the gastrocnemius does not result in foot plantar flexion).	Treat with a long-leg cast for six weeks.

HIGH-YIELD FACTS

MUSCULOSKELETAL

Table 2.10-6. Common Adult Orthopedic Injuries (continued)

INJURY	MECHANICS	TREATMENT
Knee injuries	Present with knee instability and possibly edema and hematoma. ■ **ACL:** Results from forced hyperflexion; ⊕ anterior drawer and Lachman's tests. Rule out a meniscal or MCL injury. ■ **PCL:** Results from forced hyperextension; positive posterior drawer test. ■ **Meniscal tears: Clicking or locking** may be present. Exam shows **joint line tenderness** and a ⊕ McMurray's test.	Treatment of MCL/LCL and meniscal tears is conservative unless tears are associated with symptoms or concurrent ligamentous injuries. Treatment of ACL injuries is generally surgical with graft from the patellar or hamstring tendons. Operative PCL repairs are reserved for highly competitive athletes.

(Adapted, with permission, from Le T et al. *First Aid for the USMLE Step 2,* 4th ed. New York: McGraw-Hill, 2003:266–267.)

▶ **POLYMYALGIA RHEUMATICA**

- **Pain and stiffness of the shoulder and pelvic girdle** areas with **fever,** malaise, weight loss, and minimal joint swelling.
- Patients classically have difficulty getting out of a chair or lifting their arms above their heads but have **no objective weakness.**
- Look for **anemia** and ↑↑ **ESR.**
- Treat with **low-dose prednisone** (5–20 mg/day).

▶ **FIBROMYALGIA**

- A syndrome of myalgias, weakness, and fatigue in the absence of inflammation.
- Associated with depression, anxiety, and irritable bowel syndrome (IBS); most commonly affects **women ≥ 50 years of age.**
- Suspect with 11 of 18 "**trigger points**" (see Figure 2.10-3) that, when palpated, reproduce pain. Otherwise, consider myofascial pain syndrome.
- Treat with supportive measures such as stretching and heat application. Consider hydrotherapy, transcutaneous electrical nerve stimulation (TENS), stress reduction, psychotherapy, or low-dose antidepressants.

▶ **POLYMYOSITIS**

A progressive, systemic connective tissue disease characterized by striated muscle inflammation. One-third of patients have **dermatomyositis** with coexisting cutaneous involvement. Patients may also develop myocarditis, cardiac conduction deficits, or malignancy. More commonly seen in **older women** (50–70 years of age).

SYMPTOMS/EXAM

Symmetric, progressive, **proximal** muscle weakness and pain cause the classic complaint of difficulty rising from a chair. Patients may eventually have difficulty breathing or swallowing. Dermatomyositis may present with a **heliotrope rash** (violaceous periorbital rash) and **Gottron's papules** (papules located on the dorsum of the hands over bony prominences).

Table 2.10-7. Common Pediatric Orthopedic Injuries

INJURY	CHARACTERISTICS	TREATMENT
Clavicular fracture	**Most commonly fractured long bone in children.** May be birth-related (especially in large infants) and can be associated with **brachial nerve palsies.** Usually involve the **middle third of the clavicle,** with the proximal fracture end displaced superiorly due to the pull of the sternocleidomastoid muscle.	Figure-of-eight sling versus arm sling.
Greenstick fracture	Incomplete fracture involving the cortex of only one side of the bone.	Reduction with casting. Order films at 7–10 days.
Nursemaid's elbow	**Radial head subluxation** that typically occurs as a result of being **pulled or lifted by the hand.** The child complains of pain and **will not bend the elbow.**	Manual reduction by gentle supination of the elbow at 90° of flexion. No immobilization is necessary.
Osgood-Schlatter disease	Overuse apophysitis of the tibial tubercle. Causes localized pain, especially with quadriceps contraction, in active young boys.	↓ activity for 1–2 years. A neoprene brace may provide symptomatic relief.
Salter-Harris fractures	Fractures of the growth plate in children. Classified by fracture location: ■ **I:** Physis (growth plate). ■ **II:** Metaphysis and physis. ■ **III:** Epiphysis and physis. ■ **IV:** Epiphysis, metaphysis, and physis. ■ **V:** Crush injury of physis.	Types I and II can generally be treated nonoperatively. Others, including unstable fractures, must be treated operatively to prevent complications such as leg length inequality.

(Adapted, with permission, from Le T et al. *First Aid for the USMLE Step 2,* 4th ed. New York: McGraw-Hill, 2003:268.)

DIAGNOSIS

Look for ↑ **serum creatinine, aldolase, and CPK.** EMG demonstrates fibrillations. Muscle biopsy shows inflammatory cells and muscle degeneration.

TREATMENT

High-dose **corticosteroids** generally → improved muscle strength in 4–6 weeks and can be tapered to a lower dose for maintenance therapy. If patients are unresponsive to initial treatment, immunosuppressive medication may be used. Monitor for malignancy.

▶ SCLERODERMA

■ Multisystem disease with **symmetric thickening** of the skin on the face and extremities.
■ Typically affects **women** 30–65 years of age.
■ There are two subtypes: limited and diffuse (see Table 2.10-8).

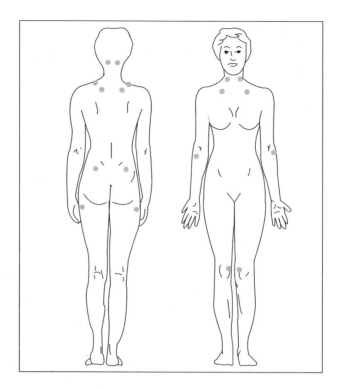

FIGURE 2.10-3. **Trigger points in fibromyalgia.**

(Reprinted, with permission, from Braunwald E. *Harrison's Principles of Internal Medicine*, 15th ed. New York: McGraw-Hill, 2001:2011.)

Table 2.10-8. **Limited vs. Diffuse Scleroderma**

	LIMITED (CREST)	DIFFUSE
Skin involvement	Distal, face only	Generalized
Progression	Slow	Rapid
Diagnosis	Anticentromere antibody	Anti-Scl-70 antibody
Prognosis	Fair	Poor
Calcinosis	+++	+
Telangiectasia	+++	+
Renal failure	0	++

CREST

Calcinosis
Raynaud's phenomenon
Esophageal dysmotility
Sclerodactyly
Telangiectasias

SECTION II

Nephrology

Glomerular Filtration Rate (GFR)

GFR provides a useful index of overall renal function and can be approximated with the creatinine clearance (CrCl):

$$\text{CrCl in mL/min} = [(U_{Cr} \text{ in mg/dL}) \times (\text{vol urine in 24 hrs in mL/day})] / [(P_{Cr} \text{ in mg/dL}) \times 1440]$$

where U_{Cr} = urine creatinine and P_{Cr} = plasma creatinine.

Alternatively, CrCl can be estimated with the Cockcroft and Gault formula:

$$\text{CrCl for males} = [(140 - \text{age}) \times (\text{weight in kg})] / (Cr \times 72)$$
$$\text{CrCl for females} = 0.85 \times (\text{GFR male})$$

A normal CrCl would be 97–137 mL/min in males and 88–128 mL/min in females.

Fractional Excretion of Sodium (Fe$_{Na}$)

$Fe_{Na} = 100 \times (U_{Na} \times P_{Cr}) / (P_{Na} \times U_{Cr})$, where U_{Na} = urinary sodium and P_{Na} = plasma sodium. See Table 2.11-1 for the interpretation of Fe_{Na} values.

Interpreting a Urinalysis (UA)

Table 2.11-2 outlines the interpretation of UA results.

▶ **HYPONATREMIA**

Serum sodium < 135 mEq/L.

SYMPTOMS/EXAM

May be asymptomatic or present with **confusion, lethargy,** muscle cramps, and nausea. Hyponatremia may progress to seizures, status epilepticus, or coma.

DIAGNOSIS

Hyponatremia is first classified by serum osmolarity (P_{osm}), as listed below. Useful tests to order here include a P_{Na}, osmolarity, total protein glucose, and lipid panel.

- **Hypertonic (P_{osm} > 295 mOsm/kg):** Hyperglycemia; hypertonic infusion (e.g., mannitol, radiocontrast).

T a b l e 2 . 1 1 - 1 . **Significance of Fe$_{Na}$ Values**

Fe$_{Na}$	CAUSES
< 1%	Prerenal
> 2%	Intrinsic renal disease

Table 2.11-2. Interpretation of UAs

TEST	INTERPRETATION
Proteinuria	A urine dip will detect only albumin, not nonalbumin proteins such as globulins and Bence Jones proteins; there must be at least 100–150 mg protein/dL (equivalent to ~ 300 mg protein/day) for the dip to become ⊕. A UA will detect albumin and nonalbumin proteins, but there must be at least 1–10 mg protein/dL for the UA to be ⊕.
Glucosuria	Indicates the possibility of hyperglycemia.
Ketonuria	Occurs with starvation, uncontrolled diabetes, and alcohol intoxication as well as postexercise and during pregnancy.
Hematuria	Will become ⊕ when myoglobin, hemoglobin, or RBCs are present in the urine.
Nitrite	Can become ⊕ with gram-negative bacteriuria.
Leukocyte esterase	Produced by WBCs in urine and suggestive of UTI.
pH	Alkalosis: *Proteus* in UTI; some strains of *Klebsiella, Pseudomonas, Providencia,* and *Staphylococcus.* Acidosis with nephrolithiasis suggests uric acid or cystine stones. Failure to acidify < pH 5.5 in the setting of metabolic acidosis suggests distal renal tubular acidosis (RTA).
Specific gravity	A rough estimate of urine osmolarity (U_{osm}).
Urobilinogen	↑ urobilinogen indicates hemolysis or hepatocellular disease. ↓ urobilinogen indicates biliary obstruction.
Bilirubin	Bilirubin in the urine suggests a conjugated hyperbilirubinemia.
Epithelial	An excessive number of epithelial cells in the urine suggests a contaminated urine sample.

Urine Sediment

FINDING	ASSOCIATION
Hyaline casts	Normal finding, but an ↑ amount suggests a prerenal condition.
RBC casts	Glomerulonephritis.
WBC casts	Pyelonephritis.
Eosinophils	Allergic interstitial nephritis.
Glomerular, "muddy brown" casts	Acute tubular necrosis (ATN).
RBCs	Indicates hematuria.
WBCs	Indicates injury to the body or urinary tract. Can be caused by infection, nephrolithiasis, neoplasm, acute interstitial cystitis, acute interstitial nephritis, strictures, and glomerulonephropathy.
Crystals	See nephrolithiasis.
Yeast, bacteria	Indicates infection if the sample is not contaminated (e.g., epithelial cells).

HIGH-YIELD FACTS

NEPHROLOGY

- **Isotonic (P_{osm} = 280–295 mOsm/kg):** Hyperlipidemia (triglycerides, chylomicrons), hyperproteinemia.
- **Hypotonic (P_{osm} < 280 mOsm/kg):** Hypotonic hyponatremia is further classified by volume status (see Table 2.11-3). Useful tests to aid in evaluation include serum BUN, creatinine, sodium, and Fe_{Na} (U_{Na}, U_{Cr}).

TREATMENT

Symptomatic hyponatremia with altered mental status or seizures requires 3% **hypertonic saline** to ↑ P_{Na} by 3–5 mEq/L over the next six hours. Concurrent furosemide may be necessary to prevent volume overload. Once the symptoms have resolved, treat the hyponatremia according to volume status. The goal in asymptomatic hyponatremia is to ↑ P_{Na} by no more than 12 mEq/L per day to prevent **central pontine myelinolysis** (flaccid paralysis, dysarthria, dysphagia). Management is tailored to volume status.

- **Hypotonic hypovolemic hyponatremia:** Fluid resuscitation with normal saline.
- **Hypotonic euvolemic hyponatremia:** Fluid restriction (free-water consumption < 1 L/day).
- **Hypotonic hypervolemic hyponatremia:** Fluid restriction with diuresis if necessary.

Syndrome of Inappropriate Antidiuretic Hormone (SIADH)

A major cause of hyponatremia due to ↑ ADH release without osmolality-dependent or volume-dependent physiologic stimuli. Causes of SIADH include the following:

- **Pulmonary:** Oat cell carcinoma, TB, pneumonia, pulmonary abscess. Consider ordering a CXR.
- **CNS:** Meningitis, brain abscess, head trauma. Consider ordering a head CT.
- **Drugs:** Clofibrate, chlorpropamide, phenothiazine, carbamazepine.
- **Ectopic ADH production:** Lymphoma, sarcoma, duodenal/pancreatic cancer.

DIFFERENTIAL

Hypothyroidism; consumption of too much water with not enough salt (psychogenic polydipsia, beer potomania).

Table 2.11-3. Classification of Hypotonic Hyponatremia by Volume Status

HYPOVOLEMIC		EUVOLEMIC	HYPERVOLEMIC
EXTRARENAL SALT LOSS (Fe_{Na} < 1%)	**RENAL SALT LOSS (Fe_{Na} > 2%)**		**EDEMATOUS STATES**
Dehydration	Diuretic use	SIADH	CHF
Diarrhea	Nephropathies	Hypothyroidism	Liver disease
Vomiting	Mineralocorticoid deficiency	Psychogenic polydipsia	Nephrotic syndrome
		Beer potomania	Advanced renal failure

DIAGNOSIS

P_{osm} < 270 mOsm/kg; U_{osm} > 100 mOsm/kg; euvolemia; normal renal, adrenal, and thyroid function.

TREATMENT

Fluid restriction (free-water consumption < 1 L/day). Add demeclocycline if response is inadequate.

► HYPERNATREMIA

Serum sodium > 145 mEq/L.

SYMPTOMS/EXAM

May present with mental status changes, weakness, focal neurologic deficits, and seizures.

DIAGNOSIS

Take a thorough history and assess the patient's volume status to determine the etiology of the hypernatremia. Check U_{osm}, P_{osm}, potassium, BUN, creatinine, calcium, and glucose.

- Hypernatremia from **hypovolemia** usually presents in the setting of dehydration when the patient has limited access to free water. U_{osm} is usually > 800 mOsm/kg. Causes include insensible losses (burns, sweating) or diarrhea.
- Hypernatremia from ↑ **sodium load** usually does **not** present with hypovolemia. Causes include overhydration with hypertonic fluids or mineralocorticoid excess (think about this if the patient has hypokalemia and hypertension).
- Hypernatremia from **renal losses** (see Table 2.11-4) usually presents in the setting of hypovolemia and a U_{osm} < 800 mOsm/kg. Consider the clinical context in the setting of the U_{osm}/P_{osm} ratio to help determine the cause.

Hypernatremia often occurs with dehydration.

Table 2.11-4. Causes of Hypernatremia 2° to Renal Losses

	ETIOLOGY	COMMENTS
Osmotic diuresis	**Causes:** Mannitol, hyperglycemia, high protein feeds, postobstructive diuresis.	U_{osm}/P_{osm} > 0.7.
Central diabetes insipidus	The pituitary does not make ADH. **Causes:** Tumor, trauma, neurosurgery, infection.	U_{osm}/P_{osm} < 0.7. U_{osm} should ↑ by 50% in response to DDAVP.
Peripheral diabetes insipidus	The kidneys are unresponsive to ADH. **Causes:** Renal failure, hypercalcemia, demeclocycline, lithium, sickle cell anemia.	U_{osm}/P_{osm} < 0.7. U_{osm} should not respond to DDAVP challenge.

TREATMENT

Treat underlying causes (e.g., DDAVP for central diabetes insipidus) and replace the free-water deficit with hypotonic saline, D_5W, or oral water depending on volume status. Correction of hypernatremia should not occur at a rate > 12 mEq/L per day to prevent cerebral swelling.

▶ HYPERKALEMIA

Serum potassium > 5 mEq/L.

SYMPTOMS/EXAM

May be asymptomatic or may present with nausea, vomiting, **intestinal colic, areflexia, weakness,** flaccid paralysis, and paresthesias. ECG findings may include **tall peaked T waves,** PR prolongation, wide QRS, loss of P waves that can progress to **sine waves,** ventricular fibrillation, and cardiac arrest (see Figure 2.11-1).

DIAGNOSIS

First, verify the hyperkalemia with a **repeat blood draw** unless the suspicion is already high. Then exclude **spurious** causes of hyperkalemia, which include hemolysis (e.g., during blood draw), fist clenching during the blood draw, extreme leukocytosis, extreme thrombocytosis, or rhabdomyolysis. Order an ECG and use the urine potassium to help determine the etiology of the hyperkalemia.

- **Urine potassium < 40 mEq/L:** Usually indicates that the hyperkalemia is caused by ↓ potassium excretion by the kidneys. Causes include renal insufficiency, drugs (e.g., spironolactone, triamterene, ACEIs, trimethoprim, NSAIDs) and mineralocorticoid deficiency (type 4 RTA). A plasma renin activity and plasma aldosterone concentration should be ordered if a mineralocorticoid deficiency is suspected.
- **Urine potassium > 40 mEq/L:** Usually indicates a nonrenal etiology. Causes include **cellular shifts** resulting from tissue injury tumorlysis, insulin deficiency, drugs (e.g., succinylcholine, digitalis, arginine, β-blockers), and **iatrogenic** factors.

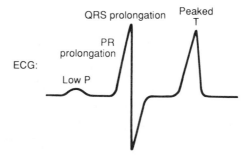

FIGURE 2.11-1. Hyperkalemia.

ECG findings include peaked T waves, PR prolongation, and a widened QRS complex. (Reproduced, with permission, from Cogan MF. *Fluid and Electrolytes.* Stamford, CT: Appleton & Lange, 1991:170.)

TREATMENT

Values > 6.5 mEq/L or ECG changes (especially PR prolongation or wide QRS) require emergent treatment. **Calcium gluconate** for cardiac cell membrane stabilization should be given immediately to prevent arrhythmias, followed by **bicarbonate** or **insulin and glucose** to temporarily shift potassium into the cells. Patients can be given **Kayexalate** and/or **furosemide** with hydration to promote potassium excretion. **Restrict potassium** in the diet and discontinue any medications that may be contributing to the hyperkalemia. Hyperkalemia refractory to the above management or patients on hemodialysis will require acute **hemodialysis.**

> **Treatment of Hyperkalemia—C BIG K**
>
> **C**alcium
> **B**icarbonate
> **I**nsulin
> **G**lucose
> **K**ayexalate

► HYPOKALEMIA

Serum potassium < 3.5 mEq/L.

SYMPTOMS/EXAM

May present with fatigue, **muscle weakness or cramps, ileus,** hyporeflexia, paresthesias, and flaccid paralysis if severe. ECG may show **T-wave flattening, U waves** (additional wave after the T wave), and ST depression followed by AV block and subsequent cardiac arrest.

DIAGNOSIS

Order an ECG and check urine potassium.

- **Urine potassium > 20 mEq/L:** Usually indicates that the kidneys are wasting potassium. Acid-base status must be examined to further stratify the etiology.
    - **Metabolic acidosis:** Type 1 RTA (e.g., amphotericin), lactic acidosis, or ketoacidosis.
    - **Metabolic alkalosis:** 1° or 2° hyperaldosteronism (check plasma renin activity and plasma aldosterone concentration), Cushing's syndrome (check 24-hour urine cortisol), diuretics (e.g., loop or thiazide), or hypomagnesemia.
    - **Variable pH:** Gentamicin.
- **Urine potassium < 20 mEq/L:** Usually indicates a nonrenal source for hypokalemia. This could be from **transcellular shift** (e.g., insulin, β_2-agonists, alkalosis, periodic paralysis) or from **GI losses** (e.g., diarrhea, chronic laxative abuse, vomiting, NG suction).

TREATMENT

Treat the underlying disorder. Administer oral and/or IV **potassium repletion.** Replace **magnesium,** as this deficiency makes potassium repletion more difficult. Monitor ECG and plasma potassium levels frequently during replacement.

► HYPERCALCEMIA

Serum calcium > 10.2 mg/dL. The most common causes are **hyperparathyroidism and malignancy** (e.g., squamous cell cancers, myeloma).

SYMPTOMS/EXAM

May present with **bones** (fractures), **stones** (kidney stones), abdominal **groans** (anorexia, vomiting, constipation), and **psychiatric overtones** (weakness, fatigue, altered mental status).

DIAGNOSIS

Order an ECG (may show a **short QT interval**), total/ionized calcium, albumin, phosphate, PTH, PTHrP (parathyroid hormone–related peptide), vitamin D (25-OH vitamin D and 1,25-OH vitamin D), TSH, serum immunoelectrophoresis, ALP, GGT, spot urine calcium, spot urine creatinine, BUN, and creatinine.

- ↑ **PTH:** Indicates that 1° hyperparathyroidism (adenoma, hyperplasia, carcinoma, MEN I/II) is the cause of the hypercalcemia. Beware of an ectopic PTH-producing tumor as well.
- **Spot urine calcium-to-creatinine ratio < 0.30:** Indicates that the kidneys are not excreting enough calcium. Causes include Addison's disease, thiazide diuretics, and familial hypocalciuric hypercalcemia.
- **Normal or low PTH:** Indicates that the cause could be excessive calcium or vitamin D intake, granulomatous disease (25-OH vitamin D is not converted into its active form, 1,25-OH vitamin D at an increased rate), malignancy that produces PTHrP, milk-alkali syndrome, multiple myeloma, or Paget's disease (where you will find an ↑ ALP in the setting of a normal GGT).

TREATMENT

Discontinue all drugs that can cause hypercalcemia; place the patient on a low-calcium diet. Patients should be well **hydrated** and given **furosemide**, which will promote calcium diuresis. Patients with symptomatic hypercalcemia or a serum calcium > 13.5 mg/dL require the administration of a **bisphosphonate**, which will ↓ serum calcium in 24–48 hours. The addition of **calcitonin** will ↓ serum calcium in 12–24 hours. **Hemodialysis** is a last resort.

> ### ▶ ACUTE RENAL FAILURE (ARF)

A ↓ in GFR (usually corresponding to an ↑ in creatinine of 0.5 mg/dL or > 50% over the baseline value) occurring over a period of hours to days. Results in the failure of the kidneys to excrete nitrogenous waste and to maintain fluid and electrolyte balance. Oliguria (defined as < 400 cc/day) is not required for ARF.

SYMPTOMS/EXAM

Patients with ARF are often asymptomatic or may present with **uremic symptoms,** which include anorexia, nausea, fatigue, malaise, asterixis, pericarditis (listen for a friction rub), or easy bleeding (uremia can cause platelet dysfunction). Examination should include checking BP, daily weights, and assessing volume status. Other findings are specific to the etiology of renal failure.

DIAGNOSIS

Order electrolytes, BUN, creatinine, urinalysis (UA), and urine eosinophils, and calculate Fe_{Na}. ARF is categorized as prerenal, intrinsic, or postrenal (see Table 2.11-5).

Causes of hypercalcemia—CHIMPANZEES

Calcium supplementation
Hyperparathyroidism
Iatrogenic/**I**mmobility
Milk-alkali syndrome
Paget's disease
Addison's disease/**A**cromegaly
Neoplasm
Zollinger-Ellison syndrome
Excess vitamin A
Excess vitamin D
Sarcoidosis

Table 2.11-5. Causes of Acute Renal Failure

PRERENAL	INTRINSIC	POSTRENAL
Hepatorenal syndrome ACE Is, NSAIDs	Interstitial: acute interstitial nephritis	Bilateral ureteral stenosis: stones, blood clot, retroperitoneal fibrosis
Renal artery stenosis	Tubular: ATN	Bladder neck: anticholinergic, tumor
All causes of shock (e.g., cardiogenic and hypovolemic)	Vascular: emboli, occlusion, vasculitis, renal vein thrombosis Glomerular	Prostate: BPH, cancer, prostatitis

- **Postrenal failure:** Caused by urinary outflow obstructions in both ureters, the bladder neck, or the prostate. Patients can present in fluid overload from urinary retention. A prostate examination is necessary to ensure that the prostate gland is not enlarged. Calculate a **postvoid residual**—ask the patient to urinate, and then insert a Foley catheter to measure the urine remaining in the bladder. A postvoid residual > 75 cc indicates that the bladder neck or the prostate is causing a postrenal obstruction. **Renal ultrasound** will detect any dilatation in the ureters.
- **Prerenal failure:** Caused by ↓ renal perfusion. Patients usually present with an $Fe_{Na} < 1\%$ and a **BUN/creatinine ratio > 20.** Commonly seen with dehydration, CHF, and liver failure. Listen for a renal artery bruit characteristic of renal artery stenosis. If the patient is not in florid CHF, a trial bolus of isotonic fluids will usually indicate shock as a cause of prerenal failure if the BUN/creatinine ratio improves after the fluids.
- **Intrinsic failure:** Usually presents with **hematuria, proteinuria, and/or casts** on the UA. Patients with glomerulonephritis present with a nephritic syndrome (RBCs, RBC casts). Patients with acute interstitial nephritis have an RUA with eosinophils, WBCs, and WBC casts. ATN presents with an $Fe_{Na} > 1\%$ and a urine sediment with pigmented granular ("muddy brown") casts and renal tubular epithelial cells. Suspect a vascular cause if predisposed patients (e.g., those with a hypercoagulable state) present with abdominal pain.

An $Fe_{Na} < 1\%$ suggests prerenal failure.

TREATMENT

All nephrotoxic medications should be discontinued. Avoid contrast studies unless they are absolutely necessary. Any medications that are excreted via the kidneys should be ↓ in accordance with the current GFR. IV fluids or furosemide should be given to keep patients euvolemic. Patients should be placed on a low-potassium diet. Monitor and correct calcium, PO_4, and potassium. Anion-gap metabolic acidosis should be treated with sodium bicarbonate to keep the pH > 7.2. Dialyze if indicated.

> *Indications for emergent dialysis— AEIOU*
>
> **A**cidosis
> **E**lectrolytes (hyperkalemia)
> **I**ngestion
> **O**verload (fluid)
> **U**remic symptoms (pericarditis, encephalopathy, bleeding, nausea, pruritus, myoclonus)

▶ ACUTE TUBULAR NECROSIS (ATN)

The most common form of intrinsic ARF due to tubular damage. Causes include the following:

- **Exogenous nephrotoxins:** Chemotherapeutic agents (cisplatin, methotrexate), aminoglycosides, amphotericin B, cephalosporins, heavy metals.

- **Endogenous nephrotoxins:** Hyperuricemia, rhabdomyolysis, massive intravascular hemolysis, Bence Jones proteins (from multiple myeloma).
- **Radiographic contrast:** Prevent with hydration and Mucomyst prior to contrast study.
- **Ischemia:** All causes of shock.

DIAGNOSIS

Usually presents with ARF, $Fe_{Na} > 1\%$, and a urine sediment with pigmented granular ("muddy brown") casts and renal tubular epithelial cells. In addition to the workup for ARF, all patients should have a serum CK and uric acid level checked.

TREATMENT

Treat as per ARF. With rhabdomyolysis, give mannitol for diuresis and bicarbonate to alkalinize the urine.

▶ HEMATURIA

Three or more RBCs/hpf on urine microscopy.

DIAGNOSIS

All patients should undergo a prostate exam to look for BPH or prostatitis as a cause of hematuria. Patients should get an UA to rule out UTI, nephrolithiasis (crystals on urine microscopy), and tubulointerstitial nephritis (urine WBC, WBC casts, and/or eosinophils). If the UA shows RBC casts or the daily urinary protein > 1 g, suspect a glomerular cause for the hematuria (see nephritic syndrome). PTT, PT, and platelets will determine if the patient has any hematologic reason for easy bleeding. A ⊕ urine cytology can be indicative of bladder cancer. If this initial workup is ⊖ or hematuria persists despite treatment, proceed as follows:

- Look for **upper tract** (kidneys and ureter) causes of hematuria by ordering an IVP, a CT urogram, or a renal ultrasound. These tests will detect any renal mass, polycystic kidneys, or hydronephrosis/hydroureter that could be 2° to nephrolithiasis.
- If no upper tract cause can be found, a cystoscopy should be ordered to look for **lower tract** causes of hematuria, such as a urethral stricture, interstitial cystitis, or cancer of the urinary system.
- If the workup is still ⊖, a **renal angiogram** should be ordered to look for any varices, aneurysms, or AVMs.
- If no cause can be found despite a full workup, patients should get an RUA and urine cytology every six months followed by a renal ultrasound every three years until the hematuria subsides.

▶ PROTEINURIA

Defined as a daily urinary protein excretion of > 150 mg. Nephrotic syndrome is severe proteinuria that is defined as a daily urinary protein excretion of > 3.5 g. Microalbuminuria is defined as a **persistent** daily urinary protein excretion of 30–300 mg in a patient with diabetes. Transient microalbuminuria can occur with infection, stress, and illness.

Generally unremarkable unless the patient has nephrotic-range proteinuria. In such instances, patients usually present with generalized edema.

DIAGNOSIS

A UA significant only for protein in the absence of known renal disease suggests **benign proteinuria**. Causes include pulmonary edema, CHF, fever, exercise, head injury, CVA, stress, orthostasis, or idiopathic benign proteinuria. Benign proteinuria will resolve when the cause is treated. For nonbenign proteinuria, obtain a 24-hour urine collection to quantify the daily urinary protein excretion. A UA, electrolytes, BUN/creatinine, urine protein electrophoresis, and serum total protein should be ordered.

- Acute or chronic **tubulointerstitial nephritis** presents with < 2 g urinary protein/24 hours and mixed low-molecular-weight proteins on urine electrophoresis. RUA usually shows WBC casts, WBCs, and/or eosinophils. Causes include infection, medications (NSAIDs, quinolones, sulfonamides, rifampin), and connective tissue diseases (SLE, sarcoidosis, Sjögren's).
- **Glomerular causes** of proteinuria usually present with > 2 g urinary protein/24 hours and primarily albumin on electrophoresis. RUA usually shows RBCs and/or RBC casts (see the discussions of nephritic and nephrotic syndromes).
- **Overflow proteinuria** usually presents with < 2 g urinary protein/24 hours and primarily light chains and low-molecular-weight proteins on urine electrophoresis. Plasma total protein is often ↑. Causes include amyloidosis, multiple myeloma, lymphoproliferative disease, hemoglobinuria, and myoglobinuria.

TREATMENT

Patients with proteinuria should be put on a low-salt and low-saturated-fat diet. Protein intake should be ~ 1 g/kg/day.

- If **hyponatremia:** Fluid restriction.
- If **peripheral edema:** Furosemide.
- If **diabetic with microalbuminuria or proteinaria:** ACEIs.
- If **benign proteinuria:** Identify and treat the underlying cause.

▶ NEPHRITIC SYNDROME

Also called glomerulonephritis. Caused by glomerular inflammation. Sudden-onset hematuria (RBC casts are the hallmark) and variable proteinuria (< 3 g/24 hours) with temporally associated ARF are characteristic. Causes are summarized in Table 2.11-6.

SYMPTOMS/EXAM

Patients may present with the classic findings of oliguria, macroscopic hematuria (smoky-brown urine), hypertension, and possibly **edema in low-pressure regions** such as the periorbital and scrotal areas.

Table 2.11-6. **Common Causes of Nephritic Syndrome**

	DESCRIPTION	HISTORY AND PE	LABS AND HISTOLOGY	TREATMENT AND PROGNOSIS
Postinfectious glomerulo-nephritis	Often associated with a recent **streptococcal infection** (group A β-hemolytic).	Oliguria, edema, hypertension, smoky-brown urine.	Low serum C3, increased antistreptolysin O (ASO) titer, **lumpy-bumpy immuno-fluorescence (IF).**	Supportive. Almost all children and most adults have complete recovery.
IgA nephropathy (Berger's disease)	**Most common type;** associated with upper respiratory or GI infections; commonly in young men.	Gross hematuria.	May see ↑ serum IgA level. Biopsy and IF will show mesangial IgA deposits.	Glucocorticoids for select patients; 20% progress to end-stage renal disease.
Wegener's granulomatosis	Granulomatous inflammation of the respiratory tract and kidney with necrotizing vasculitis; a pauci-immune form of rapidly progressive glomerulonephritis (RPGN).	Fever, weight loss, hematuria, respiratory and sinus symptoms; cavitary pulmonary lesions bleed and cause **hemoptysis.**	Presence of **c-ANCA** (cell-mediated immune response).	High-dose corticosteroids and cytotoxic agents. Patients tend to have frequent relapses.
Alport's syndrome	Hereditary glomerulonephritis; presents in boys 5–20 years old.	Asymptomatic hematuria associated with **nerve deafness** and eye disorders.	GBM splitting on electron microscopy.	Progresses to renal failure. Anti-GBM nephritis may recur after transplant.
Goodpasture's syndrome	Glomerulonephritis with pulmonary hemorrhage; peak incidence in men in their mid-20s; an immune form of RPGN.	**Hemoptysis,** dyspnea, possible respiratory failure.	**Linear anti-GBM deposits** on IF, iron-deficiency anemia, hemosiderin-filled macrophages in sputum, pulmonary infiltrates on CXR.	Plasma exchange therapy, pulsed steroids. May progress to end-stage renal disease.
Other causes	SLE, cryoglobinemia			

(Reproduced, with permission, from Le T et al. *First Aid for the USMLE Step 2,* 4th ed. New York: McGraw-Hill, 2003:463.)

Think nephritic syndrome in the setting of hematuria, hypertension, and oliguria.

DIAGNOSIS

UA will show **hematuria** and mild **proteinuria**. Patients have a ↓ GFR with ↑ BUN and creatinine. Obtain complement, ANA, ANCA, C3, C4, antistreptolysin titer, cryoglobulins, and hepatitis B and C serologies. A renal biopsy is often required to make a conclusive diagnosis.

TREATMENT

Treat hypertension, fluid overload, and uremia with salt and water restriction, diuretics, and, if necessary, dialysis. **Corticosteroids** are sometimes useful to ↓ glomerular inflammation.

▶ NEPHROTIC SYNDROME

Defined as > 3.5 g urinary protein/24 hours, albumin < 3 g/dL, and peripheral edema. Patients can also have associated hyperlipidemia and hypercoagulable states. Causes are summarized in Table 2.11-7.

DIAGNOSIS

In addition to the labs ordered for the workup of proteinuria, order a lipid panel, ANA, hepatitis B and C serologies, RPR, fasting glucose, and HIV. Consider a renal biopsy if the etiology is still not evident from the initial serologies. Roughly one-third of nephrotic syndrome cases are caused by diabetes, amyloidosis, or SLE nephropathy. The remainder are usually due to one of four 1° renal diseases: minimal change disease, focal glomerular sclerosis, membranous nephropathy, or membranoproliferative glomerulonephritis.

TREATMENT

Treat as per proteinuria, except patients with hyperlipidemia should be started on a statin. Patients developing thrombosis will need anticoagulation. Pneumovax is recommended.

▶ RENAL TUBULAR ACIDOSIS (RTA)

A net ↓ in either tubular hydrogen (H^+) secretion or bicarbonate reabsorption that results in a **non-anion-gap metabolic acidosis.** There are three main types of RTA (see Table 2.11-8). **Type IV (distal)** is the most common.

▶ NEPHROLITHIASIS

Most commonly occurs in males in the third and fourth decades of life. Risk factors include a ⊕ family history, **low fluid intake,** gout, postcolectomy/ileostomy, specific enzyme disorders, RTA, and hyperparathyroidism. Stones are most commonly calcium oxalate but may also be calcium phosphate, struvite, uric acid, or cystine (see Table 2.11-9).

SYMPTOMS/EXAM

Acute onset of severe, colicky flank pain that may **radiate to the testes or vulva** and may be associated with nausea and vomiting. Patients are unable to get comfortable and shift position frequently (as opposed to those with peritonitis, who are still).

DIAGNOSIS

UA may show gross or **microscopic hematuria** and an **altered urine pH.** Obtain a **KUB** to detect any radiopaque stones. An **IVP** can be used to detect stones that are radiolucent on KUB. **Noncontrast abdominal CT scans** may diagnose stones and other causes of flank pain. All urine should be strained, and if a stone is passed, it should be recovered and sent to the lab for analysis.

T a b l e 2 . 1 1 - 7. Causes of Nephrotic Syndrome

	DESCRIPTION	HISTORY AND PE	LABS AND HISTOLOGY	TREATMENT AND PROGNOSIS
Minimal change disease	Common in children; idiopathic etiology.	Tendency toward infections and thrombotic events.	Light microscopy appears **normal.** Electron microscopy shows **fusion of epithelial foot processes** with lipid-laden renal cortices.	Steroids; excellent prognosis.
Focal segmental glomerulosclerosis (FSGS)	Idiopathic, IVDU, HIV infection.	Typical patient is young black male with uncontrolled hypertension.	Microscopic hematuria; biopsy shows sclerosis in capillary tufts.	Prednisone, cytotoxic therapy.
Membranous nephropathy	**Most common Caucasian adult nephropathy;** an immune complex disease.	Associated with HBV, syphilis, **malaria,** and gold.	**"Spike and dome"** appearance due to granular deposits of IgG and C3 at basement membrane.	Prednisone and cytotoxic therapy for severe disease.
Diabetic nephropathy	Two characteristic forms: diffuse hyalinization and nodular glomerulo-sclerosis **(Kimmelstiel-Wilson lesions).**	Generally have long-standing, poorly controlled DM.	Thickened GBM; **increased mesangial matrix.**	Tight control of blood sugar; protein restriction; ACEIs.
Lupus nephritis	Classified as WHO types I–V. Both nephrotic and nephritic. Severity of renal disease often determines overall prognosis.	Proteinuria or RBCs on UA may be found during evaluation of SLE patients.	Mesangial proliferation; subendothelial immune complex deposition.	Prednisone and cytotoxic therapy may slow disease progression.
Renal amyloidosis	1° (plasma cell dyscrasia) and 2° (infectious or inflammatory) are the most common.	Patients may have multiple myeloma or a chronic inflammatory disease (e.g., rheumatoid arthritis, TB).	Abdominal fat biopsy; seen with **Congo red stain; apple-green** birefringence under polarized light.	Prednisone and melphalan. Bone marrow transplant may be used for multiple myeloma.
Membrano-proliferative nephropathy (MPGN)	Can also be a nephritic syndrome.	Slow progression to renal failure.	**"Tram-track"** double-layered basement membrane. Type I has subendothelial deposits; type II involves a C3 nephritic factor and ↓ C3.	Corticosteroids and cytotoxic agents may help.

(Reproduced, with permission, from Le T et al. *First Aid for the USMLE Step 2,* 4th ed. New York: McGraw-Hill, 2003:464.)

Table 2.11-8. Types of RTA

	TYPE I (DISTAL)	TYPE II (PROXIMAL)	TYPE IV (DISTAL)
Defect	H^+ secretion.	HCO_3^- reabsorption.	Aldosterone deficiency or resistance → defects in Na^+ reabsorption, H^+ and K^+ excretion.
Serum K^+	High or low.	Low.	High.
Urinary pH	> 5.3.	> 5.3 initially; < 5.3 once serum is acidic.	< 5.3.
Etiologies (most common)	Hereditary, amphotericin, collagen vascular disease, cirrhosis, nephrocalcinosis.	Hereditary, carbonic anhydrase inhibitors, Fanconi's syndrome.	Hyporeninemic hypoaldosternism with **DM,** hypertension, chronic interstitial nephritis.
Treatment	Potassium citrate.	Potassium citrate.	Furosemide, Kayexalate.
Complications	Nephrolithiasis.	Rickets, osteomalacia.	Hyperkalemia.

(Reproduced, with permission, from Le T et al. *First Aid for the USMLE Step 2,* 4th ed. New York: McGraw-Hill, 2003:467.)

Table 2.11-9. Types of Nephrolithiasis

TYPE	FREQUENCY	ETIOLOGY AND CHARACTERISTICS	TREATMENT
Calcium oxalate/ calcium phosphate	83%	Most common causes are **idiopathic hypercalciuria,** ↑ urine uric acid 2° to diet, and 1° hyperparathyroidism. Alkaline urine; radiopaque.	Hydration, thiazide diuretic.
Struvite ($Mg-NH_4-PO_4$)	9%	"Triple phosphate stones." Associated with urease-producing organisms (e.g., *Proteus*). Form staghorn calculi. Alkaline urine. Radiopaque.	Hydration; treat UTI if present.
Uric acid	7%	Associated with gout and high purine turnover states. Acidic urine (pH < 5.5). **Radiolucent.**	Hydration; alkalinize urine with citrate, which is converted to HCO_3^- in the liver.
Cystine	1%	Due to a defect in renal transport of certain amino acids (**COLA**—**C**ystine, **O**rnithine, **L**ysine, and **A**rginine). **Hexagonal crystals;** radiopaque.	Hydration, alkalinize urine, penicillamine.

(Reproduced, with permission, from Le T et al. *First Aid for the USMLE Step 2,* 4th ed. New York: McGraw-Hill, 2003:465.)

TREATMENT

Hydration and analgesia are the initial treatment; additional treatment is based on the size of the stone. Kidney stones < 5 mm in diameter can pass through the urethra; stones < 3 cm in diameter can be treated with **extracorporeal shock-wave lithotripsy** (ESWL) or percutaneous nephrolithotomy. Preventive measures include hydration and prophylactic measures that depend on stone composition.

▶ ACID-BASE DISORDERS

See Figure 2.11-2 for a description of acid-base disorders.

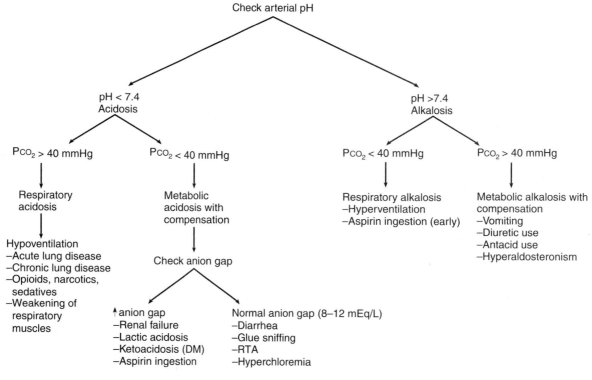

FIGURE 2.11-2. Acid–base disorders.

(Reproduced, with permission, from Le T et al. *First Aid for the USMLE Step 2*, 4th ed. New York: McGraw-Hill, 2003:455.)

SECTION II

Neurology

Acute onset of focal neurologic deficits that result from ↓ blood flow (ischemic stroke) or hemorrhage (hemorrhagic stroke) and persist for at least 24 hours.

SYMPTOMS/EXAM

- **Superior division MCA stroke:** Contralateral hemiparesis that affects the face, hand, and arm but spares the leg; contralateral hemisensory deficit in the same distribution; ipsilateral gaze preference; facial droop. If the dominant (i.e., left) hemisphere is affected, Broca's (expressive) aphasia will be seen.
- **Inferior division MCA stroke:** Contralateral homonymous hemianopsia; neglect of contralateral limbs; apraxia. If the dominant (i.e., left) hemisphere is affected, Wernicke's (receptive) aphasia will be seen.
- **Anterior cerebral artery:** Leg paresis.
- **Posterior cerebral artery:** Homonymous hemianopsia with macular sparing; prosopagnosia (inability to recognize familiar faces).
- **Basilar artery:** Coma, CN palsies, locked-in syndrome.
- **Lacunar stroke:** Pure motor or sensory deficit; dysarthria–clumsy hand syndrome; hemiparesis; facial droop.

DIFFERENTIAL

Seizure, brain mass (tumor or abscess), subdural or epidural hematoma, hypo-/hyperglycemia, multiple sclerosis, TIA.

DIAGNOSIS

- **Head CT without contrast:** To rule out a bleed.
- MRI with **diffusion-weighted imaging (DWI) and perfusion-weighted imaging (PWI):** DWI shows dying tissue; PWI shows the "penumbra," or tissue at risk of dying.
- **MR angiogram:** To evaluate vessels, including the carotids and the circle of Willis.
- **Transesophageal echocardiogram:** To evaluate for cardiac thrombi and patent foramen ovale.
- **Other:** CBC, electrolytes, coagulation studies, Hb_{A1c}, homocysteine, fasting lipids.

TREATMENT

- **Antiplatelet agents:** Aspirin has been proven to ↓ the incidence of a second event. If the patient is already on aspirin, may add clopidogrel, ticlodipine, or dipyridamole.
- **Thrombolytics:** If symptoms are of < 3 hours' duration, IV recombinant tPA should be considered provided that patients meet inclusion and exclusion criteria and the CT scan shows no bleed. In the presence of basilar artery thrombosis, patients may get intra-arterial tPA up to six hours after symptom onset.
- **Carotid endarterectomy:** If > 70% stenosis is seen on angiogram, consider surgery.
- **Anticoagulation:** Warfarin if atrial fibrillation is present or if cardiac ejection fraction is < 15%.
- Usually vascular meds, lipid-lowering agents, and antihypertensives.

Embolic strokes often occur suddenly. The deficits are usually maximal at onset. Rapid recovery favors embolism.

Thrombotic strokes often fluctuate, progressing in a stuttering fashion with some periods of improvement; symptoms are sometimes dependent on BP.

Seizures involve **excessive electrical discharge** by cortical neurons that cause focal or general neurologic symptoms.

SYMPTOMS

- **Partial seizures:** Involve only a portion of the brain. Two subtypes:
    - **Simple partial:** Do not impair consciousness; arise from a discrete region in one of the cerebral hemispheres. Manifestations may be motor (e.g., jacksonian march—progressive jerking that spreads from one limb to the next), sensory, or autonomic. Postictally, patients may have a focal neurologic deficit (i.e., Todd's paralysis) that resolves within minutes to days. An aura is the sensation patients experience from the simple partial seizure.
    - **Complex partial:** Do affect consciousness; most commonly involve the temporal lobes. Characterized by auditory or visual hallucinations, déjà vu, and automatisms (e.g., **lip smacking, chewing, picking at clothes**).
    - Both types may progress to involve the entire brain as a **generalized tonic-clonic (GTC) seizure.**
- **Generalized seizures:** Involve the entire brain. Four subtypes:
    - **Absence (petit mal):** Most common in **children**; subside by adulthood and are often familial. Involve brief, subtle episodes of impaired consciousness that last a few seconds and occur up to hundreds of times per day. EEG shows generalized spike-and-wave discharges at 3 Hz.
    - **Myoclonic:** Shocklike jerks of muscle groups.
    - **Generalized tonic-clonic (grand mal):** Tonic extension of the back and extremities, followed by 2–3 minutes of repetitive, symmetric clonic movements. There may be cyanosis, incontinence, or tongue biting. GTC is usually accompanied by postictal acidosis with low HCO_3, ↑ serum CK, and sometimes ↑ serum prolactin.
    - **Status epilepticus:** Prolonged (> 30 minutes) or repetitive seizures without a return to baseline consciousness between them. Associated with a 20% mortality rate.

EXAM

- **Fever** implies an infectious etiology or prolonged seizing.
- Look for **tongue biting** and **urinary incontinence,** which are common for generalized seizures. Also check for **neck stiffness,** which points to meningitis.

DIFFERENTIAL

- Intracranial hemorrhage, acute or **old stroke (particularly cortical), SAH,** meningitis, head injury, subdural hematoma.
- **Hyponatremia, EtOH withdrawal,** cocaine or amphetamine intoxication.
- Medications known to be associated with seizures include imipramine, meperidine, INH, metronidazole, and **fluoroquinolones.**
- **Neoplasm:** 1° CNS tumor or brain mets.

For seizures of unknown etiology, remember to "scan, stick, and wave": MRI, LP, and EEG.

Some states require up to a one-year seizure-free period before allowing seizure patients to drive.

DIAGNOSIS

- CBC, electrolytes, glucose, magnesium, calcium, ammonia, EtOH level, toxicology screen, and anticonvulsant level if the patient is currently on meds.
- An **EEG is used to help localize the focus, get a baseline, and confirm the diagnosis if in doubt.**
- If a focal deficit is present, get a CT or **MRI** of the brain.
- **If there is any evidence of infection (i.e., fever), get an LP** after confirming through imaging that there is no evidence of ↑ ICP.

TREATMENT

- **Acute:**
  - Check Airway, Breathing, and Circulation (ABCs); **intubation may be needed for airway protection.**
  - Always check **glucose level,** as it is a very common cause of convulsions. If the patient is hypoglycemic, give thiamine and then glucose. If the glucose level is normal, give lorazepam 0.1 mg/kg in 2-mg increments each over 2–3 minutes up to 8 mg.
  - If seizure continues, give **phenytoin** 15–20 mg/kg no faster than 50 mg/min. If seizure persists, consider phenobarbital coma.
- **Chronic:** Table 2.12-1 outlines pharmacotherapy for the long-term prevention of seizures.

▶ COMA

The most common causes include ischemic brain injury, traumatic brain injury, and metabolic derangements such as profound hypoglycemia.

SYMPTOMS/EXAM

Patients are unresponsive and are usually intubated. If all of the following apply, the patient is **brain dead:**

- No response to pain.
- Absence of pupillary light reflex.
- Absence of oculocephalic reflex.
- Absence of oculovestibular reflex, including response to cold caloric stimulation.
- Bilateral loss of corneal reflex.

Table 2.12-1. **First-Line Drugs for the Prevention of Seizure**

PARTIAL	TONIC-CLONIC	ABSENCE	MYOCLONIC
Carbamazepine	Valproate	Ethosuximide	Valproate
Phenytoin	Lamotrigine	Valproate	Lamotrigine
Lamotrigine	Phenytoin		Topiramate
Valproate	Carbamazepine		

- Absence of gag reflex.
- Decorticate or decerebrate posturing.
- **Roving eye** movements.

DIFFERENTIAL

- **Brain death:** Unresponsive; no brain stem reflexes; $\oplus$ **apnea test**—P_{CO_2} on ABG is at least 60 mmHg or $\uparrow$ by 20 mmHg, and there is no spontaneous breathing in the face of rising hypercarbia.
- **Locked-in syndrome:** A brain stem lesion in which the patient is quadriplegic but is fully conscious.
- Nonconvulsive status epilepticus.
- Psychogenic coma (hysterical coma).

DIAGNOSIS

- EEG to evaluate for **nonconvulsive status epilepticus.**
- LP to rule out infection or SAH.
- Urine and serum toxicology screen.
- CBC, electrolytes, and blood cultures.
- MRI of the brain.
- Angiogram.
- Transcranial Doppler ultrasound.

TREATMENT

- Manage medical causes of coma such as infection, metabolic derangement, or ischemic insults.
- Control body temperature.
- Treat seizures as indicated.

Brain death is defined as the cessation of cerebral and brain stem function.

For coma patients, always rule out nonconvulsive status epilepticus with EEG.

▶ EPIDURAL HEMATOMA

- Typically results from head trauma associated with a lateral skull fracture and **tearing of the middle meningeal artery.** A true **neurologic emergency.**
- Patients may have a **lucid interval** before onset of coma. Initial symptoms may include headache, nausea, vomiting, drowsiness, and seizures. Look for hemiparesis and **blown pupil** (fixed, dilated pupil due to herniation).
- Head CT without contrast shows a **biconvex lens-shaped hyperdensity** compressing the cerebral hemisphere (see Figure 2.12-1).
- **Prompt surgical evacuation** of blood.

▶ SUBDURAL HEMATOMA

- Typically results from blunt head trauma (commonly a fall) with resultant rupture of the bridging veins (commonly seen in **elderly** and **alcoholics**).
- Presentation includes headache, altered mental status, and hemiparesis.
- Head CT shows a **crescent-shaped,** concave hyperdensity that follows the contour of the cerebral hemisphere (see Figure 2.12-2).
- **Surgical evacuation** of blood if symptoms are present or if the lesion is $\uparrow$ in size.

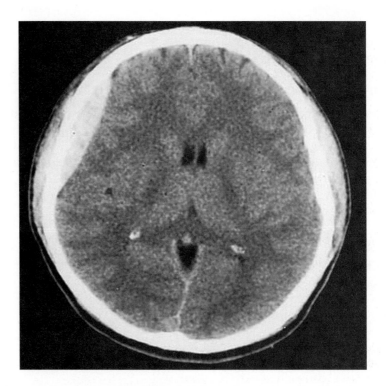

FIGURE 2.12-1. Acute epidural hematoma.

The typical lenticular shape is due to the dura, which is tightly adherent to the skull. Epidural hematomas are usually caused by disruption of the middle meningeal artery following fracture of the temporal bone. (Reproduced, with permission, from Kasper DL et al. *Harrison's Principles of Internal Medicine*, 16th ed. New York: McGraw-Hill, 2005:2450.)

▶ SPINAL CORD COMPRESSION

One of the few **neurologic emergencies.** Always **immobilize the neck** if trauma is suspected. Localize the level, image the spine, and **call neurosurgery.** Causes include the following:

- **Trauma:** Motor vehicle accidents and sports-related injuries.
- **Infection:** Epidural abscess in IV drug users; spinal TB (Pott's disease) in immunocompromised patients; vertebral osteomyelitis.
- **Neoplasm:** Metastases are most common.
- **Degenerative disease:** Cervical and lumbar disk herniations.
- **Vascular:** Infarction, epidural and subdural hematomas, and AV malformations are rare.

SYMPTOMS/EXAM

Patient presents with pain, paresthesias, and weakness. Trauma to the neck should be suspected if there is trauma to the face and body. Signs of skull fracture include the following:

- **Battle's sign** (ecchymosis over the mastoid process).
- **Raccoon sign** (periorbital ecchymosis).
- Hemotympanum and CSF rhinorrhea/otorrhea.

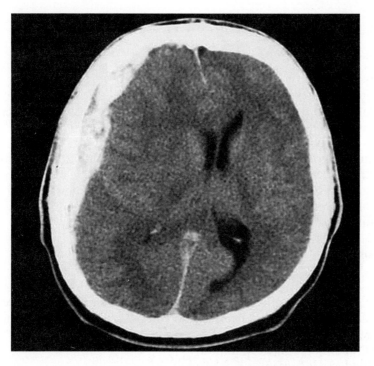

FIGURE 2.12-2. **Acute subdural hematoma in a noncontrast CT scan.**

The hyperdense clot has an irregular border with the brain and typically causes more horizontal displacement (mass effect) than might be expected from its thickness. (Reproduced, with permission, from Kasper DL et al. *Harrison's Principles of Internal Medicine*, 16th ed. New York: McGraw-Hill, 2005:2450.)

Other physical exam findings are as follows:

- **Pinprick test** to find a sensory level is the most precise and reproducible.
- **Conus medullaris involvement:** Perineal sensory loss (**saddle anesthesia**); **loss of anal wink.**
- **Cauda equina involvement:** Patchy sensory loss in the lower extremities with radicular pain and bilateral weakness.
- Radicular pain helps localize and confirm extramedullary spinal involvement.
- Abrupt onset of radicular pain, flaccid weakness, sphincter dysfunction, and a sensory level indicate cord infarction.
- **Hyporeflexia** is often present at the level of spinal cord injury with **hyperreflexia** below.

DIAGNOSIS

Spinal CT scan with contrast, **MRI/MRA** with gadolinium, or myelogram.

TREATMENT

- **Acute spinal cord injury:** Methylprednisolone 30 mg/kg IV bolus. Wait 45 minutes; then methylprednisolone 5.4 mg/kg/hr continuous infusion over the next 24 hours.
- **Spinal tumor:** Dexamethasone 100 mg IV bolus.
- Fractures, subluxations, and dislocations require surgical reduction.
- Epidural abscess requires neurosurgical decompressive laminectomy.

Always look for a sensory level when considering a spinal cord process.

Look for the following:

- **Sinus tenderness:** Indicates sinusitis.
- **Temporal artery tenderness:** Indicates temporal arteritis.
- **Conjunctival injection** (more consistent with cluster headache).
- **Cranial bruit:** Raises concern for AV malformation.
- **Neck rigidity:** Points to meningitis or SAH.
- **Kernig's sign:** ⊕ if there is pain in the neck with straightening of the flexed knee; indicates meningitis or SAH.
- **Brudzinski's sign:** ⊕ if the patient bends the knees and flexes the hips in response to passive neck flexion.
- **Papilledema:** ↑ ICP.

DIAGNOSIS

Obtain a CT scan if:

- Headache is acute and extremely severe ("**thunderclap headache**").
- Headache is progressive over days to weeks, particularly if it is not similar to previous headaches.
- Focal neurologic signs are found.
- Papilledema is present.
- Headache has morning onset or awakens the patient from sleep.

If the CT is ⊖ but SAH is still clinically suspected, an LP is necessary, as 15% of patients with an aneurysmal SAH have a ⊖ CT scan. LP will show high numbers of RBCs across all tubes collected, and xanthochromia (yellow CSF) will be present.

Migraine

SYMPTOMS

- **Migraine without aura ("common migraine"):** Recurrent headaches of 4–72 hours' duration with at least two of the following characteristics—unilateral, pulsating, severe enough intensity to limit daily activity, and aggravated by physical activity—plus one of the following: nausea, vomiting, photophobia, or phonophobia.
- **Migraine with aura ("classic migraine"):** Common migraine that also includes a homonymous visual disturbance (scintillations are called "fortification spectra"; blind spots are called "scotomata" or blurring of the vision) as well as unilateral paresthesias and, rarely, weakness.

TREATMENT

- Identify and **eliminate triggers;** this is half the battle.
- Treat according to severity:
  - **Mild:** NSAIDs plus an antiemetic such as metoclopramide.
  - **Moderate:** Abortive (**triptans** as soon as headache begins).
  - **Severe:** IV hydration, metoclopramide, dexamethasone, prochlorperazine, or ergotamine.
- **Preventive therapy:** TCAs, β-blockers, valproate.

Headache danger signs: Change in frequency or severity, fever, neurologic signs, and new-onset headaches.

Severe, sudden-onset headache should raise concern for a subarachnoid/ aneurysm rupture.

Cluster Headache

Brief, severe, **unilateral periorbital stabbing** headache. Affects men more than women; patients are usually 20–30 years of age. Attacks occur in clusters over time. Exam reveals ipsilateral lacrimation, conjunctival injection, Horner's syndrome, and nasal congestion. Responds well to 100% O_2 or low dose prednisone.

Tension Headache

A chronic disorder that begins after age 20. Presents with nonthrobbing, bilateral occipital head pain that is generally not associated with nausea, vomiting, or prodromal visual disturbances. The pain is described as a **tight band around the head.** Treat with **NSAIDs** or acetaminophen. Relaxation techniques may be helpful.

▶ GUILLAIN-BARRÉ SYNDROME (GBS)

Numbness, paresthesias, and **weakness in the distal portion of the legs, ascending** to eventually involve the face. Classically have a recent history of respiratory or GI infection (particularly *Campylobacter jejuni*).

EXAM

Look for **absent reflexes,** ↓ sensation, CN weakness (**facial nerve palsy**), proximal muscle weakness, and respiratory failure.

Absence of reflexes, ascending weakness, and recent infection—think GBS.

DIAGNOSIS

- **CBC:** May see ↑ WBC in the setting of concurrent or triggering infection.
- ESR, Lyme titer.
- **LP** typically shows ↑ protein with normal WBC levels ("**albuminocytologic dissociation**").
- **Nerve conduction study (NCS):** Look for **denervation** and **conduction block.**

TREATMENT

- **IV immunoglobulin (IVIG),** plasmapheresis, physical therapy.
- **PFTs** to monitor for **respiratory compromise.**
- Watch for **autonomic instability,** including temperature dysregulation and cardiac **arrhythmias.**

LP and EMG/NCS are crucial in diagnosing GBS.

▶ VERTIGO

Must be distinguished from lightheadedness or presyncopal sensation. Categorized as peripheral or central.

- **Peripheral:** Lesions of the labyrinth of the inner ear or the vestibular division of the acoustic nerve (CN VIII). Tends to occur intermittently and to last for brief periods; nystagmus is fatigable and causes more distress to the patient.
- **Central:**
    - Spontaneous nystagmus that cannot be suppressed with visual fixation; nystagmus that changes direction with gaze; purely vertical, horizontal,

or torsional nystagmus; saccade dysmetria (overshoot and undershoot of gaze).
- Lesions affect the brain stem vestibular nuclei or their connections. Usually acute onset, and symptoms are independent of head positioning.
- CN signs such as facial droop, dysarthria, and loss of corneal reflexes are also seen.

EXAM

- Look at the external auditory canal for vesicles (herpes zoster or **Ramsay Hunt** syndrome).
- Nystagmus:
  - Horizontal (rhythmic oscillation of the eyes, seen in both peripheral and central).
  - Rotational (peripheral).
  - Vertical (**central only**).
- Hearing loss (peripheral), diplopia (central only), limb ataxia (central only).

DIFFERENTIAL

- **Mimickers of vertigo:** Orthostatic hypotension, cardiac arrhythmia, presyncope/syncope.
- **True vertigo:**
  - Medication side effects (**furosemide, aminoglycosides**).
  - **Benign paroxysmal positional vertigo (BPPV):** Episodic attacks of severe vertigo. Self-limited; probably caused by crystals floating inside the semicircular canals brushing against the sensory cilia.
  - **Labyrinthitis/neuronitis:** Viral inflammation of CN VIII or the labyrinth; usually self-limited.
  - **Ménière's disease:** Overproduction of endolymph in the vestibular canals.
  - **Brain stem stroke:** Associated neurologic deficits are seen, including weakness, ataxia, and CN dysfunction.
  - **Schwannoma:** A mass compressing CN VIII, causing hearing loss in addition to vertigo.

DIAGNOSIS

- Neurologic exam.
- **Imaging:** Head CT without contrast; MRI of the brain with DWI.
- **Bárány** or **Dix-Hallpike maneuver:** The physician moves the patient from a sitting to a supine position, with the head rotated to one side. The test is ⊕ for BPPV if vertigo is re-created.

TREATMENT

- BPPV may respond to the **Epley maneuver** and **meclizine** 25 mg PO TID for 3–4 days along with desensitization exercises.
- If posterior circulation stroke, careful monitoring is necessary for 24–48 hours followed by stroke workup.

If there are episodic attacks of severe vertigo associated with head position, think of BPPV.

Not all that is "dizzy" is vertigo; "dizziness" can mean vertigo or lightheadedness.

Typically affects **young females.** Most commonly occurs in people residing in **northern latitudes.**

SYMPTOMS

- Visual or oculomotor; commonly blurring of vision, loss of vision, or **diplopia.**
- Weakness or **paresthesias** in a limb.
- Uncoordinated gait.
- Heat sensitivity; worsening of symptoms in a **hot shower.**

EXAM

- Hyperreflexia, **weakness,** ataxia.
- **Lhermitte's sign:** Radiating/shooting pain up or down the neck on flexion or extension.
- **Optic neuritis:** Swollen optic disk.
- **Afferent pupillary defect (Marcus Gunn pupil):** The pupil paradoxically dilates to light stimulus owing to delayed conduction.
- **Internuclear ophthalmoplegia (MLF syndrome):** The classic finding is bilateral weakness in adduction of the ipsilateral eye with nystagmus on abduction of the contralateral eye, together with incomplete or slow abduction of the ipsilateral eye on lateral gaze with complete preservation of convergence.

DIAGNOSIS

- Brain MRI with gadolinium reveals multiple focal **periventricular areas of ↑ signal,** called **Dawson's fingers** (see Figure 2.12-3).
- CSF: ↑ protein (myelin basic protein, **oligoclonal bands).**
- **Visual evoked potentials:** Show delayed conduction.

TREATMENT

- Treat acute exacerbations with corticosteroids.
- Manage relapsing-remitting disease with **interferon-β1a or 1b.**
- Glatiramer acetate, a synthetic polymer of amino acids.
- Baclofen for spasticity.

The most common form is Duchenne's muscular dystrophy, which is **X-linked,** presents by age 6, and progresses to being wheelchair-bound in childhood and to death in adolescence.

SYMPTOMS/EXAM

- **Toe walking,** waddling gait, inability to run or climb stairs.
- Proximal muscle **weakness.**
- **Gowers' sign:** In attempting to rise to standing from a supine position, patients use their arms to climb up their bodies.
- **Pseudohypertrophy** of the calves.

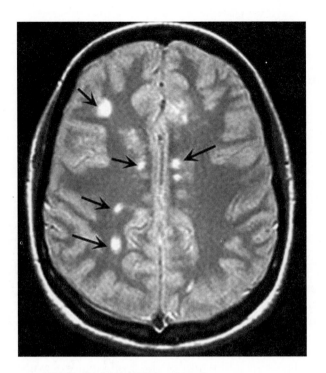

FIGURE 2.12-3. **MRI findings in multiple sclerosis.**

Multiple bright signal abnormalities in white matter, typical for multiple sclerosis. Reproduced, with permission, from Kasper DL et al. *Harrison's Principles of Internal Medicine*, 16th ed. New York: McGraw-Hill, 2005:2465.)

DIAGNOSIS

- Serum **CK** levels are ↑.
- Muscle biopsy with immunohistochemistry.
- Genetic testing for **dystrophin gene mutation.**

TREATMENT

- No definitive treatment.
- Prednisone is used to improve muscle strength but is limited in its duration.

▶ PARKINSON'S DISEASE

Characterized by **bradykinesia**—paucity of movement. Due to the striatal **deficiency of dopamine** following neuronal **degeneration within the substantia nigra.**

SYMPTOMS

- **Progressive slowness** in dressing, walking, feeding, or writing.
- Difficulty rising from a chair; hesitancy in initiating gait.
- **Frequent falls** and loss of balance.
- **Loss of facial expression (masked facies).**
- **Depression.**
- **Micrographia:** Smaller handwriting compared to previous pattern.

- **Resting tremor**
- **Bradykinesia:** Movements are slow and ↓ in amplitude. Slow blink rate; few facial expressions (masked facies).
- **Rigidity:** ↑ muscle tone, present in all directions of movement, may be **cogwheel rigidity** (rachet-like quality).
- **Loss of postural reflexes:** Patients cannot remain balanced if pushed from the front or from behind.

TREATMENT

- **Levodopa** (dihydroxyphenylalanine): A precursor amino acid to dopamine that crosses the blood–brain barrier and replenishes dopamine; gold standard of treatment.
- **Bromocriptine, pergolide, ropinirole:** Ergot derivatives with potent dopamine receptor agonist activity.
- **Surgical pallidotomy.**

Key Parkinson's signs:

- *Cogwheel rigidity*
- *Resting tremor*
- *Bradykinesia*
- *Postural instability*

► AMYOTROPHIC LATERAL SCLEROSIS (ALS)

- A chronic degenerative condition involving motor neurons in the spinal cord. Sensations and cognition are completely intact. Approximately 5–10% of cases are familial. Usually presents in **older males.**
- Patients have progressive muscular weakness, spasticity, and respiratory insufficiency.
- Look for generalized **muscle atrophy, dysarthria, tongue fasciculations,** proximal muscle weakness, and hyperreflexia. Eye movements are spared.
- EMG shows widespread denervation. Muscle biopsy shows neurogenic atrophy.
- An incurable, progressive disease. Treatment with **riluzole,** which inhibits glutamate release, has been associated with modest improvement.

► DEMENTIA

Chronic, progressive cognitive decline that interferes with daily performance in occupational and social activities. Ten percent of dementia cases are reversible. Forty to sixty percent are due to Alzheimer's disease.

SYMPTOMS

- **Impairment of recent memory** is typically the first sign, noticed by family members.
- Inability to complete recently performed tasks without difficulty (e.g., balancing the checkbook, cooking dinner).
- Disorientation first to time and then to place.
- Depression.

EXAM

- **Primitive reflexes** are present in advanced disease (e.g., palmar grasp, glabellar, rooting, palmomental).
- **Apraxia:** Inability to execute or carry out learned movements.
- **Anomia:** Inability to remember the names of things, people, or places.
- **Acalculia:** Inability to perform mathematical computations.

DIFFERENTIAL

- **Alzheimer's disease.**
- **Pick's disease:** (Frontotemporal dementia), involves personality changes).
- **Vascular/multi-infarct dementia:** Stepwise progression.
- **Normal-pressure hydrocephalus:** May also see ataxia and incontinence.
- **Alcoholism.**
- Hypothyroidism.
- **Vitamin B$_{12}$ deficiency:** May see loss of proprioception.
- **Depression:** → pseudodementia.
- Subdural hematoma.

DIAGNOSIS

- Complete neurologic exam.
- Mini-mental status exam.
- CBC, electrolytes, B$_{12}$, TSH.
- MRI of the brain.
- **Neuropsychological testing.**

TREATMENT

Current therapies are aimed at ↑ CNS ACh levels. All have limited efficacy, but some have been shown to delay admission to a nursing home by approximately six months. Treatment includes the following:

- **Acetylcholinesterase inhibitors:** Donepezil (Aricept), rivastigmine (Exelon), galantamine (Reminyl), memantine (Namenda), aglutamate receptor antagonist.
- Social support and supervision (i.e., a nursing home) if severe.

▶ WERNICKE'S ENCEPHALOPATHY

- Due to **thiamine** deficiency (vitamin B$_1$ deficiency). Most commonly seen in **alcoholics.**
- Presents with the classic **triad of ataxia, ophthalmoplegia,** and **confusion.**
- MRI may show mammillary body lesions.
- Give **thiamine IV.** Ocular deficits improve within hours. Give thiamine **before** administering glucose, as glucose is a cofactor in carbohydrate metabolism; administration of glucose may precipitate neuronal death in the absence of thiamine.

Obstetrics

All prenatal visits should document weight, BP, extremity edema, protein and glucose (urine dipstick), fundal height (> 20 weeks), and fetal heart rate. Further recommendations are as follows:

- **Weight gain:** Average-size women should gain 25–35 lbs; obese women should gain less (15–25 lbs) and thin women more.
    - The average caloric requirement is roughly 2300 kcal/day.
    - An additional 300 kcal/day is needed during pregnancy and 500 kcal/day during breast-feeding.
- **Nutrition:** ↑ requirements for protein, iron, folate, calcium, and zinc. All patients should take prenatal vitamins.
    - **Folate:** Supplement with 1 mg/day to ↓ the risk of neural tube defects. **Women with a prior history of a fetus with neural tube defects should have 4 mg/day of folate.**
    - **Iron:** Supplement with 30–60 mg/day of elemental iron in the latter half of pregnancy to prevent anemia.
    - **Calcium:** Supplement with 1500 mg/day in the later months of pregnancy and during breast-feeding.
    - **Smoking cessation.**
- **Prenatal labs:** See Table 2.13-1 for scheduled lab work during pregnancy.

Maternal Serum α-Fetoprotein (MSAFP)

- Measured between 15 and 20 weeks' gestation.
- Any result > 2.5 multiples of the mean (MoM) can signify an open neural tube defect, an abdominal wall defect, multiple gestation, incorrect dating, fetal death, or placental abnormalities.
- Sensitivity for detecting chromosomal abnormalities (**trisomy 18 and 21**) is ↑ through the addition of **estriol** and β-hCG (triple screen) to MSAFP. See Table 2.13-2 for trends in detecting genetic abnormalities.

Amniocentesis

- Performed primarily to detect possible genetic diseases or congenital malformations.
- Risks include fetal-maternal hemorrhage (1–2%) and fetal loss (0.5%).
- Amniocentesis is used:
    - In conjunction with an **abnormal triple screen.**
    - In **women > 35 years of age** (at the time of delivery).
    - In **Rh-sensitized pregnancy** to obtain fetal blood type or to detect fetal hemolysis.
    - For the evaluation of **fetal lung maturity** in the third trimester.

Chorionic Villus Sampling (CVS)

- Performed to evaluate possible genetic diseases at an earlier time than amniocentesis with comparable diagnostic accuracy.
- Done at **10–12 weeks' gestation** via aspiration of chorionic villi tissues (a precursor of the placenta).
- Risks include fetal loss (1–5%) and an association with distal limb defects.

TABLE 2.13-1. Prenatal Labs During Pregnancy

GESTATIONAL AGE (GA)	LABS TO BE OBTAINED
Initial visit	CBC, blood type, **Rh antibody screen,** sickle cell screening (in at-risk patients). UA with culture, **Pap smear,** cervical gonorrhea and chlamydia cultures. **Rubella antibody titer,** hepatitis B surface antigen, syphilis screen, PPD, HIV, +/− toxoplasmosis (for at-risk patients). Women with prior gestational diabetes should get early glucose testing.
6–11 weeks	**Ultrasound** to determine GA (more accurate than later scans).
15–19 weeks	MSAFP or preferably **triple screen** (MSAFP, estriol, β-hCG). Offer amniocentesis for those of advanced maternal age (> 35 years at delivery).
18–21 weeks	**Screening ultrasound** to survey fetal anatomy, placental location, and amniotic fluid.
26–28 weeks	**One-hour glucose challenge test;** if ≥ 140 mg/dL, follow with a three-hour glucose tolerance test. Repeat hemoglobin/hematocrit.
28 weeks	**RhoGAM** injection for Rh-negative patients. Start fetal kick counting (the patient should count 10 fetal movements under one hour every day).
32–36 weeks	Screen for **group B streptococcus** (GBS) with a rectovaginal swab. Repeat hemoglobin/hematocrit. Cervical gonorrhea and chlamydia cultures (in at-risk patients). Assess fetal position with Leopold maneuvers and ultrasound.

▶ **TESTS OF FETAL WELL-BEING**

Nonstress Test (NST)

- Fetal heart rate is monitored externally by Doppler.
- A **normal response** is an acceleration of ≥ 15 bpm above baseline lasting > 15 seconds.
- A normal or "reactive" test includes two such accelerations in a **20-minute** period.
- An abnormal or "nonreactive" NST needs a biophysical profile (see below) or a contraction stress test (see below).
- A nonreactive NST can be due to fetal sleep cycle, GA < 30 weeks, a fetal CNS anomaly, or maternal sedative or narcotic administration.

TABLE 2.13-2. Trends in Genetic Screening Markers

	NEURAL TUBE DEFECT	TRISOMY 18	TRISOMY 21
MSAFP	↑	↓	↓
Estriol	Not used	↓	↓
β-hCG	Not used	↓	↑

Contraction Stress Test (CST)

- Used to assess uteroplacental dysfunction.
- Fetal heart rate is monitored during spontaneous or induced (nipple stimulation or pitocin) contractions.
- A normal or "negative" CST has no late decelerations and is highly predictive of fetal well-being when seen with a reactive NST.
- An abnormal or "positive" CST is defined by late decelerations after 50% of contractions (minimum of three contractions) within a 10-minute period.

Biophysical Profile (BPP)

- Ultrasound is used to assess five parameters (see the mnemonic **Test the Baby, MAN**).
- A score of 2 (normal) or 0 (abnormal) is given to each of the parameters.
- A normal or "negative" test (a score of 8–10) is reassuring for fetal well-being.
- An abnormal or "positive" test (a score of ≤ 6) is worrisome for fetal compromise.

> **When performing a BPP, remember to—**
> **Test the Baby, MAN!**
>
> Fetal **T**one
> Fetal **B**reathing
> Fetal **M**ovements
> **A**mniotic fluid volume
> **N**onstress test

Fetal Heart Rate Patterns

Table 2.13-3 outlines different types of heart rate patterns seen in near-term and term fetuses.

▶ MEDICAL COMPLICATIONS OF PREGNANCY

Diabetes Mellitus (DM)

The **most common** medical complication of pregnancy. See Table 2.13-4 for a comparison of pregestational and gestational DM.

Preeclampsia/Eclampsia

- **Preeclampsia** is thought to be due to ↓ organ perfusion 2° to vasospasm and endothelial activation; it is divided into mild and severe.
- **Eclampsia** is defined as seizures in a patient with preeclampsia.

An Hb$_{A1c}$ > 8.5 prior to conception or during the first trimester will result in a higher rate of fetal malformations.

TABLE 2.13-3. Fetal Heart Rate Patterns

TYPE OF DECELERATION	DESCRIPTION	COMMON CAUSE
Early	Begins and ends at approximately the same time as maternal contractions.	Fetal head compression **(no fetal distress).**
Variable	Variable onset of abrupt slowing of fetal heart rate in association with contractions. The return is similarly abrupt in most situations.	Umbilical cord compression.
Late	Begin after the onset of maternal contractions and persist until after the contractions are finished.	**Late decelerations always indicate fetal hypoxia (fetal distress). If late decelerations are repetitive and severe, immediate delivery.**

TABLE 2.13-4. Pregestational vs. Gestational DM

	PREGESTATIONAL	GESTATIONAL
Definition	Diagnosed **prior to pregnancy.**	Diagnosed **during pregnancy.**
Risk factors	Family history; autoimmune disorders.	Obesity, family or personal history, prior gestational DM.
Diagnosis	Diagnosed prior to pregnancy.	Diagnosed if the one-hour glucose test ≥ 140 mg/dL and the follow-up three-hour glucose test has at least two ↑ levels.
Treatment	Strict control of blood glucose levels with diet, exercise, and insulin: ■ Fasting morning: < 90 mg/dL. ■ Two-hour postprandial: < 120 mg/dL.	ADA diet and regular exercise; if blood sugars are ↑ after one week, initiate insulin therapy. No oral hypoglycemic agents.
Labor	Fingersticks every 1–2 hours while in active labor with dextrose infusion +/− insulin drip to maintain tight glycemic control.	Same as with pregestational DM.
Postpartum	Continue glucose monitoring; insulin needs rapidly ↓.	Resume normal diet; no insulin required.

Complications
  Fetus
 	
  Mother
	
	Congenital malformations, stillbirth, macrosomia, hypoglycemia, birth trauma.
	Hypoglycemia, DKA, spontaneous abortion (SAB), polyhydramnios, preterm labor.
		
		Hypoglycemia from hyperinsulinemia, macrosomia, birth trauma.
		Perineal trauma from macrosomic infant; ↑ lifetime risk of mother developing DM.

■ Risk factors include nulliparity, African-American ethnicity, extremes of age, multiple gestation, renal disease, and chronic hypertension.
■ See Table 2.13-5 for key differences between mild preeclampsia, severe preeclampsia, and eclampsia.

DIAGNOSIS

■ Check UA, 24-hour urine protein and creatinine, CBC, electrolytes, BUN, creatinine, uric acid, LFTs, PT/PTT, fibrin split product and fibrinogen, and toxicology screen.
■ Determine the precise GA; consider amniocentesis to assess fetal lung maturity.
■ Diagnosis is based on **clinical findings** as described in Table 2.13-5.

HELLP syndrome:

Hemolysis
Elevated **L**iver enzymes
Low **P**latelets

TREATMENT

The **definitive** treatment is **delivery.** See Table 2.13-5 for management.

Maternal Hyperthyroidism

■ The most common etiology is Graves' disease, but it may also be caused by subacute thyroiditis, toxic nodular goiter, and toxic adenoma.

HIGH-YIELD FACTS

OBSTETRICS

TABLE 2.13-5. **Mild and Severe Preeclampsia vs. Eclampsia**

	MILD PREECLAMPSIA	**SEVERE PREECLAMPSIA**	**ECLAMPSIA**
Symptoms/exam	**SBP > 140 or DBP > 90** on two occasions. **Proteinuria** (> 0.3 g/24 hrs or 1+ on urine dipstick).	**SBP > 160 or DBP > 110** on two occasions. **Proteinuria** (> 5 g/24 hrs or > 3+ on urine dipstick). HELLP syndrome (see mnemonic). Oliguria (< 500 mL/24 hrs). Pulmonary edema.	**Seizures with the diagnosis of preeclampsia.**
Treatment	If near term, fetal lungs are mature, or preeclampsia worsens, deliver. If far from term, treat with bed rest and conservative management.	**Prophylactic magnesium sulfate (MgSO$_4$).** **BP control:** hydralazine +/– labetalol. **When stable, deliver.** **Postpartum:** Continue MgSO$_4$ for at least 24 hours after delivery. Watch for Mg$^+$ toxicity; treat with IV calcium gluconate.	**Monitor ABCs closely.** **When stable, deliver.** Seizures may occur before delivery and up to six weeks postpartum.
Complications	Fetal distress, stillbirth, placental abruption, seizure, DIC, cerebral hemorrhage.	Same as with mild preeclampsia.	Same as preeclampsia; fetal/maternal death.

- Symptoms include restlessness, heat intolerance, weight loss, frequent stools, and chest palpitations. Look for tachycardia, resting tremor, and the presence of goiter.
- **TFTs** show ↓ TSH and ↑ free T$_4$.
- Start **propylthiouracil** (PTU) until the patient becomes euthyroid; then ↓ the dose. Check TFTs every 4–6 weeks. **Subtotal thyroidectomy** in refractory or noncompliant patients.
- **Thyrotoxicosis or thyroid storm** can be precipitated by delivery, acute illness, infection, trauma, or surgery. Early recognition is key; treat with supportive care and give a large loading dose of PTU, potassium iodide, propranolol, and IV fluids.

Hyperemesis Gravidarum

- Defined as refractory vomiting → **weight loss,** poor weight gain, dehydration, ketosis from starvation, and metabolic alkalosis. Typically persists beyond 14–16 weeks' gestation.
- Risk factors include nulliparity, multiple pregnancies, and trophoblastic disease.
- Rule out molar pregnancy, hepatitis, gallbladder disease, reflux, and gastroenteritis.
- Labs will show **hyponatremia** and a hypokalemic/hypochloremic **metabolic acidosis.** Ketonuria on UA suggests starvation ketosis.

- If there is evidence of weight loss, dehydration. or altered electrolytes, **hospitalize** and give antiemetics, IV hydration, and vitamin and electrolyte replacement. Advance diet slowly and avoid fatty foods.

Postpartum Hemorrhage (PPH)

- Defined as blood loss of > 500 mL during a vaginal delivery or > 1000 mL during a cesarean section occurring before, during, or after delivery of the placenta. Table 2.13-6 summarizes common causes.
- Complications include **Sheehan's syndrome.**

Intrapartum and Postpartum Fevers

- Most commonly due to **infections** (see Table 2.13-7).
- Other causes include hematoma, atelectasis, breast engorgement, pelvic abscess, and septic pelvic thrombophlebitis.
- See the mnemonic 7 **W's** for the causes of postpartum fevers.

Mastitis

- Cellulitis of the periglandular tissue in breast-feeding mothers, typically due to *S. aureus* at about 2–4 weeks postpartum.
- Symptoms include breast pain and redness along with **high fever,** chills, and flulike symptoms. Look for **focal** breast erythema, swelling, and tenderness. **Fluctuance** indicates a breast abscess.
- Distinguish from simple breast engorgement, which can present as a swollen, firm, tender breast with low-grade fever.
- Diagnosis includes breast milk cultures and CBC.

For all uterine causes of PPH, when bleeding persists after conventional therapy, uterine/internal iliac artery ligation or hysterectomy can be lifesaving.

Breast-feeding contraindications include HIV infection, active hepatitis, and certain drugs (e.g., tetracycline, chloramphenicol, warfarin).

Treatment of mastitis includes antibiotics and continued breast-feeding.

TABLE 2.11-6. Common Causes of PPH

	UTERINE ATONY	GENITAL TRACT TRAUMA	RETAINED PLACENTAL TISSUE
Risk factors	Uterine overdistention, exhausted myometrium, uterine infection, grand multiparity.	Precipitous delivery, operative vaginal delivery, large infant, laceration.	Placenta accreta/increta/percreta, placenta previa, prior C-section, curettage, accessory placental lobe.
Diagnosis	Palpation of a soft, enlarged, "boggy" uterus.	Inspection of the cervix, vagina, and vulva for lacerations or hematoma.	Inspection of placenta and uterine cavity. Ultrasound to look for retained placenta.
Treatment	Vigorous bimanual massage. Oxytocin infusion. Methylergonovine if not hypertensive; $PGF_{2\alpha}$ if not asthmatic.	Surgical repair of the defect.	Manual removal of remaining placental tissue. Curettage with suction.

TABLE 2.13-7. Common Infections During Labor and After Delivery

	CHORIOAMNIONITIS	ENDOMETRITIS
Definition	Infection of the **chorion, amnion,** and **amniotic fluid,** diagnosed **during labor.**	Infection of the **uterus,** diagnosed **after delivery.**
Risk factors	**Prolonged rupture of membranes (ROM).** Multiple vaginal exams while in labor.	**C-section,** prolonged ROM, multiple vaginal exams while in labor.
Symptoms/exam	Fever with no other obvious source **and** one of the following: <ul><li>Fetal **or** maternal tachycardia</li><li>Abdominal tenderness</li><li>Foul-smelling amniotic fluid</li><li>Leukocytosis</li></ul>	**Two fevers within 24 hours postpartum or** any fever ≥ 38.6°C (101.5°F) without an obvious source.
Diagnosis	CBC with differential.	Pelvic exam to rule out hematoma or retained membranes. CBC with differential, UA, urine culture, and blood cultures as indicated.
Treatment	Delivery of the fetus (chorioamnionitis is **not** an indication for C-section). Antibiotics until afebrile for 24 hours.	Antibiotics until afebrile for 48 hours.

The 7 W's of postpartum fever:

Womb—
    endomyometritis
Wind—atelectasis,
    pneumonia
Water—UTI
Walk—DVT, pulmonary
    embolism
Wound—incision,
    lacerations
Weaning—breast
    engorgement,
    mastitis, breast
    abscess
Wonder drugs—drug
    fever

- Treat with **dicloxacillin** or **erythromycin.** Continue nursing or manually expressing milk to prevent milk stasis. Incision and drainage of abscess if present.

Sheehan's Syndrome (Postpartum Hypopituitarism)

- The most common cause of anterior pituitary insufficiency in adult females.
- 2° to **pituitary ischemia,** usually as a result of postpartum blood loss and hypotension.
- The most common presenting symptom is **failure to lactate** owing to ↓ prolactin levels.
- Other symptoms include lethargy, anorexia, weight loss, amenorrhea, and loss of sexual hair, but may not be recognized for many years.

▶ TERATOGENS IN PREGNANCY

- **Radiation:** Diagnostic and nuclear medicine studies pose no risk of fetal teratogenicity if overall exposure during pregnancy is < 5000 mrads (e.g., CXR = 0.1 mrad).
- **Medications:** See Table 2.13-8 for medications that are safe during pregnancy.

TABLE 2.13-8. Safe vs. Teratogenic/Unsafe Medications During Pregnancy

INDICATION	SAFE TO USE	CONTRAINDICATED
Acne	Benzoyl peroxide.	Vitamin A and derivatives (e.g., isotretinoin) → heart and great vessel defects, craniofacial dysmorphism, deafness.
Antibiotics	Penicillins, cephalosporin, macrolides	Tetracycline → discoloration of deciduous teeth. Quinolone → cartilage damage. Sulfonamide late in pregnancy → kernicterus. Streptomycin → CN VIII damage/ototoxicity.
Nausea/vomiting	Prochlorperazine, 5-HTs, promethazine	Thalidomide → limb reduction and malformation.
Bipolar disease	Need to assess risk versus benefits	Lithium (also avoid if the mother is breast-feeding) → congenital heart disease, Ebstein's anomaly.
Depression	TCAs, SSRIs.	
Diagnostic dye	Indigo carmine.	Methylene blue → jejunal and ileal atresia.
GERD	Ranitidine, cimetidine.	
Headache/migraine	Acetaminophen, codeine, caffeine.	Avoid aspirin in late pregnancy because of risk of bleeding to mother and fetus at birth. Ergotamines → abortifacient potential and theoretical risk of fetal vasoconstriction.
Hypertension	Labetalol, hydralazine, nifedipine, methyldopa, clonidine.	ACEIs and angiotensin receptor blockers → fetal renal damage, oligohydramnios.
Hyperthyroidism	PTU.	Methimazole → aplasia cutis.
Seizure	Use an anticonvulsant that works best to control maternal seizures. Folate supplementation to be started prior to conception.	Phenytoin → dysmorphic facies, microcephaly, mental retardation, hypoplasia of nails and distal phalanges, neural tube defects (NTDs). Valproic acid → craniofacial defects and NTDs. Carbamazepine → craniofacial defects, mental retardation, NTDs. Trimethadione, paramethadione → strong teratogenic potential, mental retardation, speech difficulty, abnormal facies.
Thromboembolic disease	Heparin, low-molecular-weight heparin.	Warfarin → dysmorphic facies, bony defects (chondrodysplasia).
URI	Pseudoephedrine (Sudafed), guaifenesin (Robitussin), acetaminophen, diphenhydramine, loratadine (Claritin).	
Pain	Acetaminophen, morphine, hydrocodone.	Avoid NSAIDs in late pregnancy for > 48 hours. When used over a long period, → premature closure of ductus arteriosus.

HIGH-YIELD FACTS

OBSTETRICS

TABLE 2.13-9. Causes of IUGR

FETAL CAUSES	MATERNAL CAUSES
Chromosomal abnormalities: Trisomy 21 is most common, followed by trisomies 18 and 13. **Infection: CMV is most common;** then toxoplasmosis. Placental abnormalities, uterine abnormalities, multiple gestations.	**Hypertension.** **Drugs: Cigarette** smoking is most common; also alcohol, heroin, cocaine. Malnutrition, malabsorption. Ethnic/genetic variation.

▶ OBSTETRICAL COMPLICATIONS OF PREGNANCY

Intrauterine Growth Restriction (IUGR)

- Defined as an estimated fetal weight at or below the 10th percentile for GA. See Table 2.13-9 for common causes of IUGR.
- Diagnosed by ultrasound.
- Suspect IUGR clinically if the difference between fundal height and GA is > 4 cm.
- **Focus on prevention**—e.g., smoking cessation, BP control, and dietary changes. Do ultrasound every 4–6 weeks for interval growth.

Third-Trimester Bleeding

- Describes any bleeding after 20 weeks' gestation.
- The most common causes are placental abruption and placenta previa (see Table 2.13-10).
- Other causes of bleeding include bloody show, early labor, vasa previa, genital tract lesions, and trauma (sexual intercourse).

Gestational Trophoblastic Disease (GTD)

Can range from benign (e.g., hydatidiform mole) to malignant (e.g., choriocarcinoma). Hydatidiform mole accounts for approximately 80% of cases of GTD.

SYMPTOMS/EXAM

- Suspect in patients with **first-trimester uterine bleeding** and excessive nausea and vomiting.
- Look for patients with **preeclampsia or eclampsia at < 24 weeks.**
- Other findings include uterine size greater than dates and hyperthyroidism.
- **No fetal heartbeat** is detected.
- Pelvic exam may show enlarged ovaries and possible expulsion of **grape-like molar clusters** into the vagina or blood in the cervical os.

DIAGNOSIS

- Markedly ↑ β-hCG levels (usually > 100,000 mIU/dL).
- Pelvic ultrasound shows a **"snowstorm" appearance** with no gestational sac and no fetus or heart tone present.
- CXR to look for metastases.

TABLE 2.13-10. Common Causes of Third-Trimester Bleeding

	PLACENTAL ABRUPTION	PLACENTA PREVIA	UTERINE RUPTURE
Pathophysiology	**Placental separation** from the site of uterine implantation before delivery of the fetus.	**Abnormal placental implantation** near or covering the os.	**A complete rupture includes the entire thickness of the uterine wall.**
Risk factors	**Hypertension**, abdominal/pelvic trauma, tobacco or **cocaine use,** uterine distention.	**Prior C-section,** grand multiparas, multiple gestations, prior placenta previa.	**Prior uterine scar,** trauma (e.g., motor vehicle accident), uterine anomalies.
Symptoms	**Abdominal pain; vaginal bleeding** that does **not** spontaneously cease. **Fetal distress.**	**Painless vaginal bleeding that ceases spontaneously** with or without uterine contractions. First bleeding episode usually in the second or third trimester. Usually **no fetal distress.**	**Severe abdominal pain,** usually during labor, typically at the scar site. Change in the shape of the abdomen. **Fetal distress.**
Diagnosis	**Primarily clinical.** Ultrasound to look for retroplacental hemorrhage.	**Ultrasound** for placental position.	**Primarily clinical; based on symptoms and fetal distress.**
Treatment	**Mild abruption or premature infant:** Hospitalize, fetal monitoring, type and cross, bed rest. **Moderate to severe abruption:** ABCs, type and cross, immediate delivery.	**No vaginal exams!** Stabilize patient with premature fetus. Serial ultrasound to assess fetal growth and resolution of previa. C-section if total or partial previa or the patient/infant is in distress.	**Immediate C-section** with delivery of the infant and repair of the rupture.
Complications	Hemorrhagic shock, DIC, fetal death with severe abruption.	↑ risk of placenta accreta. Hemorrhage requiring hysterectomy.	Fetal and maternal death.

TREATMENT

- D&C.
- Careful monitoring of β-hCG levels after D&C for possible progression to malignant disease; prevention of pregnancy for one year to ensure accurate monitoring of β-hCG levels.
- Treat malignant disease with chemotherapy and residual uterine disease with hysterectomy.

Oligohydramnios and Polyhydramnios

Table 2.13-11 contrasts oligohydramnios with polyhydramnios.

Oligohydramnios almost always indicates the presence of a fetal abnormality.

HIGH-YIELD FACTS

OBSTETRICS

TABLE 2.13-11. Oligohydramnios vs. Polyhydramnios

	OLIGOHYDRAMNIOS	POLYHYDRAMNIOS
Definition	Amniotic fluid index (AFI) ≤ 5 cm on ultrasound.	AFI ≥ 25 cm on ultrasound.
Causes	**Fetal urinary tract abnormalities** (renal agenesis, polycystic kidneys, GU obstruction). Chronic uteroplacental insufficiency. ROM.	Normal pregnancy, uncontrolled maternal DM, multiple gestations, pulmonary abnormalities, fetal anomalies (duodenal atresia, tracheoesophageal fistula).
Diagnosis	Ultrasound for anomalies. Rule out ROM with ferning test, Nitrazine.	Ultrasound for fetal anomalies; glucose testing for DM.
Treatment	Amnioinfusion during labor to prevent cord compression.	Depends on cause; therapeutic amniocentesis.
Complications	**Cord compression** → fetal hypoxia. Musculoskeletal abnormalities (facial distortion, clubfoot). Pulmonary hypoplasia, IUGR.	Preterm labor, fetal malpresentation, cord prolapse.

Rhesus (Rh) Isoimmunization

- When fetal Rh-⊕ RBCs leak into Rh-⊖ maternal circulation, **maternal anti-Rh IgG antibodies** can form. These antibodies can cross the placenta, react with fetal Rh-positive RBCs, and → fetal hemolysis (erythroblastosis fetalis).
- Hydrops fetalis occurs when **maternal** hemoglobin drops to < 7 g/dL.
- Inquire about prior events that may have exposed the mother to Rh-⊕ blood (ectopic pregnancy, abortion, blood transfusion, prior delivery of an Rh-⊕ child, amniocentesis, traumatic procedures during pregnancy, recent RhoGAM).

TREATMENT

- **Give RhoGAM to Rh-⊖ women:**
  - If the father is Rh-⊕, Rh status is unknown, or paternity is uncertain.
  - If the baby is Rh-⊕ at delivery.
  - If they have undergone an abortion (therapeutic or spontaneous), an ectopic pregnancy, amniocentesis, vaginal bleeding, placenta previa, or placental abruption.
- Sensitized Rh-⊖ women with titers > 1:16 should be closely monitored for evidence of fetal hemolysis with serial ultrasound and amniocentesis.
- In severe cases, intrauterine blood transfusion via umbilical vein or preterm delivery.

Premature Rupture of Membranes (PROM)

- Spontaneous ROM before onset of labor.
- Associated with low socioeconomic status, young maternal age, smoking, and STDs.
- Sterile speculum exam shows pooling of amniotic fluid in the posterior vaginal vault; look for cervical dilation.

DIAGNOSIS

- ⊕ **Nitrazine paper test:** Paper turns blue in alkaline amniotic fluid.
- ⊕ **fern test:** A ferning pattern is seen under the microscope after amniotic fluid dries on glass slide.
- AFI by ultrasound to assess amniotic fluid volume.
- Cultures and/or wet mounts to look for infectious causes.

TREATMENT

- If signs of infection are present, assume **amnionitis** (maternal fever, fetal tachycardia, foul-smelling amniotic fluid). Give antibiotics (ampicillin +/– erythromycin) and **induce labor** regardless of GA.
- If no signs of infection are present and GA is **24–32 weeks,** treat with **antibiotics** to prolong pregnancy, **steroids** for fetal lung maturation, and **tocolytics** (e.g., ritodrine, terbutaline, magnesium).
- If no signs of infection are present and GA is ≥ **33 weeks,** hospitalize and treat expectantly until labor or signs of infection.

Preterm Labor

- Labor from 20 weeks up to 36 completed weeks' gestation.
- Can → respiratory distress syndrome, intraventricular hemorrhage, retinopathy of prematurity, necrotizing enterocolitis, or fetal death.
- Patients may complain of menstrual-like cramps, uterine contractions, low back pain, pelvic pressure, new vaginal discharge, or bleeding.
- Rule out cervical incompetence (treated with cerclage) and **Braxton Hicks** contractions.

DIAGNOSIS

- Obtain an **ultrasound** to verify GA, fetal presentation, and AFI.
- Look for **regular** uterine contractions (≥ 3 contractions lasting 30 seconds each over a 30-minute period) coupled with a concurrent cervical change at < 37 weeks' gestation.

TREATMENT

- Begin with **hydration** and **bed rest.**
- Unless contraindicated, begin **tocolytic** therapy and **steroids** to accelerate fetal lung maturity.
- Give **penicillin or ampicillin** for GBS prophylaxis if preterm delivery is likely.

Fetal Malpresentation

- Defined as any presentation other than cephalic.
- Breech presentation is the most common fetal malpresentation (3% of all pregnancies). There are three subtypes (see Figure 2.13-1).

Braxton Hicks contractions are irregular and have no cervical change.

HIGH-YIELD FACTS

OBSTETRICS

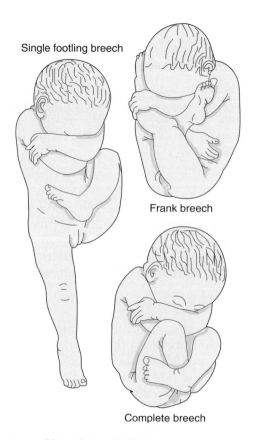

Single footling breech

Frank breech

Complete breech

FIGURE 2.13-1. Types of breech presentations.

(Reproduced, with permission, from Pernoll ML. *Benson and Pernoll's Handbook of Obstetrics and Gynecology*, 10th ed. New York: McGraw-Hill, 2001.)

DIAGNOSIS

- Perform Leopold maneuvers to identify fetal lie.
- Check an ultrasound if there is any doubt.

TREATMENT

- **Follow:** Up to 75% spontaneously change to cephalic by 38 weeks.
- **External version:** Can be attempted if persistent malpresentation after 37 weeks' gestation. Pressure is applied to the maternal abdomen to turn the infant. Risks of the procedure are placental abruption and cord compression; the infant must be monitored after the procedure, and consent must be obtained for emergent C-section.

Indications for Cesarean Section

Table 2.13-12 outlines indications for C-section.

▶ SPONTANEOUS AND RECURRENT ABORTION

Spontaneous Abortion (SAB)

- Defined as nonelective termination of pregnancy at < 20 weeks' gestation. Also known as "miscarriage."

TABLE 2.13-12. Indications for Cesarean Section

MATERNAL FACTORS	FETAL AND MATERNAL FACTORS	FETAL FACTORS
Any prior C-section regardless of uterine scar. Active genital herpes infection. Cervical carcinoma. Maternal trauma/demise.	**Cephalopelvic disproportion** (most common cause of 1° C-section). Placenta previa/placental abruption. Failed operative vaginal delivery.	Fetal malposition. Fetal distress. Cord prolapse. Erythroblastosis fetalis (Rh incompatibility).

- Occurs in 10–15% of clinically recognizable pregnancies.
- **Common causes of first-trimester bleeding:**
  - Differentiate types of SABs with symptoms, cervical exam, and ultrasound (see Table 2.13-13).
  - The differential includes normal pregnancy, postcoital bleeding, ectopic pregnancy, vaginal or cervical lesions, pedunculated myomas or polyps, and extrusion of molar pregnancy.

TABLE 2.13-13. Types of SABs

TYPE	SYMPTOMS	CERVIX/ULTRASOUND	TREATMENT
Threatened abortion	Minimal bleeding +/– cramping. Most cases are thought to be due to implantation bleed. **No products of conception (POC) are expelled.**	Closed os; normal ultrasound.	Avoid heavy activity; pelvic and bed rest.
Inevitable abortion	Cramping with profuse bleeding. **No POC are expelled.**	Open os; normal ultrasound.	Emergent D&C.
Incomplete abortion	Severe cramping and profuse bleeding. **Some POC are expelled.**	Open os; normal ultrasound.	Emergent D&C.
Complete abortion	Slight bleeding; pain has usually ceased. **All POC are expelled.**	Closed os; empty uterus on ultrasound.	None.
Missed abortion	Often no symptoms. No POC expelled.	Closed os; no fetal cardiac activity; retained fetal tissue on ultrasound.	Allow 4 weeks for POC to pass; offer medical management with misoprostol; or D&C
Septic abortion	Constitutional symptoms; malodorous discharge. Often a recent history of therapeutic abortion; maternal mortality 10–50%.	Cervical motion tenderness.	Monitor ABCs; D&C, IV antibiotics, supportive care.

All women with potential SAB should receive RhoGAM if appropriate.

TREATMENT

- Hemodynamic monitoring if significant bleeding.
- Check β-hCG to confirm pregnancy and transvaginal ultrasound to establish GA; assess fetal viability or check for remaining tissue if completed abortion.
- Check blood type and antibody screen; give RhoGAM if appropriate.

Recurrent Abortion

- Defined as ≥ 3 consecutive pregnancy losses before 20 weeks' gestation.
- Usually due to **chromosomal** or **uterine abnormalities,** but can also stem from hormonal abnormalities, infection, or systemic disease.
- Diagnosis is based on clinical and lab findings:
    - Pelvic exam (anatomic abnormalities).
    - Check cervical cultures for chlamydia and gonorrhea.
    - Perform a genetic analysis.
    - Sonohysterogram to look for uterine abnormalities.
    - Obtain TFTs, progesterone, lupus anticoagulant, and anticardiolipin antibody.
- Treatment is based on diagnosis.

SECTION II

Gynecology

Characterized by abnormalities in the frequency, duration, volume, and/or timing of menstrual bleeding (see Table 2.14-1). Most commonly due to ovulatory or anovulatory bleeding.

- **Ovulatory bleeding:**
  - Midcycle bleeding or abnormal menstrual cycles.
  - Premenstrual syndrome symptoms (weight gain, breast tenderness, dysmenorrhea).
  - More likely to have an organic cause.
- **Anovulatory bleeding:**
  - Characteristically acyclic with unpredictable onset.
  - Excessive and prolonged bleeding due to unopposed estrogen on the endometrium.
  - Most often seen in adolescent and perimenopausal women.

DIAGNOSIS

- If cycles appear **ovulatory,** diagnostic tools include transvaginal ultrasound, sonohysterogram, and D&C (gold standard) with hysteroscopy.
- If cycles appear **anovulatory,** order β-hCG, CBC, coagulation profile, and endocrine tests (FSH, LH, TSH, and prolactin). Screen for cervical cancer with a Pap smear.
- Perform an **endometrial biopsy** to screen for endometrial hyperplasia and cancer in **all women** with postmenopausal or chronic anovulatory bleeding.
- Look for anatomical causes (e.g., polyps, fibroids, gynecologic cancers) as well as nongynecologic causes (e.g., von Willebrand's disease).

TREATMENT

- Acute profuse bleeding: High-dose IV estrogen (Premarin 25 mg IV up to four doses), D&C, endometrial ablation, uterine artery embolization, hysterectomy.

TABLE 2.14-1. **Causes of Abnormal Uterine Bleeding**

NAME	DEFINITION	CAUSES
Menorrhagia	Heavy bleeding during menses.	**Leiomyoma,** endometrial hyperplasia or polyps, 1° bleeding disorders.
Metrorrhagia	Bleeding between menses.	Endometrial polyps, endometrial or cervical cancer, exogenous estrogen.
Menometrorrhagia	Heavy bleeding between and during menstrual periods.	Same as above.
Dysfunctional uterine bleeding	**A diagnosis of exclusion;** made when no anatomic lesion is found.	Proliferative endometrium caused by anovulation.
Postmenopausal bleeding	Uterine bleeding occurring one year after menopause.	Vaginal atrophy, exogenous hormones, endometrial cancer.

- Ovulatory bleeding: NSAIDs/OCPs.
- Anovulatory bleeding: OCPs.

► AMENORRHEA

Defined as either 1° or 2° amenorrhea.

- **1° amenorrhea:** Absence of menses and the lack of 2° sexual characteristics by age 14 **or** absence of menses by age 16 with or without 2° sexual characteristics. Associated with gonadal failure, congenital absence of the vagina, and constitutional symptoms.
- **2° amenorrhea:** Absence of menses for three cycles **or** for six months with prior normal menses. Etiologies include pregnancy, chronic anovulation, hypothyroidism/hyperprolactinemia, and weight loss/anorexia.

DIAGNOSIS

- **Check β-hCG** to make sure that the patient is not pregnant and that there are no structural abnormalities.
- 1° amenorrhea: See Figure 2.14-1.
- 2° amenorrhea: See Figure 2.14-2.

TREATMENT

Depends on the etiology; may include surgery, HRT, +/– drug therapy.

Always rule out pregnancy in a patient with amenorrhea.

Amenorrhea is a symptom, not a diagnosis. An etiology must be established to effectively treat amenorrhea.

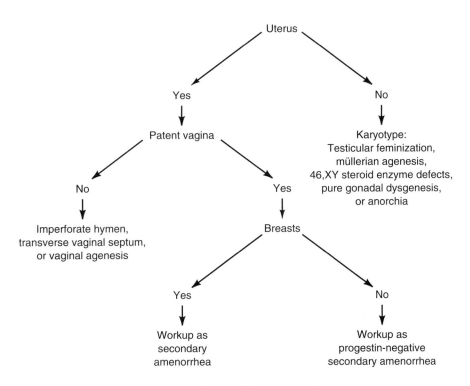

FIGURE 2.14-1. **Workup for patients with 1° amenorrhea.**

(Reproduced, with permission, from DeCherney AH, Nathan L. *Current Obstetric & Gynecologic Diagnosis & Treatment*, 9th ed. New York: McGraw-Hill, 2003:995.)

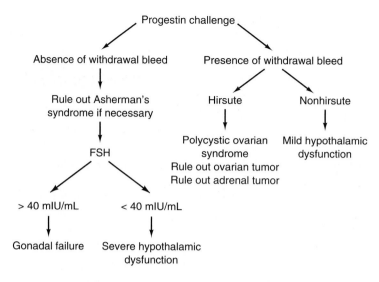

FIGURE 2.14-2. **Workup for patients with 2° amenorrhea.**

(Adapted, with permission, from DeCherney AH, Nathan L. *Current Obstetric & Gynecologic Diagnosis & Treatment*, 9th ed. New York: McGraw-Hill, 2003:996.)

▶ BENIGN BREAST DISORDERS

Include **fibrocystic change** (most common), fibroadenoma, intraductal papilloma (a common cause of bloody nipple discharge), duct ectasia, fat necrosis, mastitis, and breast abscess. See Table 2.14-2 for a list of common examples.

▶ ENDOMETRIOSIS

Abnormal growth of tissue histologically resembling the endometrium in locations other than the uterine lining, usually in the ovaries (called endometriomas or "chocolate cysts"), cul-de-sac, and bladder. Associated with premenstrual pelvic pain due to stimulation from estrogen and progesterone during the menstrual cycle.

SYMPTOMS/EXAM

- Painful menses, dyspareunia, pain with defecation or urination, infertility.
- On pelvic exam, patients may have tender nodularity along the uterosacral ligament +/– a fixed, retroflexed uterus.

DIAGNOSIS

Can be made by the history and physical, but the gold standard is surgical visualization of **"powder burn" lesions** during surgery with biopsy showing endometrial glands.

TREATMENT

Depends on the patient's symptoms, age, desire for future fertility, and stage of disease. Hysterectomy with bilateral oophorectomy **(TAH/BSO) is curative** but is not a viable option for women who wish to preserve their fertility and hormonal status. The goal for those patients is to induce a state of anovulation.

TABLE 2.14-2.   Common Benign Breast Disorders

TYPE OF BREAST DISEASE	SYMPTOMS/EXAM	TREATMENT
Fibrocystic disease	Mild to moderate pain in the breasts +/– lumps premenstrually. Multifocal, bilateral nodularity. Most common in women 35–45.	Must exclude cancer in high-risk groups; check mammogram and biopsy. Fibrocystic disease ↑ the risk of breast cancer only if cellular atypia is found.
Fibroadenoma	**The most common tumor in menstruating women** < 25 years of age. Small, firm, unilateral, nontender mass. Freely movable and slow growing.	Removal is not necessary, but surgical excision is both diagnostic and curative. Biopsy if the patient is in a high-risk group. Recurrence is common.
Intraductal papilloma	Clear, bloody, or discolored fluid from a single duct opening. Milking of the breast shows drainage from one duct opening. **Must always exclude a malignant process.**	Drainage and surgical exploration of the duct.
Fat necrosis	Local pain, erythema, and swelling of the breast. Trauma, ischemia.	Analgesia. A biopsy may be done to rule out malignancy.
Duct ectasia	Thick, white or discolored, cheesy material draining from the nipple. Ropelike induration under the areola. Obstruction, atrophy; usually after many years of nursing.	None if no infection.

- **Mild discomfort:** NSAIDs.
- **Mild to moderate pain:** NSAIDs; OCPs for six months.
- **Moderate to severe pain:** Laparoscopic surgery to excise endometriotic tissue, remove adhesions, and restore pelvic anatomy. TAH/BSO is curative (see above).

▶ DYSMENORRHEA

Defined as pain with menstrual periods that requires medication and prevents normal activity. It is divided into 1° and 2° dysmenorrhea.

- **1° dysmenorrhea:** No clinically detectable pelvic pathology. Most likely due to ↑ uterine prostaglandin production.
- **2° dysmenorrhea:** Menstrual pain due to pelvic pathology, most commonly endometriosis, adenomyosis (endometrial glands and stroma within the myometrium), myomas, or PID.

Oral Contraceptives (OCPs)

- The long-term consequences of OCP use include a ↓ in:
  - Ovarian and endometrial cancers.
  - Breast disease, but not breast cancer.
  - Dysmenorrhea.
- Contraindications to OCP use include:
  - Pregnancy.
  - Previous or active thromboembolic disease.
  - Undiagnosed genital bleeding.
  - Patients > 35 years of age who smoke.
  - Estrogen-dependent neoplasms.
  - Hepatocellular carcinoma.

Emergency Contraception

- Can be offered up to five days after unprotected intercourse; ↓ the risk of pregnancy to 1%.
- **Progestin-only regimen:** Newer, progestin-only contraceptive tablets consist of levonorgestrel 0.75 μg (the trade name is **Plan B**). It is given PO within 72 hours of unprotected intercourse and repeated 12 hours later.

▶ **VULVOVAGINITIS**

The most common outpatient gynecologic problem. During pregnancy, it can ↑ the risk of preterm labor or rupture of membranes. Vulvovaginitis can be bacterial (*Gardnerella vaginalis* → bacterial vaginosis), fungal (*Candida*), or protozoal (*Trichomonas*). Figure 2.14-3 illustrates two common causes of vulvovaginitis.

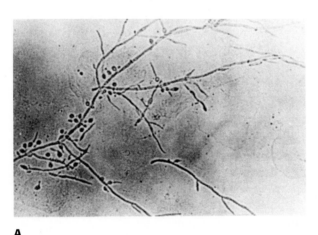
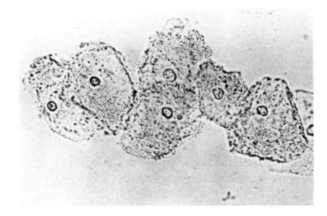

A   **B**

FIGURE 2.14-3.   Causes of vaginitis.

(A) Candidal vaginitis. Branches and budding *Candida albicans* are evident on KOH preparation of vaginal discharge. (B) *Gardnerella vaginalis*. Saline wet mount of vaginal fluid reveals granulations on vaginal epithelial cells ("clue cells") due to adherence of *G. vaginalis* organisms to the cell surface. (Reproduced, with permission, from DeCherney AH, Nathan L. *Current Obstetric & Gynecologic Diagnosis & Treatment*, 9th ed. New York: McGraw-Hill, 2003:652, 653.)

SYMPTOMS/EXAM

- Presents with ↑ vaginal discharge or a change in vaginal discharge.
- Patients also complain of vulvovaginal pruritus with or without burning and/or odor.
- Perform a complete examination of the vulva, vagina, and cervix.
- Look for vulvar edema, erythema, and discharge.

DIAGNOSIS/TREATMENT

Obtain swabs from the vagina to perform a wet mount and cultures for gonorrhea, chlamydia, and HSV, depending on the exam (see Table 2.14-3).

TABLE 2.14-3. **Common Causes of Vulvovaginitis**

	BACTERIAL VAGINOSIS (USUALLY GARDNERELLA VAGINALIS)	YEAST (USUALLY CANDIDA)	TRICHOMONAS VAGINALIS
Exam	Can be unremarkable except for discharge.	Erythema; may notice a curdlike discharge.	Malodorous discharge; the vagina and cervix can be swollen and red.
Discharge	Grayish or white, having a **fishy odor;** pronounced after intercourse.	White, curdlike discharge.	Yellow-green discharge.
Saline smear	> 20% of epithelial cells with indistinct cell margins (clue cells; see Figure 2.14-3).	Nothing.	Motile, flagellated protozoans.
KOH prep	⊕"whiff test" when KOH is placed on slide → a fishy odor.	Pseudohyphae and spores (see Figure 2.14-3).	**Nothing.**
Treatment Nonpregnant	Metronidazole.	Topical antifungal for 3–7 days or fluconazole × 1 dose.	Metronidazole.
Pregnant (second/third trimesters)ᵃ	Metronidazole.	Use only topical antifungals for seven days.	Metronidazole 2 g PO in a single dose.

ᵃ Metronidazole is not recommended in the first trimester of pregnancy owing to its teratogenic effects.

▶ POLYCYSTIC OVARIAN SYNDROME (PCOS)

- The most common cause of female hirsutism (male-pattern hair growth).
- Clinical presentation varies from mild hirsutism with regular menses to severe hirsutism, amenorrhea, and virilization.
- Typically affects women in the teenage years who are obese and hirsute.
- The cause is unknown; hyperinsulinemia with insulin resistance is usually seen.

SYMPTOMS

Look for obese woman with hirsutism, amenorrhea, infertility, obesity, acne, and diabetes or insulin resistance.

EXAM

- Evidence of hirsutism without evidence of cortisol or adrenal androgen excess.
- On pelvic exam, palpably enlarged ovaries may be felt.

DIAGNOSIS

- ↑ LH/FSH ratio (> 2); ↑ testosterone.
- An ultrasound may show ovaries with multiple small follicles but an ultrasound is no longer a recommended part of the workup to diagnose PCOS.
- Perform a glucose tolerance test to evaluate for diabetes.

TREATMENT

- Treat the specific symptoms:
    - **Infertility:** Induce ovulation with clomiphene.
    - **Hirsutism:** Start combination OCPs to suppress ovarian steroidogenesis.
- Weight loss will help with insulin resistance; treat diabetes with metformin, which may improve response to ovulation induction.

▶ MENOPAUSE

- The permanent cessation of menstruation.
- Early menopause is associated with **cigarette smoking.** Artificial menopause occurs after removal or irradiation of the ovaries.
- Postmenopausal women lose the protective effects of estrogen and are at ↑ risk for **osteoporosis** and **heart disease.**

SYMPTOMS/EXAM

- Patients may complain of menstrual irregularities, sweating, sleep disturbances, mood changes, ↓ libido, dyspareunia, cystocele, and urinary frequency/incontinence.
- Exam reveals vaginal dryness, ↓ breast size, and genital tract atrophy (see the mnemonic **HAVOC**).

Premature menopause occurs before age 40 and is often due to idiopathic premature ovarian failure.

DIAGNOSIS

- Requires **one year** without menses.
- ↑ **serum FSH** (> 30 IU/L) is suggestive.

TREATMENT

- The 1° indication for HRT is to help with **moderate to severe menopausal symptoms.**
- Contraindications include undiagnosed vaginal bleeding, active liver disease, recent MI, recent or active vascular thrombosis, and a history of endometrial or breast cancer.
- Alternatives to HRT include the following:
  - Clonidine for vasomotor instability.
  - Topical estrogens for vaginal atrophy.
  - Calcium, vitamin D, calcitonin, bisphosphonates (alendronate), and selective estrogen receptor modulators (raloxifene) for osteoporosis.
- **Guidelines for HRT use** are as follows:
  - **Use the lowest possible dose for the shortest duration to achieve treatment goals.**
  - Use combined progesterone/estrogen in women with an intact uterus; use estrogen alone in women without a uterus.
  - HRT should **not** be used for the prevention of CAD or stroke.
  - HRT is **not** recommended for the prevention of dementia.
  - Breast cancer risk is ↑ with estrogen therapy and, to a greater extent, with estrogen and progesterone therapy, beyond five years.

> **Menopause wreaks HAVOC:**
>
> **H**ot flashes (vasomotor instability)
> **A**trophy of the **V**agina
> **O**steoporosis
> **C**oronary artery disease

► URINARY INCONTINENCE

Involuntary loss of urine that can be seen objectively **and** is a social or hygienic problem. See Table 2.14-4 for an outline of stress, urge, and mixed incontinence.

SYMPTOMS/EXAM

- Voiding diaries help quantify the frequency and volume of urine as well as the amount and type of fluid taken in.
- All patients with incontinence should have a thorough neurologic exam to rule out neurologic causes.

UTI must be ruled out in all women complaining of urinary incontinence.

► ECTOPIC PREGNANCY

Any pregnancy implanted outside the uterine cavity. The most common location is the fallopian tube (95%). Risk factors include a history of PID, prior ectopic pregnancy, tubal/pelvic surgery, DES exposure in utero → abnormal tubal development, and IUD use.

SYMPTOMS/EXAM

- Patients may complain of lower abdominal or pelvic pain as well as spotting and amenorrhea.
- The abdomen may be tender to palpation +/− cervical motion tenderness and adnexal mass on bimanual exam.
- A ruptured ectopic may present with unstable vital signs, generalized abdominal pain, rebound tenderness, shoulder pain, and shock.

Any woman with abdominal pain needs a urine pregnancy test.

TABLE 2.14-4. **Types of Urinary Incontinence**

	STRESS INCONTINENCE	URGE INCONTINENCE (DETRUSOR INSTABILITY)	MIXED INCONTINENCE
History	Exertion (running) or straining (coughing, laughing).	Loss of urine with strong desire to void during a detrusor contraction. Frequency, urgency, nocturia. Urine loss from rising or lying position to standing.	Stress and urge incontinence present simultaneously.
Mechanism	Poor support or poor function of the urethral sphincter.	Involuntary detrusor muscle contractions.	A combination of both mechanisms.
Etiology	Pelvic relaxation, weakened urethral closing mechanisms, parity, cough.	Idiopathic. Neuropathy (Alzheimer's, Parkinson's, diabetes mellitus, multiple sclerosis).	As for both conditions.
Diagnosis	Demonstrable leakage with stress (cough).	Based on history. Cystometry reveals involuntary detrusor muscle contraction associated with urinary leakage.	As for both conditions.
Treatment	Pelvic floor exercises (Kegel), pessaries, biofeedback, weight loss, surgery to restore bladder neck support.	Avoid caffeinated or alcoholic beverages. **Behavioral modification** (pelvic floor exercises). Medical therapy (anticholinergic).	Based on the patient's worst symptom. Conservative methods first.

DIFFERENTIAL

Spontaneous abortion (SAB), molar pregnancy, ruptured corpus luteum cyst, PID, adnexal torsion, appendicitis, pyelonephritis, diverticulitis, regional ileitis, ulcerative colitis.

DIAGNOSIS

- An ↑ β-hCG in the absence of an intrauterine pregnancy on ultrasound is highly suspicious for an ectopic pregnancy.
    - A ⊕ serum β-hCG will not determine the location of the pregnancy.
    - An ectopic pregnancy usually has lower levels of β-hCG than expected (β-hCG levels should double every two days in a normal pregnancy). Correlate β-hCG level with gestational age (GA).
- Do an **ultrasound** to look for **intrauterine** pregnancy.
    - The sac may be visualized on:
        - Transvaginal ultrasound when β-hCG is approximately 1000–2000 mIU/mL, or at about 4–5 weeks' GA.
        - **Transabdominal** ultrasound when β-hCG is > 1800–3600 mIU/mL.
    - Fetal heart motion of the embryo can be seen after 5–6 weeks' GA.

- Definitive diagnosis is made by laparoscopy, laparotomy, or ultrasound visualization.

TREATMENT

- For **hemodynamically unstable** patients, immediate surgery is required.
- For **hemodynamically stable** patients:
  - Expectant management for asymptomatic, compliant patients with ↓ β-hCG levels or β-hCG < 200 mIU/mL, and if the risk of rupture is low.
  - Follow serial β-hCG closely with or without ultrasound studies.
  - **Methotrexate** is used for small (< 3.5 cm), unruptured ectopic pregnancies in asymptomatic women until levels are undetectable.
  - All women should be typed and screened and given **RhoGAM if Rh negative.**
  - Prevention of ectopic pregnancies includes thorough **treatment of STDs.**

↑ β-hCG in the absence of an intrauterine pregnancy on ultrasound is suspicious for an ectopic pregnancy.

▶ INFERTILITY

Inability of a couple to conceive after one year of regular intercourse without contraception. Causes include the following:
- **Male dysfunction (35%):**
  - Defects in spermatogenesis (male factor).
  - Varicoceles.
- **Female dysfunction (55%):**
  - **Ovulatory dysfunction:** Ovarian failure, prolactinoma.
  - **Uterine/tubal factors: Endometriosis,** genital tract abnormalities caused by infection, myomas, PID, congenital genital tract abnormalities.
  - **Endocrine dysfunction:** Thyroid/adrenal disease, PCOS.

Endometriosis is the leading cause of female infertility, followed by PID.

DIAGNOSIS

- Semen analysis to rule out male factors.
- Serum FSH/LH/TSH/prolactin to rule out endocrine dysfunction.
- Hysterosalpingography to rule out tubal and uterine cavity abnormalities.

TREATMENT

- Treat the underlying cause.
- Fertility rates in endometriosis can be improved by laparoscopic removal of implants.
- Ovulation can be induced with **clomiphene;** can → ovarian hyperstimulation and multiple gestations.
- Advanced reproductive technologies such as in vitro fertilization can be used for refractory cases.

Pediatrics

Developmental Milestones

Table 2.15-1 highlights major developmental milestones.

Immunizations

Table 2.15-2 summarizes the recommended timetable for childhood immunizations. Schedules vary for children who are behind and require catch-up immunizations.

Growth, development, and behavior should be assessed at every well-child check.

Routine Health Screening

Routine screening should be conducted at the following intervals:

- **Metabolic/genetic diseases:** At birth as part of newborn screening pro-

TABLE 2.15-1.   Developmental Milestones

AGE	GROSS MOTOR	FINE MOTOR	LANGUAGE	SOCIAL/COGNITIVE
2 months	Lifts head/chest when prone.	Tracks past midline.	Alerts to sound, coos.	Recognizes parent, **social smile.**
4–5 months	**Rolls** front to back, back to front (5 months).	Grasps rattle.	Orients to voice, "ah-goo," razzes.	Enjoys looking around, laughs.
6 months	**Sits unassisted.**	**Transfers objects,** raking grasp.	Babbles.	**Stranger anxiety.**
9–10 months	Crawls, pulls to stand.	Uses three-finger pincer grasp.	**Says mama/dada** (nonspecific).	Waves bye-bye, plays pat-a-cake.
12 months	Cruises (11 months), **walks alone.**	Uses two-finger pincer grasp.	Says mama/dada (specific).	Imitates actions.
15 months	Walks backward.	Uses cup.	Uses 4–6 words.	Temper tantrums.
18 months	Runs, kicks a ball.	Builds tower of 2–4 cubes.	Names common objects. Uses 8–10 words.	Copies parent in tasks (e.g., sweeping).
2 years	Walks up/down steps with help, jumps.	Builds tower of six cubes.	Uses **two-word** phrases.	Follows **two-step** commands, removes clothes.
3 years	Rides **tricycle,** climbs stairs with alternating feet (3–4 years).	Copies a circle, uses utensils.	Uses **three-word** sentences.	Brushes teeth with help, washes/dries hands.
4 years	Hops.	Copies a cross.	Counts to 10.	Cooperative play.

(Reprinted, with permission, from Le T et al. *First Aid for the USMLE Step 2,* 4th ed. New York: McGraw-Hill, 2003:380.)

Table 2.15-2. Immunizations

Vaccine	Ages Administered	Notes
Diphtheria, tetanus, acellular pertussis (DTaP)	2, 4, 6 months; 15–18 months; 4–6 years; tetanus booster at 11–12 years and then every 10 years thereafter.	Common adverse events include fever and local reactions at the injection site. Consider deferring in children with neurologic disorders.
Polio (IPV)	2, 4 months; 6–8 months; 4–6 years.	Generally well tolerated.
Hepatitis B	First given at birth OR 1–4 months; second given 4 weeks after first dose; third given 16 weeks after first dose.	In addition to receiving the vaccine, infants who may be exposed to hepatitis B perinatally may require IVIG.
H. influenzae type B (Hib)	2, 4, 6 months; 12–15 months.	Prior to the vaccine, Hib was the most common cause of bacterial meningitis in children.
Measles, mumps, rubella (MMR)	12–15 months; 4–6 years.	**Live vaccine**—avoid in immunocompromised patients.
Varicella	> 12 months.	**Live vaccine**—avoid in immunocompromised patients.
Pneumococcal conjugate vaccine	2, 4, 6 months; 12–15 months.	Children with fever, particularly those < 3 months of age, are much more likely to have a serious bacterial infection if they are unvaccinated against pneumococcus and therefore frequently require evaluation and antibiotics.

gram. Exact tests vary by state but all include testing for phenylketonuria and congenital hypothyroidism.

- **Growth parameters/development/behavior:** At each visit, every 2–6 months for the first three years, then annually.
- **Lead/anemia screening:** At 9–15 months. Lead screening should be repeated at two years of age, particularly in high-risk communities. Anemia screening repeated in menstruating adolescents.
- **Blood pressure:** Annually starting at three years of age.
- **Vision and hearing:** Subjective testing at each visit; objective vision testing annually starting at three years of age; objective hearing screening for all newborns and then annually starting at three years of age.
- **Tuberculosis:** Risk assessment at each well-child check; PPD placement for high-risk children.
- **High-risk behaviors/STD screening:** At each adolescent visit.
- **Anticipatory guidance:** Injury and violence prevention, sleep and nutrition counseling at each visit.

▶ GROWTH DEFICIENCY

Otherwise known as "failure to thrive," describes a child who is significantly underweight for age, whose weight gain is significantly slower than that of children of the same age, or who has been growing well but has "fallen off" the growth curve.

SYMPTOMS/EXAM

- A thorough feeding/nutrition history should be obtained.
- Obtain a thorough ROS to look for malabsorption and other systemic disease.
- Particular attention should be paid to social/family history—e.g., significant family stressors, CF and other genetic diseases, HIV, and inborn errors of metabolism.
- Plot height, weight, and head circumference since birth.
- Complete physical exam to look for signs of systemic disease.

DIFFERENTIAL

- Causes can be divided simply into inadequate intake, ↑ output (i.e., malabsorption), or ↑ metabolic demand.
- The most common cause is **inadequate intake,** which is often 2° to psychosocial issues with no underlying medical condition.
- Other differential diagnosis include infection, congenital heart disease, endocrine disease, lung disease, and neurologic disorders.

DIAGNOSIS

History and exam dictate the extent of workup for an organic cause, but laboratory evaluation may include CBC, electrolytes, BUN/creatinine, albumin, total protein, sweat chloride test, UA/culture, and stool for O & P.

TREATMENT

Treat the underlying cause. If no organic cause is identified on initial evaluation, initiate a calorie count and start nutritional supplementation where indicated. Hospitalization is necessary if there is evidence of neglect or severe malnourishment.

▶ **ENVIRONMENTAL HEALTH/SAFETY**

Car Seats

- Motor vehicle accidents are a major cause of death in children.
- Car seats are **required** for all children and, when used correctly, significantly reduce mortality.
- Car seats should be in the rear seat. In addition, they should be rear facing until the child is 20 lbs and 1 year of age. A car seat should never be placed in a seat with an airbag.

Trauma

- Injuries are the **leading cause of death** in children and adolescents after the first year of life; injury prevention counseling should thus be a part of each well-child visit.
- Include recommendations for **bicycle helmet use** and **water, traffic, sports, and firearm safety.**

Child Abuse

Includes physical, sexual, and emotional abuse/neglect. Diagnosis is based on a **history discordant with physical findings.**

Symptoms/Exam

- Be suspicious in any patient with multiple injuries in **various stages of healing,** irritability, or growth failure.
- Be especially concerned if there are **oddly situated bruises** (e.g., not over bony prominences), pattern injuries (e.g., immersion/cigarette burns), retinal hemorrages in infants, skeletal trauma (e.g., spiral fractures of long bones, corner fractures, posterior rib fractures), symptoms/signs of STDs/genital trauma, or intracranial hemorrhage.

Diagnosis

Clinical; based on skeletal survey, ophthalmologic exam, and neuroimaging.

Treatment

Immediate notification of child protective services (CPS). Consider hospitalization to ensure the safety of the child even if not indicated medically.

Sudden Infant Death Syndrome (SIDS)

- Defined as the sudden death of an infant < 1 year of age that remains unexplained after thorough investigation. Mechanism of death is unknown.
- Place all infants on their **backs** to sleep, as this is associated with a marked reduction in SIDS deaths.

Consider nonaccidental trauma when the history of an injury is discordant with the physical findings.

▶ NEONATOLOGY

Congenital Anomalies and Malformations

See Table 2.15-3 for common anomalies and malformations.

Neural Tube Defects

- Include anencephaly and spina bifida (myelomeningocele, meningocele).
- Associated with ↑ maternal and amniotic fluid **α-fetoprotein.** Incidence ↓ with folate ingestion during the first trimester of pregnancy.
- Anencephaly is not compatible with life. Spina bifida is treated with early surgical repair and is often associated with significant physical disability.

Assume latex allergy in spina bifida patients.

Hyperbilirubinemia/Neonatal Jaundice

Jaundice is a common neonatal problem that is usually physiologic. If severe or prolonged, occuring during the first 24 hours of life, or associated with a direct bilirubinemia, the jaundice is not physiologic, and an underlying cause must be looked for. Hyperbilirubinemia can also be toxic, with high levels resulting in a potentially fatal encephalopathy called kernicterus.

Symptoms/Exam

Search for evidence of causes of non-physiologic hyperbilirubinemia, such as infection, congenital malformations, cephalhematomas, hepatomegaly, and maternal-fetal ABO or Rh incompatibilities. Kernicterus presents with **jaundice, lethargy, poor feeding, a high-pitched cry, hypertonicity, and seizures.**

Differential

- Physiologic jaundice (see above).
- Breast milk jaundice.

Jaundice in the first 24 hours of life and direct hyperbilirubinemia are always pathologic.

TABLE 2.15-3. **Common Congenital Anomalies and Malformations**

LESION	DESCRIPTION	AGE OF PRESENTATION	SYMPTOMS	TREATMENT
Cleft lip/palate	Abnormal ridge/division of the lip/palate.	Birth.	Poor feeding; severe recurrent otitis media. May be associated with other anomalies.	Surgical repair.
Tracheoesophageal fistula	Blind esophageal pouch; fistula between the distal esophagus and trachea (most common).	Usually the first few hours of life, but other types can present later in infancy.	Copious secretions, choking, cyanosis, respiratory distress.	Suction of pouch with NG tube, reflux precautions, supportive care, surgical repair.
Abdominal wall defects	Gastroschisis (intestine extrudes through defect); omphalocele (membrane-covered herniation of abdominal contents).	Birth	Visible defect. Omphalocele often has associated anomalies, which are rare in gastroschisis.	Coverage of abdominal contents with sterile dressing, NG decompression, antibiotics, supportive care and stabilization followed by 1° or staged closure.
Intestinal atresias	Intestinal obstruction.	Antenatal or at birth.	Abdominal distention, bilious vomiting, obstipation/failure to pass meconium, polyhydramnios.	Surgical resection.
Hirschprung's disease	Absence of ganglion cells in the colon → narrowing of the aganglionic segment with dilation of the proximal normal colon.	Infancy, although can present later.	Failure to pass meconium, vomiting, abdominal distention, reluctance to feed.	Staged surgical repair with initial diverting colostomy and later resection when > 6 months old.

- **Rarer causes:** Crigler-Najjar syndrome, Gilbert's syndrome, neonatal hepatitis, biliary atresia, α_1-antitrypsin deficiency, hypothyroidism, cystic fibrosis, metabolic disease.

DIAGNOSIS

- Based on direct (conjugated) and indirect (unconjugated) bilirubin levels.
- Check a peripheral blood smear to rule out hemolysis and a Coombs' test to distinguish immune-mediated (i.e., ABO incompatibility) from non-immune-mediated (G6PD deficiency, hereditary spherocytosis) hemolytic disorders.

- If direct bilirubinemia is present, check LFTs, bile acids, sweat test, and tests for aminoacidopathies and α_1-antitrypsin deficiency.
- **If vital signs are abnormal, the patient needs a full septic workup and ICU monitoring.**

TREATMENT

Treat the underlying cause. If the level rises **above 15–20 mg/dL** or if there is a rapid rate of rise, initiate **phototherapy** (bili lights). In severe cases, exchange transfusion may be necessary.

Neonatal Respiratory Distress

Causes of neonatal respiratory distress include those listed in Table 2.15-4 along with congenital heart disease, anatomic airway anomalies, pneumothorax, neurologic abnormalities, sepsis, and pneumonia.

Neonatal Sepsis

- Serious bacterial infections are relatively common in newborn infants under one month old.
- The most common infections are bacterial sepsis, meningitis, pneumonia, and UTIs.
- Sepsis risk factors include maternal group B strep (GBS) positivity, rupture of membranes > 18 hours, maternal fever, chorioamnionitis, and premature labor.

SYMPTOMS/EXAM

- Range from fever alone at presentation to significant vital sign instability.
- Respiratory distress and poor feeding are also common presenting symptoms.

DIFFERENTIAL

The most common infectious agents include *E. coli*, GBS, and other gram-negative rods. It is also important to cover for *Listeria monocytogenes*, a less common but potentially serious cause of neonatal sepsis.

DIAGNOSIS

Full evaluation includes analysis and culture of blood, urine, and CSF. Evaluation may also include a CXR.

TREAMENT

- Begin antibiotics—**ampicillin** (to cover *Listeria*) and **gentamicin** or ampicillin and a third-generation cephalosporin (not ceftriaxone).
- Ventilatory and BP support if needed.

PREVENTION

The risk of neonatal sepsis can be reduced by screening the mother for GBS colonization with a vaginal culture at 36 weeks and prophylactically treating with intrapartum antibiotics during delivery. If no culture results are available, evaluation/treatment of the infant depends on the risk factors listed above.

Fever alone can be the presenting symptom of neonatal sepsis, so a fever in the first month of life is an indication for a full workup, admission, and antibiotics.

TABLE 2.15-4. **Common Pediatric Respiratory Disorders**

Disorder	Description	History	Exam/CXR Findings	Treatment	Complications
Respiratory distress syndrome/hyaline membrane disease	**Surfactant deficiency** → poor lung compliance and respiratory failure.	Usually occurs in **premature infants.**	↓ air movement; CXR shows ↓ lung volumes and ground-glass appearance.	Maternal antenatal steroids for prevention; surfactant administration at time of delivery; respiratory support.	Chronic lung disease.
Transient tachypnea of the newborn	**Retained fetal lung fluid** → brief, mild respiratory distress. Diagnosis of exclusion.	Term or near-term, infants; nonasphyxiated; born following short labor or often via C-section without labor.	CXR shows perihilar streaking and fluid in interlobar fissures.	Usually only mild to moderate O_2 requirement for support.	None.
Meconium aspiration syndrome	Inhalation of meconium at or near time of birth → **aspiration pneumonitis.**	**Term infants;** meconium present at time of delivery.	**Barrel chest;** coarse breath sounds; CXR shows coarse irregular infiltrates, hyperexpansion, and lobar consolidation.	Nasopharyngeal suctioning at perineum; tracheal suctioning at birth; ventilatory support.	Pulmonary hypertension.
Congenital diaphragmatic hernia	Defect in diaphragm → herniation of abdominal contents into the chest cavity; limitation of lung growth → **pulmonary hypoplasia.**	Severe respiratory distress at birth; may be diagnosed by prenatal ultrasound.	Scaphoid abdomen; CXR may show **bowel loops in chest.**	**Immediate intubation,** ventilatory support, and surgical correction after stabilization. Patients may require extracorporeal membrane oxygenation (ECMO).	Severe pulmonary hypertension. Mortality 25–40%.

Congenital Infections (TORCHeS)

Many congenital infections present with jaundice, hepatosplenomegaly, and thrombocytopenia in addition to the descriptions listed in Table 2.15-5.

Colic

- Presents with severe and paroxysmal crying that occurs mainly in the late afternoon.
- Suspect in a well-fed infant who cries > 3 hours/day, > 3 days/week for > 3 weeks.

TABLE 2.15-5. TORCHeS Infection

INFECTION	DESCRIPTION	TREATMENT	PREVENTION
Toxoplasmosis	Hydrocephalus, seizures, intracranial calcifications, and ring enhancing lesions on head CT.	Pyrimethamine, sulfadiazine, spiramycin.	Avoid exposure to cats and cat feces during pregnancy; avoid raw/undercooked meat; treat women with 1° infection.
Other	Includes HIV, parvovirus, varicella, *Listeria*, TB, malaria, and fungi.	Disease specific	For HIV-⊕ mothers, treatment of mother pre- and perinatally as well as prophylaxis of infant for six weeks after birth will ↓ transmission.
Rubella	"Blueberry muffin" rash, cataracts, hearing loss, PDA and other cardiac defects, encephalitis.	None.	Immunize mothers prior to pregnancy.
Cytomegalovirus (CMV)	Petechial rash, periventricular calcifications, microcephaly, chorioretinitis.	Ganciclovir.	Avoid exposure.
Herpes	Skin, eye, and mouth vesicles; can progress to severe CNS/systemic infection.	Acyclovir.	Perform a C-section if mother has active lesions at time of delivery. Highest risk is from mother with 1° infection.
Syphilis	Maculopapular skin rash, lymphadenopathy, "snuffles," osteitis.	Penicillin.	Treat seropositive mothers with penicillin.

- Peaks at 4–6 weeks of life; then improves without intervention.
- Management involves parental education, reassurance, and teaching of soothing skills.

▶ INFECTIOUS DISEASES

Fever of Unknown Origin (FUO)

- In all cases of FUO in infants, any identified infection should be treated with antibiotics and will likely require admission to the hospital.
- A viral infection such as a URI cannot be definitively considered a source of fever until three months of age, and therefore further evaluation is indicated.
- Deciding how to manage infants with FUO is age dependent:
  - **0–28 days:** See neonatal sepsis.
  - **1–3 months:**
    - Evaluate with CBC, UA, and urine culture.
    - If the infant is irritable or lethargic, an LP should be performed.

- If WBC is < 5 or > 15, a blood culture should be sent and the infant should be given antibiotics.
- If well appearing, the infant may be managed as an outpatient with close follow-up.
- **3–36 months:**
  - Evaluate with a UA and urine culture.
  - If the infant is well appearing and vaccinated against pneumococcus, the risk of bacteremia and/or meningitis is very low, so no further evaluation is needed.
  - If the infant is irritable or lethargic, an LP should be performed.
  - If unvaccinated against pneumococcus, a CBC should be performed to assess risk, as in the one- to three-month age range.

▶ IMMUNODEFICIENCIES

These syndromes present as recurrent or severe infections. In general they are rare, occurring with a frequency of about 1 in 10,000 (see Table 2.15-6).

- **B-cell deficiencies** are most common, generally presenting with recurrent **URIs** and **bacteremia with encapsulated organisms** (pneumococcus, *Staphylococcus, H. influenzae*) after six months of age, when maternal antibodies taper.
- **T-cell deficiencies** present earlier (1–3 months) → a broader range of infections, including **viral infection, fungal infection, and intracellular bacteria.**
- **Phagocyte** defects typically present with **mucous membrane infections** and **poor wound healing.** Catalase-⊕ (*S. aureus*) and enteric gram-⊖ organisms are common.
- **Complement deficiency** classically presents with **Neisseria infections.**

TREATMENT

- **B-cell disorders:** Generally, prophylactic antibiotic treatment. IVIG may be used in X-linked agammaglobulinemia and common variable disease.
- **T-cell disorders:** If severe, bone marrow transplantation; IVIG if humoral immunity is affected as well.
- **Phagocytic disorders:** Antibiotics; surgical debridement of wounds.

▶ KAWASAKI DISEASE (MUCOCUTANEOUS LYMPH NODE SYNDROME)

- Vasculitis of unknown etiology that predisposes to coronary artery aneurysms and later development of myocardial ischemia.
- More common in children < 5 years of age.
- More common in **Asians,** particularly Japanese.

SYMPTOMS/EXAM (SEE MNEMONIC)

Acute illness characterized by prolonged fever, bilateral conjunctivitis, swelling of the hands/feet, rash, cervical lymphadenopathy, and oropharyngeal changes ("strawberry tongue").

DIAGNOSIS

Purely a clinical diagnosis. Must have **fever for > 5 days and four or five of the other criteria** (see the mnemonic CRASH and BURN). Abnormal lab values can include ↑ **ESR/CRP** and **thrombocytosis.**

> **Kawasaki symptoms—"CRASH and BURN"**
>
> **C**onjunctivitis (bilateral, nonpurulent)
> **R**ash (truncal, nonspecific)
> **A**denopathy (at least one cervical node > 1 cm)
> **S**trawberry tongue (or any change in oropharyngeal mucosa, including injected pharynx, lip fissuring)
> **H**and/feet swelling/ desquamation
> **BURN** (fever > 5 days)

Table 2.15-6. **Pediatric Immunodeficiency Disorders**

DISORDER	DESCRIPTION	DIAGNOSIS/TREATMENT
B-cell		
X-linked (**B**ruton's) agammaglobulinemia	Profound **B**-cell deficiency in **B**oys only. May present at < 6 months of age. At risk for life-threatening *Pseudomonas* infections.	Diagnose with **quantitative Ig levels** (subclasses) and specific antidody responses.
Common variable immunodeficiency	Ig levels drop in the second to third decade of life. ↑ risk of lymphoma and autoimmune disease.	Treat with prophylactic antibiotics and IVIG.
IgA deficiency	Most common immunodeficiency. Usually asymptomatic, but recurrent infections may occur.	
T-cell		
Thymic aplasia (DiGeorge syndrome)	Presents with **tetany** (due to hypocalcemia) in the first days of life.	Diagnose with absolute lymphocyte count, mitogen stimulation response, and delayed hypersensitivity skin testing.
Ataxia-telangiectasia	Oculocutaneous telangiectasias and progressive cerebellar ataxia. A DNA repair defect.	Treat with **bone marrow transplant (BMT)** for severe disease and **IVIG** for antibody deficiency. Can do thymus transplant instead of BMT for DiGeorge. No therapy to limit progression of ataxia-telangiectasia.
Combined		
Severe combined immunodeficiency (SCID)	Severe lack of B and T cells. Patients present with frequent, severe bacterial infections, chronic candidiasis, and opportunistic organisms.	Treat SCID with **BMT** or **stem cell** transplant and IVIG for antibody deficiency. *Pneumocystis carinii* pneumonia (PCP) prophylaxis until BMT. Gene therapy may be a future option.
Wiskott-Aldrich syndrome	X-linked disorder with less severe B- and T-cell dysfunction. Patients have **eczema,** ↑ IgE and IgA, ↓ IgM, and **thrombocytopenia.**	Treatment for Wiskott-Aldrich is supportive (IVIG and aggressive antibiotic treatment of infection). Patients rarely survive to adulthood.
Phagocytic		
Chronic granulomatous disease (CGD)	X-linked or autosomal-recessive disorder with deficient superoxide production by PMNs and macrophages. Results in chronic pulmonary, GI, and urinary tract infections; osteomyelitis; and hepatitis. Anemia, lymphadenopathy, and hypergamma-globulinemia may also be present.	Diagnose with absolute neutrophil count and adhesion, chemotactic, phagocytic, and bactericidal assays. **Nitroblue tetrazolium test is diagnostic for CGD.** Treat with **daily TMP-SMX.** Judicious antibiotic use during infections. γ-interferon therapy can ↓ the incidence of serious infection.
Chédiak-Higashi syndrome	Autosomal-recessive disorder causing a defect in neutrophil chemotaxis. Syndrome includes oculocutaneous albinism, neuropathy, and neutropenia.	

(continued)

Table 2.15-6.   Pediatric Immunodeficiency Disorders *(continued)*

Disorder	Description	Diagnosis/Treatment
Complement		
C1 esterase deficiency (hereditary angioneurotic edema)	Autosomal-dominant disorder with recurrent episodes of angioedema lasting 21–72 hours and provoked by stress or trauma. Can result in life-threatening airway edema.	Diagnose with **total hemolytic complement (CH$_{50}$);** assess quantity and function of individual classical and alternative pathway components.
Terminal complement deficiency (C5–C9)	Patients are susceptible to recurrent meningococcal or gonococcal infections and, rarely, SLE or glomerulonephritis.	**Treat** C1 esterase deficiency with daily prophylactic danazol. Purified C1 esterase and FFP can be used prior to surgery.
		Treat terminal complement deficiency with meningococcal vaccine and appropriate antibiotics.

(Reprinted, with permission, from Le T et al. *First Aid for the USMLE Step 2,* 4th ed. New York: McGraw-Hill, 2003:383–384.)

TREATMENT

- Anti-inflammatory therapy, especially **high-dose aspirin** during acute illness, has been proven to ↓ the incidence of coronary abnormalities.
- Follow patients with echocardiography.
- IVIG to prevent aneurysms if necessary.

COMPLICATIONS

Myocarditis, pericarditis, **coronary artery aneurysm** predisposing to myocardial ischemia.

All patients who meet the criteria for diagnosis of Kawasaki disease should get empiric NSAIDs to prevent cardiac complications.

▶ CONGENITAL HEART DISEASE

- The incidence of congenital heart disease is approximately 1%.
- The most common lesion is VSD, followed by ASD. Most common cyanotic lesion is transposition of the great arteries (TGA).

Ventricular Septal Defect (VSD)

A congenital "hole" in the ventricular septum. Can be membranous (least likely to close spontaneously), perimembranous, or muscular.

SYMPTOMS/EXAM

- Patients may by asymptomatic at birth if the lesion is small.
- Often presents between 2–6 months of age.
- If the lesion is large with significant shunting, look for symptoms of **CHF** (shortness of breath, pulmonary edema), **frequent respiratory infections,** failure to thrive, or exercise/feeding intolerance.
- Cardiac exam may reveal **pansystolic** vibratory murmur at the **left lower sternal border,** along with a loud pulmonic S2.
- Look for signs of failure such as cardiomegaly and crackles.

DIAGNOSIS

ECG will show RVH and LVH. Definitive diagnosis is made by **echocardiogram**.

TREATMENT

- Treat cardiac failure if present. Follow small VSDs annually, since most close spontaneously.
- Surgically repair large VSDs as soon as possible to prevent pulmonary vascular disease and heart failure.

COMPLICATIONS

If a VSD remains open, **Eisenmenger's syndrome** may develop, which is characterized by **pulmonary hypertension** that → RVH and **reversal of the shunt** to right-to-left shunt, causing cyanosis. Eisenmenger's is often irreversible.

Atrial Septal Defect (ASD)

The second most common congenital heart lesion. Characterized by an opening in the atrial septum that allows the flow of blood between the atria.

SYMPTOMS/EXAM

Presents in late childhood or early adulthood: varies from asymptomatic to severe cyanosis with symptoms of failure, depending on the size of the defect. Look for patients with the following:

- **Heaving cardiac impulse** at the left lower sternal border.
- **Wide and fixed split S2.**
- Systolic ejection murmur at the **upper left sternal border.**

DIAGNOSIS

- Echocardiography with color flow Doppler is **diagnostic.**
- CXR may show cardiac enlargement and ↑ pulmonary vascularity.
- ECG shows left axis deviation.

TREATMENT

- Small defects require no treatment, but patients should be treated with **prophylactic antibiotics** prior to dental procedures.
- Surgical closure is recommended for infants presenting with **CHF.**
- Late complications include arrhythmias and RV dysfunction.

COMPLICATIONS

Shunt may reverse if pulmonary hypertension develops → Eisenmenger's syndrome.

Patent Ductus Arteriosus (PDA)

- Failure of the ductus arteriosus to close within the first few days of life → a persistent connection between the pulmonary artery and the aorta. Lesion → a **left-to-right shunt** from the aorta to the pulmonary artery.
- Risk factors include prematurity, high altitude, and maternal first-trimester rubella infection.

Patients with patent VSDs are at ↑ risk for endocarditis and septic emboli and should thus be given prophylactic antibiotics when having dental work performed.

SYMPTOMS/EXAM

Patients may be asymptomatic or may present with symptoms of heart failure, lower extremity clubbing, and dyspnea. On exam, look for a **wide pulse pressure**, a **continuous "machinery" murmur** at the second intercostal space on the left upper sternal border, a **loud S2**, and **bounding peripheral pulses.**

DIAGNOSIS

- Diagnosis is done with echocardiography showing left atrial and ventricular enlargement; may also show the PDA itself.
- ECG may show LVH; CXR may show cardiomegaly.
- Angiography shows $\uparrow O_2$ in the pulmonary artery.

TREATMENT

- Treat with **indomethacin** to close PDA.
- If indomethacin fails or if the patient is > 6–8 months old, surgical closure is required.

COMPLICATIONS

Remember that some lesions, such as transposition of the great vessels, require a patent ductus for survival.

Tetralogy of Fallot

The anatomy consists of four lesions. See the mnemonic **PROVe.**

SYMPTOMS/EXAM

Patients range from acyanotic to profoundly cyanotic depending on the severity of the pulmonic stenosis. May also present with dyspnea and easy fatigability. Look for "tet spells" in a child who needs to stop running or playing and sit. Exam reveals a **systolic ejection murmur** at the left sternal border, **RV lift,** and a **single S2.**

DIAGNOSIS

Echocardiography is diagnostic, but CXR shows a characteristic **"boot-shaped"** heart.

TREATMENT

If cyanotic, administer **PGE** at birth to keep the ductus arteriosus open. Treat "tet spells" (cyanotic spells) with O_2, knee-chest position, fluids, morphine, propranolol, and phenylephrine if severe. Definitive treatment is surgical correction.

Coarctation of the Aorta

A narrowing of the lumen of the aorta $\rightarrow \downarrow$ blood flow below the narrowing and $\uparrow$ flow above it. Risk factors include **Turner's syndrome** and male sex. Associated with a bicuspid aortic valve.

SYMPTOMS/EXAM

Patients have a range of symptoms and presentations, which may include dyspnea on exertion, syncope, or even systemic hypoperfusion/shock. Exam findings include **higher systolic blood pressure in the upper extremities than in the lower extremities**, and $\downarrow$ femoral and distal **lower extremity pulses.** There is often a late systolic murmur.

> **Tetralogy of Fallot—PROVe**
>
> **P**ulmonary stenosis (RV outflow obstruction)
> **R**VH
> **O**verriding aorta
> **V**SD

DIAGNOSIS

- Look for characteristic **CXR findings of** "rib notching" due to collateral circulation through the intercostal arteries.
- Definitive diagnosis may be made through **echocardiography** or catheterization/aortography.

TREATMENT

- Surgical correction is often successful, but recoarctation may recur.
- Balloon angioplasty is an alternative to surgical repair.
- All patients should receive endocarditis antibiotic prophylaxis even after treatment.
- Initiate repair as early as possible given the risks of heart failure, premature CAD, and intracerebral hemorrhage.

▶ GASTROINTESTINAL

Pyloric Stenosis

Hypertrophy of the pyloric canal → gastric outlet obstruction. Typically occurs at 3–4 weeks of life in term, first-born, male infants.

SYMPTOMS/EXAM

Projectile, nonbilious emesis in the first two weeks to four months of life. Infants will usually feed well initially, but the emesis ultimately → dehydration and malnutrition. On exam, look for an **epigastric olive-shaped mass** or visible gastric peristaltic waves.

DIAGNOSIS

- Electrolytes will show a **hypochloremic, hypokalemic metabolic alkalosis** 2° to emesis.
- Ultrasound is the gold standard for diagnosis and shows a **hypertrophied pylorus.**
- Barium studies show a narrow pyloric channel "string sign" or a pyloric beak.

TREATMENT

- **Correct dehydration and electrolyte abnormalities** first.
- Surgical correction with pyloromyotomy, which is usually well tolerated.
- Patients usually feed well postoperatively after a brief period of emesis.

Intussusception

Telescoping of a bowel segment into itself (see Figure 2.15-1); may → edema, arterial occlusion, gut necrosis, and death. This is the **most common** cause of bowel obstruction in the first two years of life.

SYMPTOMS

- Classically presents with the **triad** of **abdominal pain,** "currant jelly" **stools,** and **vomiting** (although all three may not be present).
- Pain is usually paroxysmal and severe, causing infants to draw their knees to their chests.
- In between episodes of pain, the child may be completely comfortable.
- Patients may also present with altered mental status (lethargy or even obtundation).

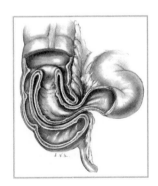

**FIGURE 2.15-1.
Intussusception.**

(Reproduced, with permission, from Way LW, Doherty GM. *Current Surgical Diagnosis & Treatment,* 11th ed. New York: McGraw-Hill, 2003:1323.)

- Between episodes of pain, the abdomen is usually nontender.
- **Look for a palpable, sausage-shaped mass.**
- Rectal exam will often show occult blood.

DIFFERENTIAL

- GI infection such as acute gastroenteritis.
- Other diagnoses include constipation, Meckel's diverticulum, and meconium ileus (infants).

DIAGNOSIS

Begin with abdominal plain films, and be sure to check an ultrasound or an **air-contrast enema.**

TREATMENT

- Start with **fluid resuscitation** and correction of electrolyte abnormalities.
- Air-contrast enema is often both **diagnostic** and **therapeutic** but is contraindicated if there are signs of strangulated bowel or perforation or if the child is "toxic" appearing.
- If enema is unsuccessful or contraindicated, **surgical reduction** is **necessary.**
- Patients need close observation for 24 hours after reduction, as intussusception may recur.

Intussusception can be both diagnosed and treated by means of an air-contrast enema.

Malrotation/Volvulus

Defined as failure of normal rotation as the gut returns to the abdominal cavity during the 10th week of gestation. This results in an incomplete fixation of mesentery to the posterior peritoneal wall, making volvulus possible, or occlusion of the superior mesenteric artery (SMA).

SYMPTOMS/EXAM

- Presents with **recurrent bilious emesis,** acute small bowel obstruction or bowel necrosis in the first three weeks of life.
- May also present later in life with signs of intermittent intestinal obstruction, malabsorption, protein-losing enteropathy, or diarrhea.

DIAGNOSIS

- **Upper GI series** shows the duodenojejunal junction on the **right side** of the spine. Contrast demonstrates "bird's beak" where gut is twisted.
- Barium enema, may show a **mobile cecum** not situated in the RLQ.

TREATMENT

- Surgical repair is indicated even in patients who are asymptomatic owing to the lifelong risk of volvulus.
- **Volvulus is a surgical emergency** owing to necrosis of gut from occlusion of the SMA.

COMPLICATIONS

The 1° complication is "short bowel syndrome," which occurs when < 30 cm of short bowel is left → malnutrition, TPN dependence, and liver failure.

Meckel's Diverticulum

A remnant of the omphalomesenteric duct that persists as an outpouching of the distal ileum. Can contain ectopic (usually gastric or pancreatic) mucosa.

SYMPTOMS/EXAM

- Often asymptomatic. Patients may present with **painless rectal bleeding** or **intussusception** (with Meckel's as the lead point).
- Exam may be unremarkable or typical of intussusception.

DIAGNOSIS

Perform a **technetium radionuclide** scan ("Meckel scan") to detect gastric mucosa. The ultimate diagnosis must be made surgically.

TREATMENT

- Stabilize the patient with hydration; transfuse if needed.
- Perform surgical exploration if symptomatic. Bowel resection may be required along with resection of diverticula depending on the location and complexity of the lesion.

> **Meckel's diverticulum rule of 2's**
>
> **2** feet proximal to ileocecal valve (most commonly)
> **2** types of ectopic tissue (gastric, pancreatic)
> **2**% of the population Males are affected **2** times as often as females
> Usually presents by age 2. About 2 inches long and 2 cm in diameter.

► PULMONARY/RESPIRATORY

Croup (Laryngotracheobronchitis)

- Acute viral inflammatory disease of the larynx/subglottic space (see Table 2.15-7).
- Most common in children three months to five years of age.
- A common etiology is parainfluenza virus (PIV) type 1, but may also be caused by other parainfluenza viruses as well as by RSV, influenza, rubeola, adenovirus, or *Mycoplasma pneumoniae*.

SYMPTOMS/EXAM

- Typical symptoms include a viral prodrome with URI symptoms.
- Other symptoms are low-grade fever, mild dyspnea, and inspiratory stridor that worsens with agitation.
- Listen for the characteristic barky cough.

DIAGNOSIS

Based on clinical findings. May see **"steeple sign"** on **lateral neck film,** formed by subglottic narrowing (see Figure 2.15-2).

TREATMENT

- **Mist therapy,** O_2, aerosolized racemic epinephrine, and corticosteroids may be useful. Avoid agitation if possible.
- Hospitalize patients with severe stridor.

Epiglottitis

- A serious and rapidly progressive infection of the epiglottis and contiguous structures that can cause **life-threatening airway obstruction.**

TABLE 2.15-7. **Characteristics of Croup, Epiglottitis, and Tracheitis**

	CROUP	EPIGLOTTITIS	TRACHEITIS
Age group	3 months to 3 years	3–7 years	3 months to 2 years
Incidence in children presenting with stridor	88%	8%	2%
Pathogen	PIV	*H. influenzae*	Often *S. aureus*
Onset	Prodrome (1–7 days)	Rapid (4–12 hours)	Prodrome (three days) → acute decompensation (10 hours)
Fever severity	Low grade	High grade	Intermediate grade
Associated symptoms	Barking cough, hoarseness	Muffled voice, drooling	Variable respiratory distress
Position preference	None	Seated, neck extended	None
Response to racemic epinephrine	Stridor improves	None	None
CXR findings	"Steeple sign" on AP films	"Thumbprint sign" on lateral film	Subglottic narrowing

(Reprinted, with permission, from Le T et al. *First Aid for the USMLE Step 2,* 4th ed. New York: McGraw-Hill, 2003:385.)

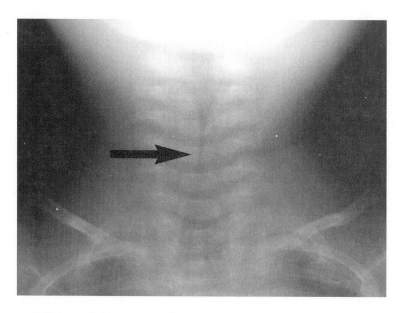

FIGURE 2.15-2. **Croup.**

The x-ray shows marked subglottic narrowing of the airway (arrow). (Reproduced, with permission, from Stone CK, Humphries RL. *Currrent Emergency Diagnosis & Treatment,* 5th ed. New York: McGraw-Hill, 2004:648.)

- Increasingly rare owing to the Hib vaccine, as the disease is most commonly caused by *H. influenzae* type B.
- Other pathogenic organisms include *Streptococcus* species and nontypable *H. influenzae*.

SYMPTOMS/EXAM

- Maintain a high index of suspicion in children with sudden-onset high fever, **dysphagia, drooling, muffled voice,** inspiratory retractions, cyanosis, and soft stridor.
- Patients may be in the **"sniffing dog" position,** with the neck hyperextended and the chin protruding.
- Can quickly progress to complete airway obstruction and respiratory arrest.

DIAGNOSIS

- Based on the clinical picture. **Do not examine the patient's throat** without an anesthesiologist present given the risk of laryngospasm and obstruction.
- Lateral neck films show the characteristic **"thumbprint sign"** of a swollen epiglottis obliterating the valleculae (see Figure 2.15-3).

TREATMENT

Keep the patient calm, **call anesthesia immediately,** and transfer the patient to the OR. Treat with **endotracheal intubation** and IV antibiotics.

Throat examination may cause laryngospasm and airway obstruction.

▶ FEBRILE SEIZURES

Fever-associated seizures that occur in children six months to six years of age. A ⊕ **family history** of febrile seizures is common. Seizures may present as two types:

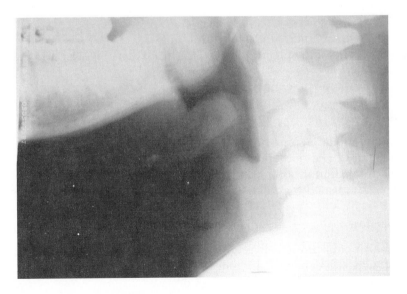

FIGURE 2.15-3. **Epiglottitis.**

The classic swollen epiglottis ("thumbprint sign") and obstructed airway are seen on x-ray. (Reproduced, with permission, from Stone CK, Humphries RL. *Current Emergency Diagnosis & Treatment,* 5th ed. New York: McGraw-Hill, 2004:1055.)

- **Simple:** A generalized seizure with short duration (< 15 minutes), one seizure/24-hour period, and quick return to normal function after seizure with no residual focal neurologic deficit.
- **Complex:** A focal seizure or focal seizure → generalized seizure, longer in duration (> 15 minutes). Patients may have > 1 seizure/24-hour period and an incomplete or slow return to normal neurologic status.

DIAGNOSIS/TREATMENT

- If the patient has a **simple febrile seizure, no further evaluation is necessary** beyond finding a source for fever in infants/young children.
- If complex, check electrolytes with glucose, blood cultures, UA, and CBC with differential.
- Perform an **LP** in all children < 1 year of age who present with seizure or in children > 1 year of age in which CNS infection is suspected.
- Obtain an **EEG** and **brain MRI** for children with complex febrile seizures.
- Treat underlying infection.

▶ ONCOLOGY

Wilms' Tumor

An embryonal tumor of renal origin and the **most common renal tumor** in children; usually seen in children 1–4 years of age. Risk factors include a family history, neurofibromatosis, aniridia, and congenital GU anomalies.

SYMPTOMS/EXAM

Patients typically have abdominal pain. There may also be **hematuria,** although this is usually microscopic. Other general symptoms include weight loss, nausea, emesis, bone pain, dysuria, and polyuria. Exam reveals a **painless abdominal/flank mass.**

ALL, is the most common solid tumors in children.

DIAGNOSIS

- Start with an abdominal CT or ultrasound.
- Assess severity and spread with CXR, chest CT, CBC, LFTs, and BUN/creatinine.
- Excisional biopsy to confirm.

TREATMENT

- Transabdominal nephrectomy.
- Postoperative chemotherapy (vincristine/dactinomycin).
- Flank irradiation in some cases.
- Prognosis is usually good but depends on staging and tumor histology.

Neuroblastoma

A tumor of neural crest cell origin most commonly affecting children < 5 years of age. Risk factors include neurofibromatosis, tuberous sclerosis, pheochromocytoma, and Hirschsprung's disease.

SYMPTOMS

Lesions can appear anywhere in the body, so symptoms vary by location. Possible presentations include **abdominal mass/distention,** anorexia, weight loss, malaise, fever, diarrhea, bone pain, irritability, or neuromuscular symptoms (if paraspinal).

EXAM

Check for an abdominal mass or tenderness. There may also be abdominal distention and hepatomegaly. Be suspicious in anyone with a skull mass. Other findings may include leg edema, hypertension, fever, pallor, and periorbital bruising.

DIAGNOSIS

- Check an abdominal CT and send 24-hour urinary catecholamines to look for ↑ VMA and HVA.
- Assess severity and spread with CXR, bone scan, CBC, LFTs, BUN/creatinine, and coagulation screen.

TREATMENT

- Localized tumors are usually cured with excision.
- Chemotherapy includes cyclophosphamide and doxorubicin.
- Radiation is often used adjunctively.
- Prognosis is improved if diagnosis is made at < 1 year of age.

SECTION II

Psychiatry

Generalized Anxiety Disorder (GAD)

Lifetime prevalence is 5%. The male-to-female ratio is 1:2; clinical diagnosis is usually made in the early 20s.

SYMPTOMS/EXAM

Characterized by **excessive and pervasive worry** about a number of activities or events that causes significant impairment or distress. Patients often seek out physicians for the somatic component of the disorder.

DIFFERENTIAL

Substance-induced anxiety disorder, anxiety disorder due to a general medical condition (e.g., hyperthyroidism), panic disorder, OCD, depression, social phobia, hypochondriasis, somatization disorder.

DIAGNOSIS

- Anxiety/worry on most days for ≥ 6 months.
- **Three or more somatic symptoms,** including restlessness, fatigue, difficulty concentrating, irritability, muscle tension, and sleep disturbance.

TREATMENT

- Pharmacologic therapy with venlafaxine, SSRIs, buspirone, and TCAs.
- Benzodiazepines offer faster relief, but tolerance and dependence may occur.
- Psychotherapy and relaxation training are important adjuncts.

Obsessive-Compulsive Disorder (OCD)

Lifetime prevalence is 2–3%. Typically presents in late adolescence or early adulthood.

SYMPTOMS/EXAMS

- Obsessions are **persistent, intrusive thoughts, impulses, or images** that are recognized as a product of the patient's own mind. Common themes are contamination and fear of harm to self or others.
- Compulsions are **conscious, repetitive behaviors** (e.g., hand washing) or mental acts (e.g., counting) that the patient feels driven to perform in order to ↓ anxiety from an obsession.

DIFFERENTIAL

Other anxiety disorders, Tourette's syndrome (multiple motor and vocal tics), depression, schizophrenia, obsessive-compulsive personality disorder (lacks severe functional impairment), medical conditions (e.g., brain tumor, temporal lobe epilepsy).

DIAGNOSIS

Obsessions and/or compulsions that are recognized at some point as **excessive or unreasonable** (in adults), cause marked distress, and are time-consuming (> 1 hour/day).

Pharmacotherapy (e.g., SSRIs or clomipramine) and **behavior therapy** (e.g., exposure and response prevention).

Panic Disorder

More common in women; mean age of onset is 25. Lifetime prevalence is 1.5–3.5%. Panic disorder is often accompanied by **agoraphobia,** a fear of public places.

SYMPTOMS/EXAM

Presents as **panic attacks**—discrete periods of intense fear or discomfort in which ≥ 4 of the following symptoms develop abruptly and peak within 10 minutes: palpitations, sweating, trembling, shortness of breath, chest pain, nausea, dizziness, numbness, depersonalization, and fear of losing control.

DIFFERENTIAL

Medical conditions (e.g., angina, hyperthyroidism, hypoglycemia), substance-induced anxiety disorder, other anxiety disorders.

DIAGNOSIS

Recurrent, unexpected panic attacks, followed by at least **one month** of worry about attacks.

TREATMENT

- Cognitive-behavioral therapy (CBT).
- Pharmacotherapy with SSRIs, TCAs, and MAOIs.
- Benzodiazepines (e.g., alprazolam and clonazepam) are effective for immediate relief but have dependence and abuse potential.

Phobias (Social and Specific)

Lifetime prevalence is 10% (the most common mental disorder).

SYMPTOMS/EXAM

Persistent, excessive, or unreasonable fear and/or avoidance of an object or situation that → significant distress or impairment. Exposure to the object or stimulus often → **panic attacks.**

DIFFERENTIAL

Other anxiety disorders, depression, avoidant and schizoid personality disorders, schizophrenia, appropriate fear, normal shyness.

DIAGNOSIS

- **Social phobia** is characterized by unreasonable, marked, and persistent **fear of scrutiny and embarrassment in social or performance situations.**
- **Specific phobia** is immediately **cued by an object or a situation** (e.g., animals, heights).
- In adults, the **duration is ≥ 6 months.**

TREATMENT

- CBT and pharmacotherapy (e.g., SSRIs, benzodiazepines, β-blockers) are effective for social phobias.
- **Behavioral therapy,** often using exposure and desensitization, is best for specific phobia.

Post-Traumatic Stress Disorder (PTSD)

The lifetime prevalence is 8%.

SYMPTOMS/EXAM

- Characteristic symptoms develop following **exposure to a traumatic event** that involved actual or threatened death or serious injury and evoked intense fear, helplessness, or horror.
- Watch for survival guilt, personality change, substance abuse, depression, and suicide.

DIFFERENTIAL

- **Acute stress disorder:** The same symptoms as PTSD, but lasts < 1 month and must occur within one month of a trauma.
- **Adjustment disorder with anxiety:** Emotional or behavioral symptoms within three months of a stressor; lasts < 6 months.
- **Other:** Depression, OCD, acute intoxication or withdrawal, factitious disorders, malingering, borderline personality disorder.

DIAGNOSIS

Symptoms must persist for > 1 month and must include the following:

- Reexperiencing of the event (e.g., nightmares).
- Avoidance of trauma-related stimuli.
- ↑ arousal (e.g., hypervigilance, exaggerated startle).

TREATMENT

- Pharmacotherapy with TCAs (e.g., imipramine and amitriptyline), SSRIs, MAOIs, anticonvulsants, lithium, propranolol, and buspirone.
- CBT and group therapy are also effective.

Anxiolytic Medications

- Benzodiazepines:
  - Used for anxiety, alcohol withdrawal, insomnia, anesthesia, seizures, and muscle spasms.
  - **Rapid onset of action.**
  - Cons include risk of abuse, tolerance, dependence, and withdrawal.
  - **Augments sedation and respiratory depression** from other CNS depressants (e.g., alcohol).
  - P-450 inhibitors (e.g., cimetidine, fluoxetine) ↑ levels; carbamazepine and rifampin ↓ levels.
- Buspirone:
  - A 5-HT$_{1A}$ partial agonist.
  - Used to treat GAD and to augment depression/OCD therapy. Not used for panic disorder.

- Few side effects and no tolerance, dependence, or withdrawal.
- Slow onset of action and lower efficacy than benzodiazepines.
- Do not use with MAOIs.
- Zolpidem:
  - Nonbenzodiazepine for insomnia.
  - Rapid onset.
  - Rare withdrawal.

▶ MOOD DISORDERS

Major Depressive Disorder

Untreated episodes can last ≥ 4 months, and recurrence risk is 50% after only one episode. **The male-to-female ratio is 1:2.** Lifetime prevalence is 10–25% for females (the highest risk is in childbearing years) and 5–12% for males. Onset may occur at any age, but average age of onset is in the mid-20s. Not uncommonly associated with a stressor. Up to 15% die by suicide.

SYMPTOMS/EXAM

Symptoms are described by the mnemonic **SIG E CAPS.**

DIFFERENTIAL

- **Dysthymia:** Milder, chronic depressed state for ≥ 2 years.
- **Bereavement:** No severe impairment/suicidality; usually improves in two months.
- **Adjustment disorder with depressed mood:** Fewer symptoms; occurs within three months of stressor; lasts < 6 months.
- **Other:** Substance-induced mood disorder (e.g., illicit drugs, β-blockers), mood disorder due to a medical condition (e.g., hypothyroidism), dementia.

DIAGNOSIS

- Characterized by ≥ 1 major depressive episodes.
- Requires at least **five signs/symptoms,** one of which must be **depressed mood or loss of interest/pleasure.**
- Symptoms last ≥ **2 weeks,** causing significant dysfunction or impairment.

TREATMENT

- **Pharmacotherapy:** Effective in 50–70% of patients, but requires 3–4 weeks to take effect. Continue treatment for at least six months.
- **Electroconvulsive therapy (ECT):**
  - Safe and highly effective.
  - Best for refractory or catatonic depression; may also be used for acute mania or acute psychosis.
  - Adverse effects include postictal confusion, arrhythmias, headache, and **retrograde amnesia.**
  - Relative contraindications include intracranial mass, aneurysm, and recent MI/stroke. Pregnancy is **not** a contraindication.
- **Psychotherapy:** Combined with antidepressants, **more effective than either alone.**

Antidepressant Medications

- **SSRIs:** Fluoxetine, sertraline, paroxetine, citalopram, escitalopram, fluvoxamine.

> **SYMPTOMS OF DEPRESSION— SIG E CAPS**
>
> **S**leep (hypersomnia or insomnia)
> **I**nterest (loss of interest or pleasure in activities)
> **G**uilt (feelings of worthlessness or inappropriate guilt)
> **E**nergy (↓)
> **C**oncentration (↓)
> **A**ppetite (↑ or ↓)
> **P**sychomotor agitation or retardation
> **S**uicidal ideation

Depression has associated impaired cognition, often called "pseudodementia."

Seasonal affective disorder, typified by recurrent fall/winter depression, is treated with bright-light therapy.

Depressed patients may also have psychotic symptoms of hallucinations and delusions, which should be treated with an antipsychotic in addition to an antidepressant.

TCAs are the most lethal antidepressants in overdose.

TCA toxicity– Tri-C's

Convulsions
Coma
Cardiac arrhythmias

Cheese and red wine can precipitate a hypertensive crisis in those taking MAOIs.

- First-line therapy for depression and many anxiety disorders.
- Well tolerated, effective, and relatively safe in overdose.
- Side effects include **sexual dysfunction,** nausea, diarrhea, anorexia, headache, anxiety, tremor, and sleep disturbance.
- Can ↑ warfarin levels because of P-450 interactions.
- **TCAs:** Nortriptyline, desipramine, imipramine, amitriptyline, clomipramine, doxepin.
  - Block the reuptake of norepinephrine (NE) and serotonin.
  - Levels ↑ when used with SSRIs because of P-450 competition.
  - Anticholinergic side effects are common (e.g., dry mouth, constipation). Other adverse effects include orthostatic hypotension, sedation, weight gain, and cardiac toxicity (**check baseline ECG**).
  - Useful for chronic pain and migraines. OCD responds to clomipramine.
- **MAOIs:** Phenelzine, tranylcypromine, isocarboxazid.
  - Common side effects include orthostatic hypotension, insomnia, weight gain, edema, and sexual dysfunction.
  - May cause **tyramine-induced hypertensive crisis.** Dietary restrictions include certain cheeses, fish, cured meats, and alcoholic beverages.
  - Potentially fatal **serotonin syndrome** (diarrhea, agitation, autonomic instability, myoclonus, seizures, delirium) if combined with SSRIs, TCAs, meperidine, fentanyl, and indirect sympathomimetics (found in **OTC cold remedies**).
- **Mirtazapine:**
  - An α_2-antagonist that enhances NE and 5-HT.
  - Side effects include sedation, weight gain, and ↑ cholesterol. Little effect on sexual function.
- **Bupropion:**
  - May act via dopamine (DA) reuptake inhibition.
  - First-line therapy for depression and smoking cessation.
  - Effective for patients with sexual side effects from other antidepressants.
  - No weight gain or orthostatic hypotension. **Lowers seizure threshold.**
- **Venlafaxine:**
  - Main action is 5-HT and NE reuptake inhibition.
  - Used for major depression and GAD, with faster response than SSRIs.
  - Adverse effects include **diastolic hypertension (monitor BP),** insomnia, nervousness, sedation, sexual dysfunction, anticholinergic effects, and nausea.
- **Nefazodone and trazodone:**
  - Primarily inhibits 5-HT reuptake.
  - Nefazodone is not associated with sexual dysfunction.
  - Trazodone is associated with **priapism.** Used for insomnia therapy, owing to its sedative effect.

Suicide

- Eighth leading overall cause of death in the United States.
- Occurs in those with depressive disorders, substance abuse, schizophrenia, and other mental disorders. Look for **prior suicide attempts and a family history of suicide.**
- The suicide rate for 15- to 24-year-olds is ↑; suicide is the third leading cause of death in that age group.
- **Suicide rates ↑ with age.** The highest rate of suicide is in those ≥ 75 years of age.

- Women attempt suicide more frequently than men, but **men actually complete suicide > 4 times as often as women.**
- More whites commit suicide than other racial groups.
- Marriage lessens the risk of suicide.
- **Hospitalize** an acutely suicidal patient.

Always assess suicide risk in patients with depression.

Bipolar Disorder

Prevalence is 1%, and the male-to-female ratio is 1:1. A family history of bipolar illness significantly ↑ risk. Up to 10–15% die by suicide.

SYMPTOMS/EXAM

- Manic episode:
  - **One week** of abnormally and persistently **elevated, expansive, or irritable mood.**
  - At least three of the following (four if mood is irritable):
    - Inflated self-esteem or grandiosity
    - ↓ need for sleep
    - Pressured speech
    - Flight of ideas/racing thoughts
    - Distractibility
    - ↑ goal-directed activity/psychomotor agitation
    - Excessive involvement in pleasurable activities
- Hypomanic episode:
  - At least four days of manic symptoms as outlined above.
  - Does **not** cause marked functional impairment, require hospitalization, or present with psychotic features.
- Mixed episode:
  - Patients meet the criteria for both manic and depressive episodes for at least one week.

DIFFERENTIAL

- **Cyclothymic disorder:** Chronic cycles of mild depression and mania over two years.
- **Other:** Substance-induced mood disorder, schizophrenia, schizoaffective disorder, personality disorders, medical conditions (e.g., temporal lobe epilepsy, hyperthyroidism).

DIAGNOSIS

- **Bipolar I disorder:** One or more mixed or manic episodes. Depressive episodes are common but are not required for diagnosis.
- **Bipolar II disorder:** One or more major depressive episodes and at least one hypomanic episode.

TREATMENT

- **Acute mania:** Mood stabilizers, antipsychotics, benzodiazepines, ECT.
- **Bipolar depression:** Mood stabilizers +/− antidepressants. Start mood stabilizers first to avoid inducing mania. ECT is also effective.

Mood Stabilizers

- **Lithium:**
  - The mainstay of treatment of bipolar disorder. Effective in mania and in augmenting antidepressants.

Treatment of lithium toxicity
may require hemodialysis.

- Has a **narrow therapeutic index** and requires serum level monitoring.
- Adverse effects include thirst, polyuria, fine tremor, weight gain, diarrhea, nausea, acne, and hypothyroidism. **Monitor renal and thyroid function.**
- Toxicity includes **coarse tremor, ataxia,** vomiting, confusion, seizures, and arrhythmias.
- **Valproic acid:**
  - First-line agent; effective in rapid cyclers ($\geq$ 4 episodes/ year).
  - Side effects include sedation, weight gain, hair loss, tremor, ataxia, and GI distress.
  - Pancreatitis, thrombocytopenia, and fatal hepatotoxicity are uncommon.
  - Monitor platelets, LFTs, and serum drug level.
- **Carbamazepine:**
  - Second-line agent with adverse effects of nausea, sedation, rash, and ataxia.
  - Hepatic toxicity, hyponatremia, and bone marrow suppression occur rarely. Stevens-Johnson syndrome is rare but potentially fatal.
  - Monitor blood counts, transaminases, and electrolytes. Drug interactions complicate its use.
- **Other anticonvulsants (lamotrigine, gabapentin, topiramate):**
  - Efficacy is not well documented.
  - Do not require blood level monitoring and do not cause weight gain.
  - Lamotrigine is gradually titrated owing to the potential for rash and its association with Stevens-Johnson syndrome.

▶ PSYCHOTIC DISORDERS

Schizophrenia

Lifetime prevalence is 1%. Peak onset is at 18–25 years for men and 25–35 years for women. Few patients have a complete recovery. Suicide rate is 10%. The incidence of substance abuse is $\uparrow$, and > 75% of patients are smokers.

SYMPTOMS/EXAM

At least two of the following that have been active $\geq$ 1 month, with **continuous signs for $\geq$ 6 months:**

- Delusions
- Hallucinations
- Disorganized speech
- Grossly disorganized or catatonic behavior
- Negative symptoms (affective flattening, avolition)

DIFFERENTIAL

- **Brief psychotic disorder:** Symptoms < 1 month; often follows a psychosocial stressor; associated with a better prognosis.
- **Delusional disorder: Nonbizarre delusions for $\geq$ 1 month** in the absence of other psychotic symptoms; often chronic.
- **Schizoaffective disorder:** Mood symptoms are present for a significant portion of the illness, but psychotic symptoms have been present without mood episode.
- **Schizophreniform disorder:** The same criteria as for schizophrenia, but with a **duration < 6 months.**

- **Other:** Mood disorder with psychotic features; substance-induced psychosis (e.g., amphetamines) or drug withdrawal (e.g., alcoholic hallucinosis); psychosis due to a general medical condition (e.g., brain tumor), delirium, or dementia.

TREATMENT

Pharmacotherapy with antipsychotics (neuroleptics). Hospitalize when the patient is a danger to self or others. Psychosocial treatments, individual supportive psychotherapy, and family therapy help prevent relapse.

Antipsychotic Medication

- **Typical antipsychotics:** Act through DA receptor blockade; used for psychotic disorders and acute agitation. Cheap and effective. **High-potency agents (haloperidol,** fluphenazine) → more extrapyramidal symptoms. **Low-potency agents** (thioridazine, chlorpromazine) → more sedation, anticholinergic effects, and hypotension. Key side effects include the following:
  - **Extrapyramidal symptoms (EPS):** See Table 2.16-1.
  - **Hyperprolactinemia:** Amenorrhea, gynecomastia, galactorrhea.
  - **Anticholinergic effects:** Dry mouth, urinary retention, constipation.
  - **Neuroleptic malignant syndrome:** Fever, muscle rigidity, autonomic instability, and delirium; ↑ CPK, WBC, and LFTs. To treat, stop the neuroleptic and give dantrolene/bromocriptine and IV fluids.
  - **Other:** Cardiac arrhythmias, weight gain, sedation.
- **Atypical antipsychotics:** Currently first-line treatment for schizophrenia. Act through 5-HT$_2$ and DA antagonism. Benefits are fewer EPS and anticholinergic effects as well as improved efficacy for treatment-refractory patients. May cause **sedation, weight gain, type 2 DM, and QT prolongation.**
  - **Risperidone, olanzapine, quetiapine, ziprasidone, aripiprazole:** All are commonly used.

TABLE 2.16-1.   Extrapyramidal Symptoms and Treatment

SYMPTOM	DESCRIPTION	TREATMENT
Acute dystonia	Involuntary muscle contraction or spasm (e.g., torticollis, oculogyric crisis).	Give an anticholinergic (benztropine) or diphenhydramine. To prevent, give prophylactic benztropine with an antipsychotic.
Akathisia	Subjective/objective restlessness.	↓ neuroleptic and try β-blockers (propranolol). Benzodiazepines or anticholinergics may help.
Dyskinesia	Pseudoparkinsonism (e.g., shuffling gait, cogwheel rigidity).	Give an anticholinergic (benztropine) or DA agonist (amantadine). ↓ dose of neuroleptic or discontinue (if tolerated).
Tardive dyskinesia	Stereotypic oral-facial movements. Likely from DA receptor sensitization. Often irreversible (50%).	Discontinue or ↓ dose of neuroleptic, attempt treatment with more appropriate drugs, and consider changing neuroleptic (e.g., to clozapine or risperidone). **Giving anticholinergics or ↓ neuroleptic may initially worsen tardive dyskinesia.**

- Clozapine: Reserved for treatment-refractory patients. May → **agranulocytosis (requires weekly CBCs).**

Enduring patterns of inner experience and behavior that deviate from cultural standards, are pervasive and inflexible, begin in adolescence or early adulthood, are stable over time, and → distress or impairment (see Table 2.16-2).

Somatization Disorder

- **Pain symptoms at ≥ 4 sites** that are not intentionally produced and cannot be explained by an organic etiology.
- Onset before the age of 30; much more prevalent in women.

Conversion Disorder

- **Sensory symptoms, motor deficits, or "pseudoseizures"** that are not intentionally produced and cannot be explained by an organic etiology.
- Relation to a **stressful event** suggests association with psychological factors.

Table 2.16-2. **Signs and Symptoms of Personality Disorders**

CLUSTER	DISORDERS	CHARACTERISTICS	CLINICAL DILEMMA/STRATEGY
Cluster A: **"weird"**	Paranoid	Distrustful, suspicious; interpret others' motives as malevolent.	Patients are suspicious and distrustful of doctors and rarely seek medical attention.
	Schizoid	Isolated, detached "loners." Restricted emotional expression.	Be clear, honest, noncontrolling, and nondefensive. Avoid humor. Maintain emotional distance.
Cluster B: **"wild"**	Borderline	Unstable mood/relationships, feelings of emptiness. Impulsive.	Patients change the rules, demand attention, and feel they are special.
	Histrionic	Excessively emotional and attention seeking. Sexually provocative.	Will manipulate staff and doctor ("splitting").
	Narcissistic	Grandiose, need admiration, sense of entitlement. Lack empathy.	Be firm: Stick to treatment plan. Be fair: Do not be punitive or
	Antisocial	Violate rights of others, social norms, laws. Impulsive. Lack remorse.	derogatory. Be consistent: Do not change rules.
Cluster C: **"worried and wimpy"**	Obsessive-compulsive	Preoccupied with perfectionism, order, control. Inflexible morals, values.	Patients are controlling and may sabotage their treatment. Words may be inconsistent with actions.
	Avoidant	Socially inhibited, rejection sensitive. Fear being disliked or ridiculed.	Avoid power struggles. Give clear recommendations, but do not push
	Dependent	Submissive, clingy, need to be taken care of. Difficulty making decisions.	patients into decisions.

Hypochondriasis

- Preoccupation over > 6 months with **fear of having a serious disease,** based on misinterpretation of symptoms.
- Not reassured by negative medical evaluation, but symptoms are not delusions.

Body Dysmorphic Disorder

- Preoccupation with an **imagined defect** in appearance.
- Multiple visits to surgeons and dermatologists are common.

Factitious Disorder

- Symptoms are intentionally put forth or **actively produced to assume a sick role.**
- More common in men and in health care workers.
- **Munchausen's syndrome** involves predominantly physical symptoms and can be "by proxy" (usually produced in a child by a parent).

Malingering

Fabrication of symptoms for **external motivations** (money, food, shelter).

May be familial. Often associated with mood disorders, substance abuse, and GAD. Attacks may be triggered by strong emotion.

SYMPTOMS/EXAM

- Excessive daytime sleepiness.
- Daytime **sleep attacks** with abnormal REM sleep.
- May have hypnagogic (just before sleep) or hypnopompic (just before awakening) hallucinations.

Cataplexy is the sudden onset of sleep.

TREATMENT

Amphetamines (**methylphenidate**) or nonamphetamine stimulants (modafinil).

Substance Abuse/Dependence

The lifetime prevalence of substance abuse is about 20%. Roughly 40% of the population report having used ≥ 1 illicit substances in their lifetimes. Comorbid psychiatric disorders are common.

SYMPTOMS

Symptoms are as follows (see also Table 2.16-3):

- **Substance abuse:** Failure to meet obligations, substance use during hazardous activities, substance-related legal problems, or continued use despite social problems.
- **Substance dependence:** Tolerance, withdrawal, ↑ use, desire to ↓ use, significant amount of time spent obtaining substance, withdrawal from activities.

TABLE 2.16-3.   Signs and Symptoms of Intoxication and Withdrawal

DRUG	INTOXICATION	WITHDRAWAL
Alcohol	Disinhibition, emotional lability, slurred speech, ataxia, aggression, hypoglycemia, blackouts (retrograde amnesia), coma.	Tremor tachycardia, hypertension, malaise, nausea, seizures, DTs, agitation, hallucinations.
Opioids	CNS depression, nausea, vomiting, constipation, **pupillary constriction,** seizures, respiratory depression (life threatening in overdose). Naloxone/naltrexone will block opioid receptors and reverse effects (beware of antagonist clearing before opioid, particularly with long-acting opioids such as methadone).	Anxiety, insomnia, anorexia, diaphoresis, dilated pupils, fever, rhinorrhea, piloerection, nausea, stomach cramps, diarrhea, yawning.
Amphetamines	Psychomotor agitation, impaired judgment, tachycardia, **pupillary dilation,** hypertension, paranoia, angina, hallucinations, sudden death. Treat with haloperidol for severe agitation and symptom-targeted medications.	Post-use "crash" with hypersomnolence, depression, malaise, severe craving, suicidality.
Phencyclidine hydrochloride (PCP)	Belligerence, psychosis, violence, impulsiveness, psychomotor agitation, fever, tachycardia, **vertical/ horizontal nystagmus,** ataxia, delirium. Give benzodiazepines for severe symptoms; otherwise reassure.	Recurrence of intoxication symptoms due to reabsorption in the GI tract; sudden onset of severe, random violence.
LSD	Marked anxiety or depression, delusions, visual hallucinations, flashbacks, pupillary dilation. Give benzodiazepines or traditional antipsychotics for severe symptoms.	
Marijuana	Euphoria, slowed sense of time, impaired judgment, social withdrawal, ↑ appetite, dry mouth, conjunctival injection, hallucinations, anxiety, paranoia, amotivational syndrome.	
Barbiturates	Low safety margin, respiratory depression.	Anxiety, seizures, delirium, life-threatening cardiovascular collapse.
Benzodiazepines	Interactions with alcohol, amnesia, ataxia, somnolence, mild respiratory depression.	Rebound anxiety, seizures, tremor, insomnia, hypertension, tachycardia.
Caffeine	Restlessness, insomnia, diuresis, muscle twitching, arrhythmias.	Headache, lethargy, depression, weight gain.
Nicotine	Restlessness, insomnia, anxiety, arrhythmias.	Irritability, headache, anxiety, weight gain, craving, tachycardia.

HIGH-YIELD FACTS

PSYCHIATRY

Check urine and serum toxicology; seek out collateral information from friends and family, since use is often underreported. Offer HIV testing; check LFTs and consider hepatitis testing.

TREATMENT

Group therapy, Narcotics Anonymous, recovery housing; hospitalization may be necessary for acute withdrawal. Consider methadone maintenance for opiate dependence.

Alcohol Abuse

Roughly 10% of women and 20% of men have met the criteria for alcohol abuse in their lifetimes, and 3–5% of women and 10% of men have met the criteria for alcohol dependence. Family history ↑ risk. The common causes of death in these patients are suicide, cancer, heart disease, and hepatic disease.

EXAM

Screen with the CAGE questions (see the **CAGE** mnemonic). Monitor vital signs for tachycardia and ↑ BP associated with withdrawal. Look for stigmata of liver disease, such as palmar erythema or spider angiomata. Lab tests may reveal macrocytosis and an ↑ AST and GGT.

TREATMENT

- Rule out medical complications; correct electrolyte abnormalities and hydrate.
- Start **benzodiazepine taper** (e.g., chlordiazepoxide) for withdrawal symptoms.
- Give multivitamins and folic acid; give **thiamine** before glucose to prevent Wernicke's encephalopathy.
- Individual or group counseling, **Alcoholics Anonymous,** disulfiram, naltrexone.

COMPLICATIONS

GI bleeding (e.g., gastritis, varices, Mallory-Weiss tears), **pancreatitis, liver disease,** delirium tremens (DTs), alcohol-induced psychosis, peripheral neuropathy, cerebellar degeneration, **Wernicke's encephalopathy** (ataxia, confusion, ophthalmoplegia), **Korsakoff's syndrome** (anterograde amnesia).

▶ **EATING DISORDERS**

Anorexia Nervosa

Females account for 90% of cases. Peak incidences are at age 14 and age 18. There is an ↑ risk in first-degree relatives. Mortality from suicide or medical complications is 10%. Major depression is a common comorbid condition.

SYMPTOMS

Classified as **restricting type** (excessive dieting or exercising), **binge-eating type,** or **purging type** (vomiting, laxatives, diuretics). Presents with the following:

- **Refusal to maintain normal body weight** (> 85% ideal body weight).
- Intense fear of weight gain.

Alcohol use is related to 50% of all homicides and automotive fatalities.

CAGE questions

1. Have you ever felt the need to **C**ut down on your drinking?
2. Have you ever felt **A**nnoyed by criticism of your drinking?
3. Have you ever felt **G**uilty about drinking?
4. Have you ever had to take a morning **E**ye opener?

More than one "yes" answer makes alcohol abuse likely.

DTs are a medical emergency with an untreated mortality rate of 20%. Administer IV lorazepam.

Anorexic patients deny health risks associated with their behavior, making them resistant to treatment.

HIGH-YIELD FACTS

PSYCHIATRY

- Distorted body image.
- Amenorrhea (three missed cycles).

EXAM

Measure height and weight. Check CBC, electrolytes, TFTs, and ECG. Look for **lanugo** (fine body hair), dry skin, lethargy, bradycardia, hypotension, and peripheral edema.

TREATMENT

Monitor caloric intake and **focus on weight gain,** with hospitalization as necessary. Individual, family, and group psychotherapy are helpful. SSRIs (fluoxetine) have been used successfully.

Bulimia Nervosa

Unlike anorexic patients, bulimic patients are at or above their expected weight.

Affects 1–3% of young adult females. Prognosis is better than for anorexia nervosa. Associated with an ↑ frequency of affective disorders, substance abuse, and borderline personality disorder.

SYMPTOMS

Behaviors occur twice a week for ≥ 3 months:

- **Binge eating** with sense of lack of self-control.
- **Compensatory behavior to prevent weight gain** (e.g., self-induced vomiting, laxatives, diuretics, overexercise).

EXAM

Same as for anorexia nervosa. Look for **poor dentition, enlarged parotid glands, scars on dorsal hand surfaces** (from finger-induced vomiting), and **hypokalemia.**

TREATMENT

CBT is the most effective treatment. **Antidepressants** are useful even in nondepressed patients.

SECTION II

Pulmonary

▶ PULMONARY FUNCTION TESTS (PFTs)

The two measurements used most often are FEV_1 (forced expiratory volume in one second) and FVC (forced vital capacity).

- An FEV_1/FVC ratio of < 70% indicates **obstruction**.
- An FVC of < 80% is consistent with **restriction**.

Obstructive Lung Diseases	Restrictive Lung Diseases
▪ COPD	▪ Obesity
▪ Asthma	▪ Kyphosis
▪ Chronic bronchitis	▪ Inflammatory and fibrosing lung disease
▪ Bronchiectasis	▪ Interstitial lung disease

Other points to keep in mind when looking at a set of PFTs (see Table 2.17-1) are as follows:

- Total lung capacity (TLC) will be ↓ in **restrictive** processes and ↑ in **obstructive** processes.
- DL_{CO} is defined as the diffusing capacity of carbon monoxide and measures the gas exchange ability of the capillary-alveolar interface.

▶ HYPOXIA

Defined as a room-air O_2 saturation of < 88% or a PaO_2 of < **55 mmHg** on ABG measurement. Think about the **cause of hypoxia** in order to determine the next step:

- **Ventilation-perfusion (V/Q) mismatch:**
  - Examples include asthma, COPD, and pneumonia.
  - **Responds to O_2.**
  - ↑ **alveolar-arterial (A-a) gradient.**
- **Shunt physiology:**
  - Think about acute respiratory distress syndrome (**ARDS**), massive pulmonary embolus (**PE**), patent foramen ovale, or patent ductus arteriosus (**PDA**).
  - This typically **does not respond to O_2.**
  - ↑ **A-a gradient.**
- **Hypoventilation:**
  - Commonly **oversedation** from medications.
  - **Responds to O_2.**
  - **Normal A-a gradient.**

*Hypoxia due to shunt physiology **will not** correct with supplemental O_2*

Hypoxia can → apnea in infants, so be sure to use supplemental O_2 to maintain O_2 saturations.

TABLE 2.17-1. **PFTs in Common Settings**

	FEV₁/FVC	TLC	DL_CO
Asthma	↓	Nl	Nl to ↑
COPD	↓	↑	Nl to ↑
Fibrotic disease	Nl to ↑	↓	↓
Extrathoracic restriction	Nl	↓	Nl

- ↓ diffusion:
  - Think about interstitial lung diseases.
  - ↑ A-a gradient.
  - Very low DL_{CO}.
- High altitude:
  - Normal A-a gradient.
  - Responds to O_2.

TREATMENT

Always treat hypoxic patients with adequate amounts of O_2 to maintain saturations of > 90% or PaO_2 of > 60 mmHg. Definitive treatment entails removing the underlying cause of the hypoxia.

Think of methemoglobinemia in a patient with a low O_2 saturation on pulse oximetry but normal PaO_2 on ABG. Treatment is with methylene blue.

▶ BRONCHIOLITIS

Involves inflammation in smaller airways and occurs most often in infants from two months to one year of age. **RSV** accounts for the vast majority of cases. Other viral causes include influenza, parainfluenza, and adenovirus.

SYMPTOMS

Patients are typically **infants.** Symptoms begin as those of a **URI** (sore throat, runny nose) and **progress** over the next 3–7 days to lower respiratory symptoms (cough, wheezing).

EXAM

Patients may have cough, fever, **tachypnea,** and **intercostal retractions.** Look for cyanosis, expiratory wheezing, and crackles.

DIAGNOSIS

- Look for **hyperinflation** of the lungs on CXR with flattening of the diaphragms.
- RSV may be diagnosed with **ELISA** or fluorescent antibody test.

TREATMENT

- **Supplemental O_2** (oxygen tent).
- Aerosolized **albuterol.**
- In cases of RSV, use **ribavirin** in patients with severe disease or underlying cardiac or pulmonary problems.

Intubate infants with ↑ PCO_2 levels or ↑ O_2 requirements.

▶ CYSTIC FIBROSIS (CF)

An autosomal-recessive disorder with mutations located in the CFTR gene, which → abnormal transfer of sodium and chloride. Multiple exocrine glands and cilia in various organs become dysfunctional. The **most common** genetic disease in the United States and among **Caucasians.**

SYMPTOMS

Patients typically present in childhood or adolescence. Look for patients with **recurrent pulmonary infections,** sinusitis, **bronchiectasis,** and **pancreatic insufficiency** (diabetes, malabsorption, steatorrhea).

- Infants may present with **meconium ileus** or **intussusception.**
- Adult males may have **aspermia**, and females may have **miscarriages.**

EXAM

Patients may have short stature. Lung exam often reveals **wheezing, crackles,** or **squeaks. Clubbing** may be present. During acute exacerbations, look for accessory muscle use.

DIAGNOSIS

- Diagnosis is made with sweat chloride test— > **60 mEq/L** under age 20; > 80 mEg/L for others.
- Genetic testing can confirm the presence of gene mutation.

TREATMENT

- Manage the symptoms of disease with **mucolytics** (DNase), **bronchodilators, pancreatic enzymes,** and **chest PT.**
- Patients need supplemental **fat-soluble vitamins (A, D, E, K)** owing to fat malabsorption.
- May need **chronic antibiotics,** including **inhaled tobramycin** (to cover for *Pseudomonas*).
- Consider bilateral **lung transplant.**

COMPLICATIONS

Associated with both **pseudomonal** and **staphylococcal** infections.

▶ ASTHMA

Asthma consists of reversible inflammation of the airways. Patients may be atopic (the classic triad is eczema, wheezing, and seasonal rhinitis).

SYMPTOMS

- Look for **intermittent wheezing,** coughing, or shortness of breath.
- Symptoms may be seasonal or may occur after exposure to **triggers** (URIs, dust, pets, cold air) or with exercise.

EXAM

- Determine the severity of the attack by assessing **mental status, ability to speak in full sentences,** presence of cyanosis, use of accessory muscles, and, of course, vital signs.
- Look for wheezing or rhonchi along with a prolonged expiratory phase. Patients with severe exacerbations may have ↓ **wheezing.** These patients will need prompt assessment of their gas exchange (with ABG) and aggressive treatment (see below).

DIFFERENTIAL

Not all that wheezes is asthma! Rule out foreign-body aspiration, laryngeal spasm or irritation, GERD and CHF. In patients with chronic cough, think about allergic rhinitis. Differentiate asthma from COPD and chronic bronchitis with PFTs (see below).

Think of GERD in a patient with chronic cough that worsens when lying supine.

DIAGNOSIS

- CXR may show **flat diaphragms,** suggesting air trapping, but can also be normal.
- Definitive diagnosis is made by demonstration of obstruction on PFTs:
  - **$FEV_1/FVC < 80\%$ and**
  - **Reversibility** with bronchodilators as defined by an ↑ **in FEV_1 or FVC by 12% and** 200 mL.
  - **Methacholine challenge** testing in a monitored setting can be used to confirm the diagnosis.

A ⊖ methacholine challenge excludes asthma.

TREATMENT

Treatment is as follows (see also Table 2.17-2):

- Remove triggers (remember to include smoking cessation!).
- Chronic treatment will depend largely on severity:
  - For **mild intermittent** symptoms, use **short-acting β-agonists** (albuterol).
  - For **moderate** symptoms, use low-potency **inhaled corticosteroids** or a mast cell stabilizer (cromolyn sodium) and a **short-acting β-agonist** as a **rescue** therapy.
  - For more **severe** symptoms, add a **long-acting β-agonist** (salmeterol) **and** a high-potency **inhaled corticosteroid** (fluticasone). Short-acting β-agonists are useful as rescue.
  - If this does not work, add systemic corticosteroids (prednisone) or a leukotriene antagonist (montelukast).
- For an **acute** asthma exacerbation, recognizing the severity of the attack and instituting the correct therapy are the keys to treatment:
  - Initiate **short-acting β-agonist** (albuterol) therapy (nebulizer or MDI).
  - Administer **systemic corticosteroids** such as methylprednisolone or prednisone.
  - Begin **inhaled corticosteroids** as well.

Inhaled corticosteroids are safe for use in pregnancy.

HIGH-YIELD FACTS

PULMONARY

TABLE 2.17-2. Medications for Chronic Treatment of Asthma

TYPE	SYMPTOMS (DAY/NIGHT)	FEV₁	Medications
Severe persistent	Continual Frequent	≤ 60%	High-dose inhaled corticosteroids + long-acting inhaled β₂-agonists. Possible PO steroids. PRN short-acting bronchodilator.
Moderate persistent	Daily > 1 night/week	60–80%	Low- to medium-dose inhaled corticosteroids + long-acting inhaled β₂-agonists. PRN short-acting bronchodilator.
Mild persistent	> 2/week but < 1/day > 2 nights/month	≥ 80%	Low-dose inhaled corticosteroids. PRN short-acting bronchodilator.
Mild intermittent	≤ 2 days/week ≤ 2 nights/month	≥ 80%	No daily medications. PRN short-acting bronchodilator.

(Reprinted, with permission, from Le T et al. *First Aid for the USMLE Step 2,* 4th ed. New York: McGraw-Hill, 2003:431.)

- Follow patients closely with **peak flows** and tailor your therapy to the response.
- Chronic antibiotics (without evidence of infection), anticholinergics, cromolyn, and leukotriene antagonists are generally **not useful** in this setting.

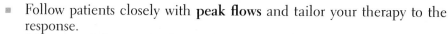

► **CHRONIC OBSTRUCTIVE PULMONARY DISEASE (COPD)**

This disease process is actually a mixture of emphysema and chronic bronchitis and generally involves destruction of lung parenchyma. This results in decreased elastic recoil, which in turn → air trapping. **TLC** ↑ due to a **rise** in the **residual volume (RV)**. Chronic bronchitis is defined as excess mucus production for three consecutive months for two years.

SYMPTOMS

Look for cough, dyspnea, wheezing, and a **history of smoking.** Dyspnea is usually progressive. In advanced disease, weight loss may be present.

EXAM

- **Emphysema ("pink puffer"):** ↓ breath sounds, minimal cough, dyspnea, pursed lip breathing, hypercarbia/hypoxia late, barrel chest.
- **Chronic bronchitis ("blue bloater"):** Rhonchi, productive cough, cyanotic but with mild dyspnea, hypercarbia/hypoxia early, frequently overweight with peripheral edema.
- **Look for clubbing.**
- Patients may also have evidence of **cor pulmonale** (right heart failure from pulmonary hypertension).

DIAGNOSIS

- PFTs may suggest the diagnosis in a patient who smokes.
- **FEV$_1$/FVC < 80%.**
- **No improvement** with bronchodilators.
- ↓ **DL$_{CO}$** occurs in more advanced disease.
- ↑ **TLC.**

CXR shows hyperlucent, **hyperinflated** lungs with **flat diaphragms** and narrow cardiac silhouette (see Figure 2.17-1).

TREATMENT

Chronic COPD

- Mainstays of treatment are inhaled β-agonists (**albuterol**) and **anticholinergics (ipratropium).**
- **O$_2$ therapy** is indicated for patients with an O$_2$ saturation of < 88% **or a PaO$_2$ of < 55 mmHg.**
- **Smoking cessation is key.**
- Inhaled corticosteroids **do not** play a major role unless there is significant reversible airway disease on PFTs.
- Remember to **vaccinate** patients with COPD against **influenza** (yearly) and **pneumococcal pneumonia** (at least once).

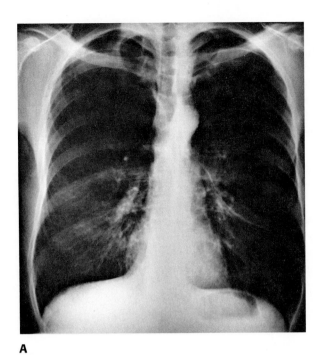

A

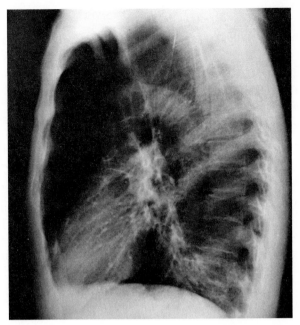

B

FIGURE 2.17-1. **COPD.**

Note the hyperinflated and hyperlucent lungs, flat diaphragms, increased AP diameter, narrow mediastinum, and large upper lobe bullae on AP (A) and lateral (B) CXRs. (Reproduced, with permission, from Stobo JD et al. The *Principles and Practice of Medicine*, 23rd ed. Stamford, CT: Appleton & Lange, 1997:135.)

Acute COPD Exacerbation

- Check a **CXR** to look for causes of the exacerbation (pneumonia, CHF).
- Administer O_2 to maintain a saturation of 90–95% (no need to go higher!).
- Initiate inhaled β-**agonist** (albuterol) and **anticholinergics** (ipratropium).
- **Systemic steroids** (prednisone) may ↓ length of hospital stay and should be tapered over 3–7 days.
- **Empiric antibiotics** with coverage of *Streptococcus, H. influenzae,* and *Moraxella* (such as a macrolide or quinolone) **are indicated** in the acute setting.
- Spirometry in the acute setting is **not helpful** in guiding therapy.

Always treat hypoxic patients with O_2! CO_2 retention won't kill the patient, but hypoxia will.

▶ PLEURAL EFFUSION

Effusions are characterized as either transudative or exudative based on composition.

SYMPTOMS/EXAM

- Patients are usually short of breath and may complain of pleuritic chest pain. Some may be asymptomatic or have symptoms of an underlying process (e.g., CHF, pneumonia, cancer).
- Exam reveals ↓ **breath sounds, dullness** to percussion, and ↓ tactile fremitus on the side with the effusion.

A thoracentesis is indicated on any effusion > 10 mm thick (or about 100 mL) on CXR.

Always do a pleural biopsy if you suspect TB. Send the fluid for cytology if you suspect malignancy.

Suspect PTX with shortness of breath and chest pain + underlying COPD, CF, chest procedures (e.g., central lines), or trauma.

The differential for shortness of breath/chest pain includes PTX, MI, PE, and dissection.

DIAGNOSIS

■ Thoracentesis. Obtain the following assays on the pleural fluid to aid in management: Gram stain and culture, acid-fast bacilli (AFB), total protein, serum LDH, glucose, triglycerides, cell count with differential, and pH. You will also need serum total protein and LDH values (see Table 2.17-3).

■ If the fluid is **transudative,** no further workup is needed; focus on treating the underlying cause (e.g., diuresing the patient). If it is **exudative,** refer to Table 2.17-4 to help determine the cause.

TREATMENT

■ If the CXR shows an effusion > 10 mm thick (or about 100 mL), always do a **thoracentesis.** This may be therapeutic (to relieve dyspnea) as well as diagnostic.

■ **Indications for chest tube (any one of these)** are as follows:
  ■ Pleural WBC count > 100,000 or frank pus.
  ■ Glucose < 40.
  ■ pH < 7.00.

COMPLICATIONS

■ An untreated pleural effusion may quickly become infected and turn into an empyema.

■ Over time, effusions may become loculated and require video-assisted thoracoscopy (VATS) drainage or surgical decortication.

■ The major complications of thoracentesis include pneumothorax and bleeding (remember, the neurovascular bundle runs along the inferior side of the rib).

▶ PNEUMOTHORAX (PTX)

Defined as air that becomes trapped in the pleural space. This can be from traumatic, spontaneous, or iatrogenic causes. Spontaneous PTX can be due to underlying lung pathology such as COPD or CF.

SYMPTOMS/EXAM

Look for patients who develop acute shortness of breath and pleuritic chest pain. Look for **tachypnea,** ↓ tactile fremitus, ↓ breath sounds and **tympany** on percussion on the side involved, and tracheal deviation toward the affected side.

DIAGNOSIS

CXR will reveal the diagnosis. Look for a distinct lack of lung markings within the PTX, along with collapse of the lung on that side (see Figure 2.17-2.). Tracheal deviation may be present (especially with tension).

Table 2.17-3. **Thoracentesis Findings in Transudative and Exudative Pleural Effusions**

	PLEURAL/SERUM PROTEIN (RATIO)	PLEURAL/SERUM LDH (RATIO)	PLEURAL LDH
Transudative	< 0.5 *and*	< 0.6 *and*	< 200
Exudative	> 0.5 *or*	> 0.6 *or*	> 200

Table 2.17-4. Assays for Exudative Fluid and Their Associated Differential Diagnosis

Pleural Assay	Value	Differential
Glucose	< 60	Empyema or parapneumonia, TB, RA, malignancy.
WBC	> 10,000	Empyema or parapneumonia, RA, malignancy.
RBC	> 100,000	Gross blood—think of trauma, PE.
Cellular differential	Lymphocytes PMNs Eosinophils	TB, sarcoid, malignancy. Empyema, PE. Bleeding, pneumothorax.
pH	< 7.20	Complicated effusion or empyema.
Triglycerides	> 150	Diagnostic of chylothorax.

TREATMENT

- Insertion of a chest tube is required in patients with a pneumothorax > 30% PTX.
- Smaller PTXs may be managed simply with supplemental O₂ and observation.
- Treat pain with morphine and NSAIDs.
- For patients with recurrent PTX, consider pleurodesis.

Tension Pneumothorax

In this emergent complication of PTX, defects in the chest wall act as a one-way valve. This allows air to be drawn into the pleural space and become

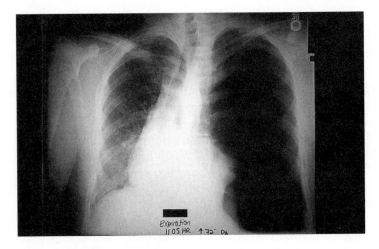

FIGURE 2.17-2. Tension pneumothorax.

Note the hyperlucent lung field (1), hyperexpanded lower diaphragm (2), collapsed lung (3), tracheal deviation (4), mediastinal shift (5), and compression of the opposite lung (6) on AP CXR. (Reproduced, with permission, from Le T et al. *First Aid for the USMLE Step 2*, 4th ed. New York: McGraw-Hill, 2003:441.)

A tension PTX is an emergency! If you suspect this, don't wait for imaging; insert a needle to decompress the chest.

trapped. The result is **rapid decompensation,** hypotension, and circulatory collapse → **shock.**

- Common scenarios to think of tension PTX include **penetrating trauma,** positive-pressure ventilation, and COPD.
- Diagnostic clues include those of a **PTX** along with **tachycardia, hypotension,** ↑ O₂ requirements, and ↑ JVP.
- If you suspect that the patient has a tension PTX, **don't wait for imaging!** Insert a needle to decompress the chest and then insert a chest tube.

▶ PULMONARY EMBOLUS (PE)

Remember **Virchow's triad** when thinking of risk factors for DVT and PE:

- **Stasis:** Immobility, CHF, obesity, ↑ CVP.
- **Endothelial injury:** Trauma, surgery, recent fracture, prior DVT.
- **Hypercoagulable state:** Pregnancy, OCP use, coagulation disorder, malignancy, burns.

SYMPTOMS

Think about PE or DVT in **any patient with risk factors** and complaints of leg pain or swelling, acute-onset chest pain (especially pleuritic), shortness of breath, or syncope.

EXAM

Findings on exam include tachypnea, tachycardia, cyanosis, loud P2 or S2, ↑ JVP, and signs of right heart failure. Patients may occasionally have hemoptysis or a low-grade fever.

DIFFERENTIAL

Most signs and symptoms of PE are nonspecific, so be sure to think about other entities that can present this way, including **acute MI, pneumonia, CHF,** and **aortic dissection.**

DIAGNOSIS

Consider PE in any hospitalized patient who has dyspnea.

See Figure 2.17-3 for a diagnostic algorithm. Initial assessment should include the following:

- **ABG,** which may show a 1° respiratory alkalosis and ↑ A-a gradient.
- **CXR** findings can include the following:
    - **Normal** (most common!).
    - Wedge-shaped infarct (Hampton's hump).
    - Oligemia in the affected lobe (Westermark's sign).
    - Pleural effusion.
- **ECG** may reveal an S wave in lead I, a Q wave in lead III, and T-wave inversion in lead III (not very sensitive or specific).
- The **pretest probability** of PE will help determine the diagnostic utility of the V/Q scan. If either the pretest probability or the V/Q scan results are intermediate, some type of confirmatory testing will be needed.
- In a nonhospitalized patient, a negative D-dimer assay, when combined with some form of imaging, may help rule out DVT with good negative predictive value.

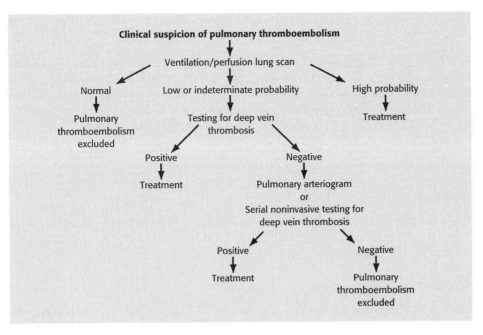

FIGURE 2.17-3. Diagnostic approach to pulmonary embolism.

(Reproduced, with permission, from Tierney LM et al. *Current Medical Diagnosis & Treatment: 2004.* New York: McGraw-Hill, 2003: ___.)

- **CT angiography,** if available, may also be useful as a confirmatory test when the V/Q scan is indeterminate.
- **Pulmonary angiography** is still considered the **gold standard** to diagnose PE and may be needed if other testing is intermediate.

TREATMENT

- Treat patients with DVT or PE with anticoagulation.
  - Initially use **IV heparin or low-molecular-weight heparin.**
  - Patients who are not anticoagulated adequately within 24 hours have a high rate of recurrence.
  - Patients should then be transitioned to warfarin therapy, with a goal INR of 2.0–3.0.
- In patients with documented large **central PEs** (saddle PEs) and hypotension or shock, administer **tPA** along with heparin. The duration of therapy will vary with risk factors:
  - For patients with a **first event** and **reversible** or time-limited risk factors (e.g., surgery, pregnancy), treat for at least **3–6 months.**
  - Consider **lifelong anticoagulation** in patients with **chronic risk factors** (malignancy, paraplegia, recurrent DVTs, or PEs).
- In patients who cannot safely be anticoagulated, an IVC filter may be useful. Although these filters can ↓ the risk of PE, they are associated with a **higher risk** of recurrent DVT.

Don't forget to order DVT prophylaxis for all your hospitalized patients!

ARDS is a common problem in the ICU and is a significant cause of mortality. It can be 2° to a range of underlying conditions with a similar end result of **widespread inflammation** in the lung parenchyma → **pulmonary edema** and alveolar damage. **Smokers** and patients with **cirrhosis** are at higher risk for developing ARDS. Common etiologies are as follows:

- **Direct:** Pneumonia, aspiration.
- **Indirect:** Sepsis, transfusions, pancreatitis, trauma.

SYMPTOMS

Look for a patient with risk factors, usually in an **ICU setting**. Patients will be hypoxic and difficult to oxygenate, requiring intubation in order to maintain an acceptable PaO_2.

DIAGNOSIS

Patients will be hypoxic in spite of maximal O_2 therapy and typically have **diffuse bilateral pulmonary infiltrates** on CXR without evidence of volume overload (e.g., **normal capillary wedge pressure**). Look at the PaO_2/FiO_2 **ratio** (ratio of the arterial O_2 level on ABG divided by the fraction of inhaled O_2 the patient is on). A ratio of > 200 is consistent with ARDS.

Think of ARDS in a patient with a PaO_2/FiO_2 ratio < 200.

TREATMENT

Patients will typically require intubation and mechanical ventilation for management of hypoxia. **Low tidal volumes** (6 mL/kg) →↓ risk of barotrauma and permissive hypercapnia (i.e., letting the PCO_2 rise), and use of **positive end-expiratory pressure (PEEP)**. Look for the **underlying cause** and focus treatment on that, as you are stabilizing the patient and treating hypoxia.

Defined as a radiodense lesion seen on chest imaging that is **< 3 cm in diameter**. Most commonly, SPNs are detected on routine CXRs in patients who are otherwise **asymptomatic.**

Appearance of laminar or "popcorn" calcification within an SPN likely represents a benign hamartoma.

DIAGNOSIS

Benign processes include histoplasmosis, coccidioidomycosis, TB, and hamartoma. Characteristics and risk factors include the following:

- **Very fast** or **no growth** on serial imaging two years apart.
- **Diffuse, central, or laminar "popcorn" calcification pattern.**
- Patients who are **lifelong nonsmokers, are < 35 years of age,** and have **no history of malignancy.**

Malignant lesions include lung cancer or metastases. Characteristics and risk factors include the following:

- Size **> 2 cm.**
- **Spiculated** (i.e., ragged edges).
- Upper lobe location.
- Patients who are **smokers, > 40 years of age,** or have a **prior diagnosis of cancer.**

TREATMENT

Start by looking at old radiographs to determine age and change in size. Lesions with > 1 malignant feature should be further evaluated. Consider obtaining a **PET scan** as an initial step to determine whether the lesion is metabolically active. If the PET scan is ⊖, the lesion may be followed with **serial studies**. If the PET scan is ⊕, **surgical excision** of the nodule is preferred.

► SARCOIDOSIS

Idiopathic illness characterized by **noncaseating granuloma** formation in various organs. Most patients have pulmonary involvement.

SYMPTOMS

Typical features include **fever, cough, malaise, weight loss, dyspnea,** and **arthritis** (particularly of knees and ankles).

DIFFERENTIAL

Sarcoidosis is a **diagnosis of exclusion,** so be sure to rule out other diseases that present similarly, such as **TB, lymphoma,** fungal infection, idiopathic pulmonary fibrosis, HIV, and berylliosis.

DIAGNOSIS

Look for **bilateral hilar lymphadenopathy** on CXR and/or infiltrates. PFTs will show a **restrictive** pattern. Patients may also have **hypercalcemia.** Tissue biopsy will show **noncaseating granulomas without organisms.**

TREATMENT

Therapy includes systemic **corticosteroids** such as prednisone. Gear other medications toward control of symptoms such as cough or wheezing.

> **Features of sarcoidosis— GRUELING**
>
> **G**ranulomas
> **R**heumatoid arthritis
> **U**veitis
> **E**rythema nodosum
> **L**ymphadenitis
> **I**nterstitial fibrosis
> **N**egative PPD
> **G**ammaglobulinemia

► OBSTRUCTIVE SLEEP APNEA (OSA)

Characterized by recurrent episodes of upper airway collapse during sleep → **intermittent hypoxia and recurrent arousals.**

SYMPTOMS

Patients and their bed partners may complain that they **snore.** Patients may also have **excessive daytime sleepiness,** neurocognitive impairment, morning headache, unrefreshing sleep, or impotence. They may report choking or gasping during sleep and may have witnessed apnea episodes at home.

EXAM

Patients are typically **obese** and **hypertensive.** They may also have a **large neck circumference.** Look for **retrognathia** and large tonsils. Many patients also have peripheral edema.

DIFFERENTIAL

Rule out other causes of excessive daytime sleepiness, including **obesity-hypoventilation syndrome,** narcolepsy, and restless leg syndrome.

DIAGNOSIS

Overnight polysomnography (sleep study) is the gold standard for diagnosis. Severity is measured by the apnea-hypopnea index (AHI), defined as the number of apneas and/or hypopneas per hour of sleep. **AHI > 5** is diagnostic of OSA.

TREATMENT

Encourage weight loss. Definitive treatment is with **continuous positive airway pressure (CPAP)** to keep the airways open during sleep. Surgery such as uvulopalatopharyngoplasty (UPPP) is effective in 40–50% of cases.

COMPLICATIONS

Patients with OSA are at ↑ risk of **motor vehicle accidents** as well as for developing **hypertension, LV dysfunction, pulmonary hypertension,** and insulin resistance.

High-Yield CCS Cases

► HOW TO USE THIS SECTION

In this section are 100 **minicases** reflecting the types of clinical situations encountered on the actual CCS. Each case consists of **columns** that start on the left-hand page and end on the right-hand page with the **Final Diagnosis.** As you read each column, ask yourself what you should do and/or think next (see Table 3.1). If no results are given for a test, assume that is **normal.** To get the most out of these minicases, we **strongly** recommend that you do at least a few of the CCS cases on the USMLE CD-ROM (or from the USMLE Web site) to get a feel for the case flow and key decision points. This will allow you to place the minicases in context. Happy studying!

Table 3.1. Approaching the CCS Minicases

WHEN READING . . .	ASK YOURSELF . . .
History	What should I be looking for on VS and PE? Do I need to stabilize the patient or do an emergency procedure before doing a PE?
Physical exam	What are the most likely diagnoses that explain the patient's presentation?
Differential	What are the initial diagnostic tests and treatment that should be done? Does the patient need to be transferred to another location (e.g., from the ER to the ICU)? Does the clock need to be advanced?
Initial management	What additional workup and management should occur? Can the patient be discharged or transferred to another setting?
Continuing management	What should be done in follow-up, including long-term disease management, health maintenance, patient counseling, etc.? Should any treatment or monitoring be stopped?
Follow-up	What is the final diagnosis?

Headache

CASE 1

HX	PE	DDX
21 yo F presents with a severe headache. She has a history of throbbing left temporal pain that lasts for 2–3 hours. Before these episodes start, she sees flashes of light in her right visual field and feels weakness and numbness on the right side of her body for a few minutes. The headaches are often associated with nausea and vomiting. She has a family history of migraine.	VS: T 37°C (99.2°F), P 70, BP 120/80, RR 15, O$_2$ sat 100% room air Gen: NAD Lungs: WNL CV: WNL Abd: WNL Ext: WNL Neuro: WNL	• Cluster headache • Intracranial neoplasm • Migraine (complicated) • Partial seizure • Pseudotumor cerebri • Tension headache • Trigeminal neuralgia

CASE 2

HX	PE	DDX
29 yo F presents with several episodes of bilateral bandlike throbbing pain in her frontal-occipital region that last between 30 minutes and a few hours. She usually experiences these episodes when she is either tired or under stress. She denies any associated nausea, vomiting, phonophobia, photophobia, or aura. She also feels pain and stiffness in her neck and shoulder.	VS: Afebrile, P 70, BP 120/80, RR 15 Gen: NAD Lungs: WNL CV: WNL Abd: WNL Ext: WNL Neuro: WNL	• Cluster headache • Intracranial neoplasm • Meningitis • Migraine headache • Pseudotumor cerebri • Sinusitis • Tension headache

CASE 3

HX	PE	DDX
65 yo F presents with a severe intermittent headache in the right temporal lobe together with blurred vision in her right eye and pain in her jaw during mastication.	VS: T 37°C (99°F), P 85, BP 140/85, RR 18, O$_2$ sat 100% room air Gen: NAD HEENT: Tenderness on temporal artery palpation Neck: No rigidity Lungs: WNL CV: WNL Abd: WNL Ext: WNL Neuro: WNL	• Cluster headache • Intracranial neoplasm • Meningitis • Migraine • Temporal arteritis (giant cell arteritis) • Tension headache • Trigeminal neuralgia

INITIAL MGMT	CONTINUING MGMT	F/U

Emergency room W/U
- CT—head
- CBC
- Chem 8
- ESR

Rx
- IV normal saline
- IV promethazine, prochlorperazine, or meto-clopramide
- ASA, NSAIDs, or acetaminophen
- Caffeine
- IM sumatriptan (if patient does not improve)

F/U
- Follow up in one month
- Prophylactic therapy if the migraine recurs—e.g., β-blockers, antidepressants (SSRIs, TCAs), anticonvulsants (valproic acid, gabapentin), calcium channel blockers

Final Dx - Migraine (complicated)

INITIAL MGMT	CONTINUING MGMT	F/U

Office W/U
- CT—head
- CBC with differential
- Chem 8
- ESR

Rx
- Cold compresses
- Acetaminophen
- NSAIDs

F/U
- Follow up in one month
- Relaxation exercises

Final Dx - Tension headache

INITIAL MGMT	CONTINUING MGMT	F/U

Emergency room STAT
- IV normal saline
- Prednisone

Emergency room W/U
- CBC
- Chem 8
- CT—head: ⊖
- CXR: ⊖
- ESR: ↑↑
- CRP: ↑↑

Ward W/U
- Ophthalmology consult
- Temporal artery biopsy: ⊕ for temporal arteritis
- ESR every morning

Rx
- Continue prednisone until ESR normalizes; then taper

F/U
- Discharge home
- Continue low-dose maintenance prednisone
- ESR in two weeks
- Adequate dietary calcium and vitamin D if steroids are to be used chronically

Final Dx - Temporal arteritis (giant cell arteritis)

CASE 4

HX	PE	DDX
25 yo M presents with a high fever, severe headache, and photophobia.	VS: T 39°C (103°F), P 95, BP 150/85, RR 18, O₂ sat 100% room air Gen: Moderate distress Neck: Nuchal rigidity Lungs: WNL CV: WNL Abd: WNL Ext: WNL Neuro: ⊕ Kernig's and Brudzinski's signs	• Encephalitis • Intracranial or epidural abscess • Meningitis • Migraine • Sinusitis • Subarachnoid hemorrhage

CASE 5

HX	PE	DDX
60 yo M with a past medical history of hypertension presents with severe headache, nausea, and vomiting. The patient states that he stopped taking his metoprolol because he thought that he did not need it anymore.	VS: T 37°C (99.3°F), P 100, BP 220/120, RR 20, O₂ sat 95% room air Gen: Severe distress HEENT: Funduscopy reveals papilledema Lungs: WNL CV: WNL Abd: WNL Ext: WNL Neuro: WNL	• Cluster headache • Intracranial hemorrhage • Intracranial neoplasm • Malignant hypertension • Migraine • Partial seizure

INITIAL MGMT	CONTINUING MGMT	F/U
Emergency room STAT • IV normal saline • Blood culture • LP-CSF: ↑ WBCs, ↑ protein, ↓ CSF/blood glucose ratio, gram-⊕ cocci, ↑ opening pressure • Ceftriaxone + vancomycin • IV dexamethasone **Emergency room W/U** • CBC: ↑ WBC count • Chem 8 • CT—head: ⊖ • CXR: ⊖ **Rx** • Acetaminophen	**Ward W/U** • CSF culture: ⊕ for *S. pneumoniae* • Blood culture: ⊖ **Rx** • Continue ceftriaxone + vancomycin + steroids	• Improved within 48 hours • Discharge home • Follow up in one month

Final Dx - Bacterial meningitis

INITIAL MGMT	CONTINUING MGMT	F/U
Emergency room STAT • O_2 • IV labetalol • BP in both arms • CT—head: White matter changes consistent with hypertension • ECG: LVH • CXR **Emergency room W/U** • Cardiac/BP monitoring • CPK-MB, troponin × 3: ⊖ • CBC • Chem 8 • UA	**ICU W/U** • Continuous cardiac monitoring • Lipid profile • Echocardiography: EF < 45% **Rx** • Labetalol or metoprolol if good control previously • ACEI (low EF) • HCTZ	• Transfer to the floor • Counsel patient re medication compliance • Discharge home • Follow up in one week

Final Dx - Hypertensive emergency

Altered Mental Status/Loss of Consciousness

CASE 6

HX	PE	DDX
84 yo F brought in by her son complains of forgetfulness (e.g., forgets phone numbers, loses her way home) along with difficulty performing some of her daily activities (e.g., bathing, dressing, managing money, answering the phone). The problem has gradually progressed over the past few years.	VS: P 90, BP 120/60, RR 12 Gen: NAD Lungs: WNL CV: WNL Abd: WNL Ext: WNL Neuro: On mini-mental status exam, patient cannot recall objects, follow three-step commands, or spell "world" backward; cranial nerves intact; strength and sensation intact	• Alzheimer's disease • B_{12} deficiency • Chronic subdural hematoma • Depression • Hypothyroidism • Intracranial tumor • Neurosyphilis • Pressure hydrocephalus • Vascular dementia

CASE 7

HX	PE	DDX
79 yo M is brought in by his family complaining of a seven-week history of difficulty walking accompanied by memory loss and urinary incontinence. Since then he has had ↑ difficulty with memory and more frequent episodes of incontinence.	VS: P 92, BP 144/86, RR 14 Gen: NAD Lungs: WNL CV: WNL Abd: WNL Ext: WNL Neuro: Difficulty with both recent and immediate recall on mini-mental status exam; spasticity and hyperreflexia in upper and lower extremities; problem initiating gait (gait is shuffling, broad-based, and slow)	• Alzheimer's disease • B_{12} deficiency • Chronic subdural hematoma • Frontal lobe syndromes • Huntington's disease • Intracranial tumor • Meningitis • Normal pressure hydrocephalus • Parkinson's disease • Vascular dementia

CASE 8

HX	PE	DDX
The on-call physician is called to see a 46 yo M patient because of seizures. The patient was admitted to the surgical ward two days ago, after emergency trauma surgery. The nurse reports that the patient was anxious, agitated, irritable, and tachycardic last night. Later on, the nurse noted nausea, diarrhea, sweating, and insomnia. The patient had tremors, startle response, and hallucinations earlier tonight.	VS: T 37°C (99°F), P 133, BP 146/89, RR 22, O_2 sat 92% room air Gen: Sweating; cigarette burns on hands; multiple tattoos and rings Chest: WNL Abd: Hepatomegaly Ext: Evidence of recent surgery Neuro: Tremor, confusion, delirium, clouded sensorium, and evidence of peripheral neuropathy	• Alcohol withdrawal • Amphetamine psychosis • Delirium • Sedative withdrawal • Systemic lupus erythematosus

INITIAL MGMT	CONTINUING MGMT	F/U

Office W/U
- CBC
- Chem 14
- TSH
- Serum B$_{12}$
- Serum folic acid
- VDRL/RPR
- CT—head

Rx
- Donepezil

- Patient counseling
- Support group
- Advance directives
- Family counseling

Final Dx - Alzheimer's disease

INITIAL MGMT	CONTINUING MGMT	F/U

Emergency room W/U
- CBC
- Chem 8
- LFTs
- TSH
- LP
- Serum B$_{12}$
- Serum folic acid
- CT—head: Enlarged lateral ventricles with no prominence of cortical sulci

Rx
- Large-volume LP

Ward W/U
- Neurosurgery consult
- Neurology consult
- Ventriculoperitoneal shunt

- Advance directives
- Family counseling
- Supportive care

Final Dx - Normal pressure hydrocephalus

INITIAL MGMT	CONTINUING MGMT	F/U

Ward W/U
- CBC: MCV 110 fL
- Chem 8: Hypokalemia, hypomagnesemia
- Urine toxicology
- LFTs: GGT 40 U/L
- CT—head: Cerebral atrophy, no subdural hematoma

Rx
- Thiamine before IV D$_5$W NS
- Pyridoxine
- Folic acid
- IV diazepam
- Atenolol
- Replete K and Mg

Ward W/U
- Chem 8: Corrected hypokalemia, hypomagnesemia

Rx
- IV normal saline
- IV diazepam
- Atenolol
- Naltrexone (for maintenance therapy if indicated)

- Follow up in four weeks
- Patient counseling
- Smoking cessation
- Dietary supplements
- Addiction unit consult
- Social work consult

Final Dx - Alcohol withdrawal

HIGH-YIELD CASES

CASE 9

HX	PE	DDX
24 yo M is brought to the ER in a drowsy state. His wife reports that he was working at home when he suddenly stiffened, fell backward, and lost consciousness. While he was lying on the ground, he was noted to have no respiration for about one minute, followed by jerking of all four limbs for about five minutes. He was unconscious for another five minutes.	VS: T 37°C (98.2°F), P 90, BP 120/80, RR 12 Gen: NAD Lungs: WNL CV: WNL Abd: WNL Ext: WNL Neuro: In a state of confusion and lethargy but oriented; no focal neurologic deficits	• Alcohol withdrawal • Cardioembolic stroke • Frontal lobe epilepsy • Migraine headache • Psychiatric conditions • Seizures • Syncope • Vascular conditions

CASE 10

HX	PE	DDX
72 yo M is brought to the ER complaining of syncope. He underwent a coronary artery bypass graft (CABG) three years ago. He reports fatigue and dizziness over the past five days. The patient's fall was broken by his wife, and as a result he has no head trauma. His wife reports loss of consciousness of about three minutes' duration. Prior to the syncopal episode, the patient recalls a prodrome of lightheadedness. His medications include propranolol, digoxin, and diltiazem.	VS: T 37°C (98.1°F), P 35, BP 114/54, RR 15 Gen: NAD Lungs: WNL CV: Irregular S1 and S2, bradycardia Abd: WNL Ext: WNL Neuro: Alert and oriented; CN II–XII intact; 5/5 motor strength in all extremities	• Aortic stenosis • Asystole • Dilated cardiomyopathy • Heart block • MI • Myocarditis • Myopathies • Restrictive cardiomyopathy • Vasodepressor/vasovagal response

INITIAL MGMT	CONTINUING MGMT	F/U
Emergency room W/U • CBC • Chem 8 • LFTs • ABG • Serum calcium, magnesium, phosphate • ECG • EEG • CT—head • MRI—brain • UA • Urine toxicology	**Ward W/U** • Continue IV • O_2 **Rx** Neurology consult	• Follow up in 3–4 weeks • Patient counseling • Family counseling • Advise patient to use seat belts • Advise patient not to drive

Final Dx - Grand mal seizure (complex tonic-clonic seizure)

INITIAL MGMT	CONTINUING MGMT	F/U
Emergency room W/U • IV normal saline • CBC • Chem 8 • LFTs • ECG: Third-degree AV block • Cardiac enzymes • Serum troponin I • Serum calcium, magnesium, phosphate • CXR • UA • O_2 • Continuous cardiac monitoring **Rx** • Temporary transvenous cardiac pacemaker • Withhold AV nodal agents	**ICU W/U** • Continuous cardiac monitoring • ECG • Lipid profile • Echocardiography **Rx** • Lipid-lowering agents • Cardiology consult • Cardiac catheterization, angiocardiography • Permanent cardiac pacemaker	• Cardiac rehabilitation program • Smoking cessation • Counsel patient to limit alcohol intake • Counsel patient not to drive • Low-fat, low-sodium diet

Final Dx - Complete heart block

CASE 11

HX	PE	DDX
25 yo F with no significant past medical history is brought to the ER after having been found unresponsive with an empty bottle lying next to her.	VS: T 38°C (99.8°F), P 50, BP 110/50, RR 9, O_2 sat 92% room air Gen: Drowsy HEENT: Pinpoint pupils Lungs: WNL CV: Bradycardia Abd: WNL Ext: WNL Neuro: Opens eyes to painful stimuli Limited PE with ABCs	• Acetaminophen overdose • Narcotic overdose • TCA overdose

CASE 12

HX	PE	DDX
60 yo M was found unconscious by his wife, who called the paramedics. She left him in bed at 7 A.M. to go to her volunteer job. When she returned for lunch at 1 P.M., she found an empty bottle of amitriptyline next to him. When paramedics arrived, he was noted to be in respiratory distress and was transferred to the ER.	VS: T 38°C (101°F), P 110, BP 95/45, RR 35, O_2 sat 89% on 100% face mask Gen: Acute distress; shallow, rapid breathing HEENT: Dilated pupils Lungs: WNL CV: Tachycardia Abd: WNL Neuro: Opens eyes to painful stimuli **Limited PE**	• Anticholinergic toxicity • TCA intoxication

INITIAL MGMT	CONTINUING MGMT	F/U

Emergency room STAT
- Suction airway
- Fingerstick blood sugar
- IV normal saline
- IV naloxone: Patient responded
- Dextrose 50%
- IV thiamine
- ABG

Emergency room W/U
- CBC
- ECG
- Urine toxicology
- UA
- Serum acetaminophen
- Chem 13
- PT/PTT, INR
- Serum lactate
- CXR, PA
- Cardiac enzymes

ICU W/U
- Gastric lavage: Pill fragments
- Continuous monitoring: Patient started to become drowsy again (monitor events)

Rx
- IV naloxone: Patient responded
- Psychiatry consult
- Suicide precautions

- Monitor for at least 24 hours

Final Dx - Narcotic overdose

INITIAL MGMT	CONTINUING MGMT	F/U

Emergency room STAT
- Intubate

Emergency room W/U
- Cardiac/BP monitoring
- Chem 14
- CBC
- ABG
- Serum lactate
- Serum osmolality
- Blood ketones
- Urine toxicology: $\oplus$ for TCAs
- ECG: Widened QRS
- Serum magnesium
- CXR, PA
- Cardiac enzymes
- CT—head

Rx
- IV D_5W 0.9 NS
- Thiamine
- Central line placement
- NG tube gastric lavage
- Activated charcoal
- IV bicarbonate

ICU W/U
- Continuous monitoring of urine output q 1 h
- Continuous BP monitoring
- Continuous cardiac monitoring
- Neuro check

Rx
- Cardiology consult
- Lidocaine for TCA-induced ventricular arrhythmias
- IV magnesium sulfate, one time

- Psychiatry consult

Final Dx - Tricyclic antidepressant (TCA) intoxication

HIGH-YIELD CASES

Fatigue/Weakness

CASE 13

HX	PE	DDX
68 yo M presents following a 20-minute episode of slurred speech, right facial drooping and numbness, and weakness of the right hand. His symptoms had totally resolved by the time he got to the ER. He has a history of hypertension, diabetes mellitus, and heavy smoking.	VS: T 37°C (98°F), P 75, BP 150/90, RR 16, O_2 sat 100% room air Gen: NAD Neck: Right carotid bruit Lungs: WNL CV: WNL Abd: WNL Ext: WNL Neuro: WNL	• Intracranial tumor • Seizure • Stroke • Subdural or epidural hematoma • Transient ischemic attack

CASE 14

HX	PE	DDX
40 yo F presents with numbness, lower extremity weakness, and difficulty walking. She reports having had a URI approximately two weeks ago. She says that her weakness started from her lower limbs to her hip and then progressed to her upper limbs. She also complains of lightheadedness on standing and shortness of breath.	VS: Afebrile, P 115, BP 130/80 with orthostatic changes, RR 16 Gen: NAD Lungs: WNL CV: WNL Ext: WNL Neuro: Loss of motor strength in lower limbs; absent DTRs in patella and Achilles tendon; sensation intact	• Conversion disorder • Guillain-Barré syndrome • Myasthenia gravis • Paraneoplastic neuropathy • Poliomyelitis • Polymyositis

INITIAL MGMT	CONTINUING MGMT	F/U
Emergency room STAT • Assess ABCs • O$_2$ • IV normal saline • CT—head **Emergency room W/U** • Continuous cardiac and BP monitoring • ECG • CBC • Chem 8 • CXR • PT/PTT, INR • Neurology consult **Rx** • ASA	**Ward W/U** • Repeat neurologic exam • Continuous cardiac and BP monitoring • Telemetry • Lipid profile, Hb$_{Alc}$ • Echocardiography: EF 60% • Carotid duplex: > 75% stenosis in right carotid artery **Rx** • Vascular surgery consult • Patient is scheduled for elective carotid endarterectomy • ASA	• Counsel patient re smoking cessation, exercise • Treat hypertension • Treat diabetes • Diabetic diet • Diabetic teaching • Treat cholesterol • Low-fat, low-sodium diet

Final Dx - Transient ischemic attack (TIA)

INITIAL MGMT	CONTINUING MGMT	F/U
Emergency room W/U • CBC • Chem 8 • TSH • ESR • CRP • RF • VDRL • Serum B$_{12}$ • Serum folic acid • Nerve conduction study: Slow conduction • ECG • Serum CPK • MRI—brain • MRI—spine • CXR • LP: ↑ CSF protein • HIV testing, ELISA • Spirometry	**Ward Rx** • Immunoglobulins • Plasmapheresis • Rehabilitative medicine consult • Neurology consult • Immunology consult • Spirometry	• Follow up in 3–4 weeks • Patient counseling • Family counseling • Advise patient to use seat belts

Final Dx - Guillain-Barré syndrome

CASE 15

HX	PE	DDX
40 yo F presents with fatigue, weight gain, sleepiness, cold intolerance, constipation, and dry skin.	VS: T 36°C (97°F), BP 100/60, HR 60 Gen: Obese Skin: Dry HEENT: Scar on neck from previous thyroidectomy Lungs: WNL CV: WNL Neuro: Delayed relaxation of DTRs	• Anemia • Depression • Diabetes • Hypothyroidism

CASE 16

HX	PE	DDX
16 yo M complains of myalgia, fatigue, and sore throat. He also reports loss of appetite and nausea but no vomiting. He reports that his girlfriend recently had similar symptoms that lasted a few weeks.	VS: T 38°C (101°F), P 85, BP 125/80, RR 18 Gen: Maculopapular rash HEENT: Posterior and auricular lymphadenopathy and pharyngitis with diffuse exudates and petechiae at junction of hard and soft palates Lungs: WNL CV: WNL Abd: Soft, nontender; mild hepatosplenomegaly Ext: WNL Neuro: WNL	• CMV • Hepatitis • Infectious mononucleosis • 1° HIV infection • Streptococcal pharyngitis • Toxoplasmosis

CASE 17

HX	PE	DDX
40 yo F complains of feeling tired, hopeless, and worthless. She also reports depressed mood, inability to sleep, and impaired concentration. She has been missing work. She denies any suicidal thoughts or attempts and denies having hallucinations. She has no history of alcohol or drug abuse and has not lost a loved one within the last 12 months. She is married and has one child and a supportive husband.	VS: P 70, BP 120/60, RR 12 Gen: NAD Lungs: WNL CV: WNL Abd: WNL Ext: WNL Neuro: WNL	• Adjustment disorder • Anemia • Anxiety • Cancer • Chronic fatigue syndrome • Dementia • Depression • Fibromyalgia • Hypothyroidism

INITIAL MGMT	CONTINUING MGMT	F/U

Office W/U
- CBC
- Chem 14
- TSH: ↑
- FT_4: ↓
- ECG
- Lipid profile
- Depression index

Rx
- Thyroxine

F/U
- Check TSH after one month

Final Dx - Hypothyroidism

INITIAL MGMT	CONTINUING MGMT	F/U

Office W/U
- CBC: ↑ WBC count
- Peripheral smear: Atypical lymphocytes
- Chem 14: ↑ SGOT and SGPT
- ESR
- CRP
- Mono test: ⊕
- Serum EBV titer: ↑

Rx
- Acetaminophen or NSAIDs
- Hydrate; patient counseling

F/U
- Follow up in two weeks with CBC
- Advise patient to rest at home
- Avoid sports

Final Dx - Infectious mononucleosis

INITIAL MGMT	CONTINUING MGMT	F/U

Office W/U
- CBC
- Chem 14
- TSH
- Urine/serum toxicology

Rx
- Suicide contract
- SSRI (e.g., sertraline) or
- SNRI (e.g., mirtazapine)
- Psychiatry consult

F/U
- Follow up in one week
- Supportive psychotherapy
- Exercise program
- Patient counseling

Final Dx - Major depression

HIGH-YIELD CASES

Cough/Shortness of Breath

CASE 18

HX	PE	DDX
2 yo M is brought in by his mother because of sudden-onset shortness of breath and cough. He had a URI four days ago. Earlier in the day he was playing with peanuts with his brother. His immunizations are up to date.	VS: T 37°C (98°F), P 110, BP 80/50, RR 38, O_2 sat 99% room air Gen: Respiratory distress; using accessory muscles HEENT: WNL Neck: WNL Lungs: Inspiratory stridor; ↓ breath sounds in right lower base CV: Tachycardia Abd: WNL	• Angioedema • Asthma • Croup • Epiglottis • Foreign-body aspiration • Laryngitis • Peritonsillar abscess • Pneumonia • Retropharyngeal abscess

CASE 19

HX	PE	DDX
75 yo F presents with chest pain and shortness of breath. She reports having fallen five days ago and has a long cast for her femoral fracture.	VS: Afebrile, BP 120/75, HR 100, RR 24 Gen: Respiratory distress HEENT: WNL Lungs: Rales, wheezing, ↓ breath sounds in left lower lung CV: Loud P2 and splitting of S2 Abd: WNL	• CHF • Lung cancer • MI • Pericarditis • Pneumothorax • Pulmonary embolism • Syncope

CASE 20

HX	PE	DDX
5 yo M is brought to the ER with a harsh barking cough. He has a history of URIs with coryza, nasal congestion, and sore throat. His symptoms have been present for about a week.	VS: T 38°C (101°F), BP 110/65, HR 100, RR 22 Gen: Pallor and mild respiratory distress with intercostal retraction and nasal flaring HEENT: WNL Lungs: Stridor, hoarseness, barking cough CV: WNL Abd: WNL	• Bacterial tracheitis • Croup • Diphtheria • Epiglottitis • Measles • Peritonsillar abscess • Retropharyngeal abscess

INITIAL MGMT	CONTINUING MGMT	F/U

Emergency room STAT
- CXR, PA and lateral
- XR—neck
- CBC
- Bronchoscopy: Foreign body is removed and patient improves

Rx
- Consider IV methylprednisolone before removal of the foreign body

F/U:
- Follow up in two weeks

Final Dx - Foreign-body aspiration

INITIAL MGMT	CONTINUING MGMT	F/U

Emergency room W/U
- IV normal saline
- NPO
- CBC
- Chem 14
- ABG: Hypoxia and hypocapnia
- CXR: Left lower lobe atelectasis, Hampton's humps
- CT of the chest: pulmonary embolism
- ECG
- DVT U/S: Venous DVT
- Heparin IV and warfarin

Ward W/U
- Continuous cardiac and BP monitoring
- Pulmonary medicine consult
- PT/PTT/INR

Rx
- Discontinue heparin two days after INR is therapeutic
- Warfarin

F/U:
- Follow up in two weeks with PT/INR
- Chest physical therapy
- Warfarin
- Rehabilitative medicine consult

Final Dx - Pulmonary embolism

INITIAL MGMT	CONTINUING MGMT	F/U

Emergency room W/U
- O_2
- CBC
- Chem 8
- Throat culture
- XR—neck: Subglottic narrowing
- Direct laryngoscopy

Ward Rx
- Humidified air
- Epinephrine
- Dexamethasone

F/U:
- Follow up in one month
- Family counseling

Final Dx - Croup

CASE 21

HX	PE	DDX
75 yo M presents with shortness of breath on exertion along with cough and blood-streaked sputum. He reports progressive malaise and weight loss together with loss of appetite over the past six months. He smokes 40 packs of cigarettes per year.	VS: Afebrile, BP 130/85, HR 90, RR 15 Gen: WNL Chest: Barrel-shaped chest, gynecomastia Lungs: Rales, wheezing, ↓ breath sounds, dullness on percussion in left upper lung CV: WNL Abd: Mild tenderness in RUQ with mild hepatomegaly Ext: Finger clubbing; dark-colored, pruritic rash on both forearms	• Lung cancer • Lymphoma • Sarcoidosis • Tuberculosis

CASE 22

HX	PE	DDX
60 yo M presents with ↑ dyspnea, sputum production, and a change in the color of his sputum to yellow over the past three days. He is a smoker with a history of COPD.	VS: T 38°C (100.6°F), P 90, BP 130/70, RR 28, O_2 sat 92% on 2-L NC Gen: Moderate respiratory distress Lungs: Rhonchi at left lower base; diffuse wheezing CV: WNL Abd: WNL Ext: WNL	• Bronchitis • Congestive heart failure • COPD exacerbation • Lung cancer • Pneumonia • URI

INITIAL MGMT	CONTINUING MGMT	F/U

Office W/U
- CBC: ↓ hemoglobin
- Chem 8
- LFTs: ↑ transaminase
- ABG
- ESR: ↑
- CXR: Infiltrate and nodules in upper left lobe
- Sputum cytology: Adenocarcinoma
- Sputum culture
- PPD: ⊖
- CT—chest: Left upper lobe mass

Office W/U
- PFTs
- Oncology consult
- Surgery consult
- Dietary consult
- Bronchoscopy with biopsy
- CT—abdomen and pelvis
- CT—head
- Antiemetic medication

- Smoking cessation
- Patient counseling
- Family counseling
- Follow up in 3–4 weeks with CXR and CBC
- Counsel patient to limit alcohol intake

Final Dx - Lung cancer

INITIAL MGMT	CONTINUING MGMT	F/U

Emergency room STAT
- O_2
- IV normal saline
- IV steroids
- Albuterol by nebulizer
- Atrovent by nebulizer
- Sputum culture
- Blood culture

Emergency room W/U
- CBC: ↑ WBC count
- CXR: Left lower lobe infiltrate
- ECG
- ABG
- Peak flow: < 200 L/min
- Sputum Gram stain: Gram-⊕ cocci
- Chem 8

Rx
- Third-generation cephalosporin + azithromycin vs. levofloxacin or gatifloxacin IV

Ward W/U
- Peak flow: 300 L/min
- FEV_1: 2 L
- Sputum culture: ⊕ for S. *pneumoniae* sensitive to levofloxacin
- Blood culture: ⊖

Rx
- Change to levofloxacin
- Change IV prednisone

- Taper prednisone over the next two weeks
- Smoking cessation
- Consider pneumonia vaccine and flu shot

Final Dx - Chronic obstructive pulmonary disease (COPD) exacerbation/Pneumonia

CASE 23

HX	PE	DDX
50 yo Mexican immigrant M presents with cough productive of bloody sputum accompanied by night sweats, weight loss, and fatigue of three months' duration.	VS: T 38°C (100°F), BP 130/85, HR 90, RR 22 Gen: Pallor Lungs: ↓ breath sounds in upper lobes of both lungs CV: WNL Abd: WNL	• Bronchiectasis • Fungal lung infection • Lung cancer • Lymphoma • Sarcoidosis • TB • Vasculitis

CASE 24

HX	PE	DDX
55 yo M presents with cough that is exacerbated when he lies down at night and improves when he props his head up on three pillows. He also reports worsening exertional dyspnea for the past two months (he now has dyspnea at rest). He has had a 25-pound weight gain since his symptoms began. His past medical history is significant for hypertension, an MI five years ago, hyperlipidemia, and smoking.	VS: P 70, BP 120/70, RR 28, O_2 sat 86% room air Gen: Moderate respiratory distress Neck: JVD Lungs: Bibasilar crackles CV: S1/S2/S3 RRR, 3/6 systolic murmur at apex Abd: WNL Ext: +2 bilateral pitting edema	• Congestive heart failure • COPD exacerbation • MI • Pericardial tamponade • Pulmonary embolism • Pulmonary fibrosis • Renal failure

INITIAL MGMT	CONTINUING MGMT	F/U

Emergency room W/U
- CXR: Infiltrate/nodules in upper lobes
- AFB sputum/culture × 3 days: ⊕ stain
- Sputum Gram stain and culture
- PPD: 16 mm
- CBC
- Chem 14
- HIV testing
- CT—chest: Infiltrates and cavity consistent with TB

Rx
- Respiratory isolation
- Transfer to the ward

Ward W/U
- Social worker consult

Rx
- INH + rifampin + pyrazinamide + ethambutol
- Vitamin B$_6$

- Sputum culture and smear at three months
- LFTs
- Ophthalmology consult
- Family education
- Family PPD placement
- Report case to the local public health department

Final Dx - Tuberculosis (TB)

INITIAL MGMT	CONTINUING MGMT	F/U

Emergency room STAT
- O$_2$
- IV
- IV furosemide
- CXR: Pulmonary edema
- ECG: Old Q wave in anterior leads

Emergency room W/U
- Cardiac/BP monitoring
- CPK-MB, troponin q 8 h
- CBC
- Chem 8: K 3.4
- Serum calcium, magnesium, phosphate

Rx
- IV KCl
- Daily weight
- Discontinue any β-blockers
- SQ heparin
- Low-fat, low-sodium diet

Ward W/U
- TSH
- Lipid profile
- Echocardiography: Hypokinesia in anterior wall; EF 20%
- Chem 8: K 3.7

Rx
- Fluid restriction
- Lisinopril
- Atorvastatin
- ASA
- Digoxin
- Spironolactone
- Change IV furosemide
- Restart β-blockers (when euvolemic)

- Cardiac rehabilitation
- Counsel patient re smoking cessation, hypertension, exercise, relaxation, and lipids
- Follow up in one week
- Refer to cardiology; with ischemic cardiomyopathy and EF < 30%, patients may benefit from an automatic implantable cardiac defibrillator (AICD)

Final Dx - Congestive heart failure (CHF) exacerbation

CASE 25

HX	PE	DDX
5 yo F presents with shortness of breath. She has a history of recurrent pulmonary infection and fatty, foul-smelling stool. She has also shown failure to thrive and has a history of meconium ileus.	VS: T 38°C (101°F), BP 110/65, HR 110, RR 24 Gen: Pallor, mild respiratory distress, low weight and height for age, dry skin HEENT: Nasal polyps Lungs: Barrel-shaped chest, rales, dullness and ↓ breath sounds over lower lung fields CV: WNL Abd: Abdominal distention, hepatosplenomegaly	• Asthma • Cystic fibrosis • Failure to thrive • Malabsorption syndrome • Sinusitis

CASE 26

HX	PE	DDX
65 yo F with a history of hypertension and diabetes mellitus presents with LUQ pain accompanied by fever and a productive cough with purulent yellow sputum.	VS: T 38°C (101°F), P 105, BP 130/75, RR 22, O_2 sat 95% room air Gen: NAD Neck: WNL Lungs: ↓ breath sounds and rhonchi on left side CV: Tachycardia Abd: Tenderness in LUQ	• Bronchitis • Infectious mononucleosis • Lung abscess • Lung cancer • Pneumonia • Pyelonephritis • Spleen abscess

INITIAL MGMT	CONTINUING MGMT	F/U

Emergency room W/U
- CBC: ↓ hemoglobin
- Chem 8: ↑ sugar, ↓ albumin
- ABG: Hypoxia
- CXR: Hyperinflation
- Sputum Gram stain and culture
- O_2

Ward W/U
- PFTs
- Sweat chloride test: ⊕
- Pancreatic enzymes
- 24-hour fecal fat
- Dietary consult
- Genetics consult
- Cystic fibrosis specialist
- Pulmonary medicine, pediatrics consults

Rx
- IV normal saline
- O_2
- IV piperacillin
- Albuterol, inhalation

- Follow up in two months
- Chest physical therapy
- Regular multiple vitamins
- Influenza vaccine
- Pneumococcal vaccine
- Family counseling

Final Dx - Cystic fibrosis (CF)

INITIAL MGMT	CONTINUING MGMT	F/U

Office W/U
- CBC: ↑ WBC count
- Chem 8
- UA
- Sputum Gram stain: Gram-positive cocci
- Sputum culture: Pending
- CXR: Left lower lobe infiltrate
- U/S—abdomen

Ward W/U
- Sputum culture: ⊕ for *Streptococcus pneumoniae*

Rx
- IV normal saline
- PO levofloxacin
- Chest physiotherapy
- Tylenol
- SQ heparin

- Discharge home
- Continue PO levofloxacin × 14 days

Final Dx - Pneumonia

CASE 27

HX	PE	DDX
25 yo HIV-⊕ M presents with shortness of breath, malaise, dry cough, fatigue, and fever.	VS: T 38°C (101°F), BP 110/65, HR 110, RR 24 Gen: Pallor, mild respiratory distress, generalized lymphadenopathy HEENT: Oral thrush Lungs: Intercostal reaction; rales and ↓ breath sounds over both lung fields CV: WNL Abd: Soft, nontender; hepatosplenomegaly Ext: Reddish maculopapular rash	• CMV • Interstitial pneumonia • Kaposi's sarcoma • Legionellosis • *Mycobacterium avium-intracellulare* • *Pneumocystis carinii* pneumonia • TB

Chest Pain

CASE 28

HX	PE	DDX
40 yo F presents with sudden onset of 8/10 substernal chest pain that began at rest, has lasted for 20 minutes, and radiates to the jaw. The pain is accompanied by nausea. The patient has a prior history of hypertension, hyperlipidemia, and smoking.	VS: P 80, BP 130/60, RR 14, O₂ sat 99% room air Gen: Moderate distress Lungs: WNL CV: WNL Abd: WNL Ext: WNL	• Angina • Aortic dissection • Costochondritis • GERD • MI • Pericarditis • Pneumothorax • Pulmonary embolism

INITIAL MGMT	CONTINUING MGMT	F/U

Office W/U
- CBC
- CD4: 200
- Chem 8
- ABG: Hypoxia
- Sputum Gram stain and culture
- Sputum AFB smear
- Bronchial washings—*Pneumocystis* stain (bronchoscopy is a prerequisite along with thoracic surgery consult): ⊕
- CXR: Bilateral interstitial infiltrate
- PPD: ⊖

Office W/U
- LFTs
- VDRL
- Anti-HCV
- HBsAg
- Anti-HBc
- Serum *Toxoplasma* serology

Rx
- TMP-SMX or pentamidine (if patient cannot tolerate TMP-SMX)
- Prednisone
- Begin highly active antiretroviral therapy (HAART)

- Regular follow-up visits
- LFTs
- Influenza vaccine
- Pneumococcal vaccine
- Counsel patient re safe sex practices
- HIV support group
- Patient counseling
- Family counseling

Final Dx - *Pneumocystis carinii* pneumonia (PCP)

INITIAL MGMT	CONTINUING MGMT	F/U

Emergency room STAT
- O_2
- Chewable aspirin
- SL nitroglycerin
- IV normal saline
- IV morphine
- ECG: T-wave inversions

Emergency room W/U
- Cardiac/BP monitoring
- CPK-MB, troponin q 8 h: ⊖
- CBC
- Chem 14
- PT/PTT
- CXR

ICU W/U
- ECG
- Lipid profile
- TSH
- Echocardiography: EF 60%
- Stress test: ⊕

Rx
- Enoxaparin
- ASA
- Clopidogrel
- β-blocker (atenolol)
- ACEI (enalapril)
- Atorvastatin
- Cardiology consult
- Cardiac catheterization

- Cardiac rehabilitation
- Counsel patient re smoking cessation, hypertension, exercise, relaxation, and lipids
- Advise patient to rest at home
- Low-fat, low-sodium diet

Final Dx - Unstable angina

HIGH-YIELD CASES

CASE 29

HX	PE	DDX
58 yo M was working in his office 30 minutes ago when he suddenly developed right-sided chest discomfort and shortness of breath. He has a prior history of asthma and emphysema.	VS: P 123, BP 101/64, RR 28, O_2 sat 91% room air Gen: Cyanosis, severe respiratory distress Lungs: No breath sounds on right side with hyperresonance on percussion CV: Tachycardia; apical impulse displaced to the left Abd: WNL **Limited PE**	• Angina • Aortic dissection • Asthma exacerbation • Pneumothorax • Pulmonary embolism • Tension pneumothorax

CASE 30

HX	PE	DDX
34 yo F presents with stabbing retrosternal chest pain that radiates to the back. The pain improves when she leans forward and worsens with deep inspiration. She had a URI one week ago.	VS: T 37°C (99.2°F), P 80, BP 130/70, RR 16, O_2 sat 98% room air Gen: NAD Neck: WNL Lungs: WNL CV: S1/S2, pericardial friction rub Abd: WNL Ext: WNL	• Angina/MI • Aortic dissection • Costochondritis • Esophageal rupture • GERD • Pericarditis • Pneumothorax • Pulmonary embolism

CASE 31

HX	PE	DDX
48 yo F presents with palpitation and anxiety. She reports that she feels hot and has to run the air conditioner all the time. She also reports hand tremors. She has lost 10 pounds over the past few months despite her good appetite.	VS: P 113, BP 145/85, RR 20 Gen: Mild respiratory distress, dehydration, sweaty palms and face, warm skin, hand tremor HEENT: Exophthalmos with lid lag, generalized thyromegaly, thyroid bruit Lungs: WNL CV: Tachycardia Abd: WNL Ext: Edema over the tibia bilaterally	• Anxiety • Atrial fibrillation • Early menopause • Hyperthyroidism • Mitral valve prolapse • Panic attack • Withdrawal syndrome

INITIAL MGMT	CONTINUING MGMT	F/U

Emergency room STAT
- IV normal saline
- O_2
- Needle thoracostomy
- Chest tube
- CXR: Collapsed right lung, mediastinal shift to left
- IV morphine

Emergency room W/U
- Cardiac/BP monitoring
- ECG: Sinus tachycardia
- CBC
- Chem 14
- PT/PTT

Ward W/U
- Thoracic surgery consult
- CXR: Inflated right lung

Rx
- Morphine
- Chest tube to water seal and vacuum device

Ward
- Pleurodesis if indicated

Final Dx - Tension pneumothorax

INITIAL MGMT	CONTINUING MGMT	F/U

Emergency room W/U
- Continuous cardiac and BP monitoring
- Stat ECG: Diffuse ST elevation, PR depression
- CPK-MB, troponin × 3
- CBC
- Chem 7
- CXR: No cardiomegaly
- ESR

Rx
- ASA or NSAIDs
- Start IV
- O_2

Ward W/U
- Discontinue continuous monitoring
- Echocardiography: Minimal pericardial effusion

Rx
- Reassure patient
- ASA

- Discharge home
- Follow up in two weeks

Final Dx - Pericarditis

INITIAL MGMT	CONTINUING MGMT	F/U

Office W/U
- CBC
- BMP
- Thyroid studies (T_4, T_3RU, T_3, TSH): ↑ T_3/T_4, ↓ TSH
- Serum thyroid autoantibodies: ⊕
- ECG
- CXR
- Nuclear scan—thyroid: ↑ uptake

Rx
- Propranolol
- Methimazole
- PTU

Office W/U
- Endocrinology consult

- Check thyroid studies in one month
- Patient counseling

Final Dx - Hyperthyroidism

CASE 32

HX	PE	DDX
65 yo M presents with sudden onset of severe tearing anterior chest pain that radiates to the back. He is anxious and diaphoretic. He has a history of long-standing hypertension.	VS: T 36°C (97°F), BP 195/110 right arm, 160/80 left arm, HR 100, RR 30, O_2 sat 98% room air Gen: Acute distress Lungs: WNL CV: Tachycardia, S4, diastolic decrescendo heard best at left sternal border Abd: WNL Ext: Unequal pulse in both arms **Limited PE**	• Aortic dissection • MI • Pericarditis • Pulmonary embolism

CASE 33

HX	PE	DDX
34 yo F is brought to the ER after a car accident. She is gasping for air and complains of weakness, chest pain, and dizziness.	VS: Afebrile, BP 100/50, HR 115, RR 22, pulsus paradoxus Gen: Confusion, cyanosis, respiratory distress Neck: ↑ JVP, engorged neck veins, Kussmaul's sign Lungs: WNL CV: Muffled heart sounds, ↓ PMI Abd: WNL Ext: WNL	• Aortic dissection • Cardiogenic shock • MI • Pericardial tamponade • Pericarditis • Pneumothorax • Pulmonary embolism

INITIAL MGMT	CONTINUING MGMT	F/U

Emergency room STAT
- ASA
- O_2
- IV normal saline
- SL nitroglycerin
- CXR: Widened mediastinum
- IV-β blockers
- ECG: LVH
- IV morphine

Emergency room W/U
- Cardiac/BP monitoring
- CPK-MB, troponin × 3: ⊖
- CBC
- Chem 8
- TEE: Aortic dissection type A or
- CT—chest with IV contrast: Aortic dissection

Rx
- Thoracic surgery consult

ICU W/U
- Continuous cardiac and BP monitoring
- Blood type and cross-match
- PT/PTT, INR

Rx
- Continuing IV β-blockers
- Emergent surgery

- Diet and lifestyle modifications
- Lipid/BP management

Final Dx - Aortic dissection

INITIAL MGMT	CONTINUING MGMT	F/U

Emergency room W/U
- O_2
- IV normal saline
- NPO
- Pulse oximetry
- ECG: Tachycardia, low voltage, nonspecific ST- and T-wave changes
- CPK-MB
- CBC
- Chem 8
- ABG
- Coagulation profile
- Blood type and crossmatch
- CXR: Cardiomegaly
- Echocardiography: Tamponade
- Pericardiocentesis

ICU W/U
- Continuous cardiac and BP monitoring
- ECG
- Echocardiography
- CXR
- Cardiac surgery consult
- ABG

Rx
- NPO to liquid
- O_2
- Follow up in two weeks

- CXR
- Echocardiography
- Patient counseling

Final Dx - Pericardial tamponade

CASE 34

HX	PE	DDX
28 yo F presents with palpitation, chest pain, nausea, and dizziness that last for almost 5–6 minutes. She has had several attacks over the past few weeks. During these episodes, she becomes diaphoretic and occasionally has diarrhea. In the course of some of her attacks, she describes feeling as if she might die.	VS: P 90, BP 125/75, RR 20 Gen: Mild respiratory distress, dehydration, sweating, cold hands HEENT: WNL Lungs: WNL CV: WNL Abd: WNL Ext: WNL	• Anxiety • Asthma attack • Atrial fibrillation • Early menopause • Hyperthyroidism • Hyperventilation • Hypoglycemia • Mitral valve prolapse • Panic attack • Pheochromocytoma • Pulmonary embolus • Substance abuse

CASE 35

HX	PE	DDX
32 yo F presents with occasional palpitation, chest pain, and dizziness. She also reports shortness of breath and chest tightness during her attacks.	VS: P 90–200 (variable), BP 125/75, RR 20 Gen: Mild cyanosis HEENT: WNL Lungs: Bibasilar crackles CV: Irregularly irregular, tachycardia Abd: WNL Ext: WNL	• Anxiety • Atrial fibrillation • Hyperthyroidism • Hyperventilation • Mitral valve prolapse • Panic attack

INITIAL MGMT	CONTINUING MGMT	F/U

Office W/U
- CBC
- Chem 8
- UA
- Urine toxicology: ⊖
- TFTs
- ECG
- CXR

Rx
- Reassure patient
- Benzodiazepines (e.g., alprazolam, lorazepam, clonazepam) or
- SSRIs

- Outpatient follow-up in four weeks
- Psychiatry consult
- Patient counseling
- Behavioral modification program
- Relaxation exercises

Final Dx - Panic attack

INITIAL MGMT	CONTINUING MGMT	F/U

Emergency room W/U
- IV normal saline
- O_2
- CBC
- Chem 8
- TFTs
- ECG: Atrial fibrillation
- CXR: Pulmonary vascular congestion
- Echocardiography: Enlarged left atrium

Rx
- Synchronous cardioversion
- Amiodarone (give prior to DC cardioversion if possible)
- Propranolol
- Heparin

ICU W/U
- ECG
- Continuous cardiac monitoring
- Continuous BP monitoring
- Warfarin
- ASA

- Follow up in two weeks
- Patient counseling

Final Dx - Atrial fibrillation

Abdominal Pain

CASE 36

HX	PE	DDX
38 yo M presents with RUQ abdominal pain of 48 hours' duration. He reports that the pain radiates to his right groin and scrotal area and comes in waves of severe intensity that prevent him from finding a comfortable resting position.	VS: T 36°C (96°F), BP 130/85, HR 100, RR 22 Gen: In pain Lungs: WNL CV: Tachycardia Abd: Soft, nontender, no distention, tenderness in right flank, no peritoneal signs, ⊕ BS Rectal exam: WNL, guaiac ⊖	• Gastroenteritis • Nephrolithiasis • Pancreatitis • Perforated duodenal ulcer • Retrocecal appendicitis

CASE 37

HX	PE	DDX
60 yo M presents with generalized weakness, left flank discomfort, nausea, and constipation of two weeks' duration. He has lost 20 pounds over the past four months.	VS: T 37°C (99.2°F), P 90, BP 120/60, RR 18 Gen: NAD Lungs: WNL CV: WNL Abd: ↓ BS, left flank tenderness with deep palpation Rectal exam: WNL Ext: WNL Neuro: WNL	• Colorectal cancer • Renal cell carcinoma • Renal obstruction (BPH) • UTI

CASE 38

HX	PE	DDX
32 yo F presents with two days of progressive flank pain, urinary frequency, and a burning sensation during urination. She also reports associated fever and shaking chills.	VS: T 39.1°C (102°F), BP 130/85, HR 86, RR 18 Gen: Mild discomfort with exam Lungs: WNL CV: Tachycardia Abd: ⊕ BS, mild suprapubic tenderness, no peritoneal signs Back: Mild CVA tenderness on the left Pelvic: WNL Rectal exam: WNL, guaiac ⊖	• Acute cervicitis • Acute cystitis • Acute pelvic inflammatory disease • Acute pyelonephritis • Acute urethritis • Ectopic pregnancy • Nephrolithiasis

INITIAL MGMT	CONTINUING MGMT	F/U
Emergency room W/U • CBC: ↑ WBC count • Chem 8 • Serum amylase, lipase • UA: Microscopic hematuria • Urine culture • KUB: Radiopaque 3-mm stone • CT—kidney: $\oplus$ **Rx** • IM morphine • Counsel patient re oral hydration • NSAIDs	• Serum calcium, magnesium, phosphate • Serum uric acid • Urine strain • Stone analysis: Calcium oxalate	• ↑ fluid intake • Follow up in four weeks • Patient counseling • Counsel patient to limit alcohol intake • Counsel patient to limit caffeine intake • Smoking cessation

Final Dx - Nephrolithiasis

INITIAL MGMT	CONTINUING MGMT	F/U
Office W/U • CBC: Hemoglobin 9.0 • Chem 14: Ca 15, BUN 40, creatinine 2.0 • UA: $\oplus$ for RBCs • CXR • U/S—complete abdominal: Left renal mass • Admit to ward **Rx** • IV normal saline • Bisphosphonate (pamidronate)	**Ward W/U** • Intact PTH: ↓ • Chem 7: Ca 10, BUN 20, creatinine 1.5 • CT—abdomen and chest: Left renal mass • Renal mass biopsy • Bone scan • CT—head • Ferritin, TIBC, serum iron **Rx** • Oncology consult • Surgery consult	

Final Dx - Renal cell carcinoma

INITIAL MGMT	CONTINUING MGMT	F/U
Office W/U • CBC: ↑ WBC count • Chem 8 • UA: WBC, bacteria, nitrite $\oplus$ • Urine culture: Pending • Urinary β-hCG: $\ominus$ • U/S—renal **Rx** • Ciprofloxacin (fluoroquinolone)	**Office W/U** • Urine culture: $\oplus$ for *E. coli*	• Follow up in 3–5 days • Patient counseling • Counsel patient re medication compliance • Counsel patient to limit alcohol intake

Final Dx - Pyelonephritis

CASE 39

HX	PE	DDX
10 yo African-American M presents with sudden onset of jaundice, dark-colored urine, back pain, and fatigue. He was started on TMP-SMX for an ear infection a few days ago. He has a family history of blood disorders.	VS: T 38°C (99.8°F), P 90, BP 110/50, RR 14 Gen: NAD Skin: Jaundice HEENT: Icterus, pallor Lungs: WNL CV: WNL Abd: WNL Ext: WNL	• Autoimmune hemolytic anemia • DIC • G6PD deficiency • Sickle cell anemia • Spherocytosis • Thalassemias • TTP

CASE 40

HX	PE	DDX
58 yo alcoholic M presents with a one-day history of sharp epigastric pain that radiates to his back. He is nauseated and has vomited several times. He also complains of anorexia. The patient reports heavy alcohol use over the past 2–3 days. He has no previous history of peptic ulcer disease.	VS: T 38.2°C (101°F), BP 138/68, HR 110, RR 22 Gen: WD/WN but agitated, lying on bed with knees drawn up Lungs: ↓ breath sounds over left lower lung CV: Tachycardia Abd: Tender and distended with ↓ BS	• Acute cholecystitis • Acute gastritis • Acute pancreatitis • Aortic dissection • Cholelithiasis • Intestinal perforation • MI • Perforated duodenal ulcers • Pneumonia

INITIAL MGMT	CONTINUING MGMT	F/U

Office W/U
- CBC stat and q 12 h: ↓↓ hemoglobin, ↓↓ hematocrit
- Peripheral smear: Bite cells, fragment cells
- Chem 14: ↑ indirect bilirubin
- PT/PTT, INR

Rx
- Discontinue TMP-SMX

Ward W/U
- Reticulocyte count: ↑
- LDL: ↑
- Haptoglobin: ↓
- UA
- G6PD assay: Consistent with G6PD deficiency
- Type and cross two units of packed RBCs

Rx
- Start IV
- IV normal saline
- Transfuse two units of packed RBCs

- Discharge home
- Follow up in two months
- Educate patient/family

Final Dx - G6PD deficiency

INITIAL MGMT	CONTINUING MGMT	F/U

Emergency room W/U
- IV normal saline
- NPO
- Monitor, continue BP cuff
- NG tube suction
- ECG: No evidence of ischemia
- CBC
- Chem 14
- Serum amylase, lipase: ↑
- ABG
- O$_2$
- Pulse oximetry
- LFTs
- Serum calcium
- AXR, upright
- CXR

Rx
- NG tube
- IV meperidine

Ward W/U
- Monitor, continue BP cuff
- Continue NPO
- U/S—liver, gallbladder and bile duct, pancreas
- PT/PTT
- CT—abdomen
- Surgery consult
- GI consult
- Advance diet as tolerated

- Follow up in seven days
- Patient counseling
- Counsel patient to cease alcohol intake
- Smoking cessation

Final Dx - Acute pancreatitis

CASE 41

HX	PE	DDX
1-day-old M born at home is brought to the ER because of bilious vomiting, irritability, poor feeding, lethargy, and an acute episode of rectal bleeding.	VS: T 38°C (100°F), P 170, BP 69/44, RR 43, O$_2$ sat 89% room air Skin: Evidence of poor perfusion Chest: WNL CV: WNL Abd: Distention; evidence of intestinal obstruction **Limited PE**	• Duodenal web • Intestinal atresia • Malrotation with volvulus • Meconium plug/ileus • Necrotizing enterocolitis

CASE 42

HX	PE	DDX
21-month-old M is brought to the ER because of intermittent abdominal pain that causes him to become still while drawing up his legs. He also presents with irritability and vomiting that initially was clear but then became bilious. The child seemed lethargic between the pain episodes. In the ER, the child passes some dark red stool.	VS: T 38.5°C (101°F), P 157, BP 81/59, RR 35, O$_2$ sat 93% room air Skin: No evidence of purpura Chest: WNL CV: WNL Abd: Soft and mildly tender; examination of RUQ fails to identify presence of bowel; ill-defined mass in the RUQ **Limited PE**	• Intoxication • Intussusception • Metabolic disease • Neurologic disease • Small bowel obstruction • Volvulus

INITIAL MGMT	CONTINUING MGMT	F/U

Emergency room STAT
- IV normal saline
- O_2
- ABG: Metabolic acidosis

Emergency room W/U
- CBC: ↑ WBC count, mildly ↓ hemoglobin
- Chem 8
- AXR: Airless rectum; large gastric bubble
- CXR: No evidence of diaphragmatic hernia

Rx
- NG tube suction
- IV bicarbonate (to correct acidosis if pH < 7.0)
- Pediatric surgery consult

Ward W/U
- Upper GI series: Bird's-beak, corkscrew appearance of proximal jejunum
- Barium enema: Cecum in RUQ

Rx
- NG tube suction
- IV normal saline

- Follow up in 48 hours
- Family counseling

Final Dx - Malrotation with volvulus

INITIAL MGMT	CONTINUING MGMT	F/U

Emergency room STAT
- IV normal saline
- O_2

Emergency room W/U
- CBC: ↑ WBC count
- Chem 14
- ABG: Metabolic acidosis
- AXR: Distended bowel with air-fluid levels; mass in right abdomen
- U/S—abdomen: Compatible with intussusception

Rx
- NG tube suction
- Barium enema: Coiled-spring appearance; disorder is relieved by air insufflation
- Pediatric surgery consult

Ward W/U
- AXR: Gastric bubble; no air-fluid levels
- ABG: Derangements being resolved

Rx
- D/C NG tube suction
- IV normal saline
- Advance diet

- Follow up in 48 hours
- Family counseling

Final Dx - Intussusception

CASE 43

HX	PE	DDX
27-month-old M presents to the ER with seizures, irritability, anorexia, altered sleep patterns, emotional lability, ↓ play activity, and vomiting. His mother states that the family has been living for about a year in an old, poorly maintained building that has only recently begun to undergo renovation. Since she was laid off at the battery plant, the family has been considering moving out of town.	VS: T 37°C (99°F), P 129, BP 89/61, RR 20, O$_2$ sat 92% room air Neuro: Lethargy, ataxia, seizures Remainder of physical examination is noncontributory (except for some conjunctival pallor)	• Lead toxicity • Metabolic disease • Neurologic disease • Nonmetal intoxication • Other heavy metal toxicity

CASE 44

HX	PE	DDX
7-day-old alert M presents to a clinic with jaundice that started two days ago. The baby was born at term via an uneventful vaginal delivery and started breast-feeding after some delay. The mother states that she took the baby to the doctor's office at that time and that the baby's bilirubin was 14 mg/dL. The mother does not take any drugs. She is very concerned that the baby's jaundice is not improving and asks if the baby has kernicterus.	VS: T 37°C (99°F), P 129, BP 80/51, RR 29, O$_2$ sat 94% room air PE: WNL except for jaundice Neuro: WNL	• Breast-feeding jaundice • Crigler-Najjar syndrome • Gilbert's disease • Hereditary spherocytosis • Physiologic hyperbilirubinemia

CASE 45

HX	PE	DDX
31 yo M comes to the office complaining of midepigastric pain that usually begins 1–2 hours after eating and sometimes awakens him at night. He also has occasional indigestion. He is taking an antacid for his problem. He denies melena or hematemesis.	VS: T 37.1°C (99°F), BP 130/75, HR 100, RR 16 Gen: Pallor, no distress Lungs: WNL CV: WNL Abd: Epigastric tenderness Rectal exam: WNL	• Acute gastritis • Diverticulitis • GERD • Pancreatic disease • Peptic ulcer disease • Viral gastroenteritis

INITIAL MGMT	CONTINUING MGMT	F/U
Emergency room W/U • CBC: Hemoglobin 9 g/dL; MCV 75, blood smear reveals coarse basophilic stippling in RBCs • Chem 8 • Serum lead: 70 µg/dL • UA: Glycosuria • Erythrocyte protoporphyrin: ↑ • Serum toxicology: ⊖ **Rx** • IV normal saline • IM EDTA	**Ward Rx** • IV normal saline • Serum lead • IM EDTA (if necessary) • Family counseling	• Follow up in seven days • Family counseling • Lead paint assay in home

Final Dx - Lead intoxication with encephalopathy

INITIAL MGMT	CONTINUING MGMT	F/U
Office W/U • CBC: WNL, smear WNL • Direct Coombs' test: Noncontributory • Serum bilirubin: ↑ indirect bilirubin • TSH: WNL	**Office W/U** • Breast-feeding suppression test: Bilirubin levels ↓ on cessation of breast-feeding; levels ↑ again when breast-feeding restarted **Rx** • ↑ breast feedings • +/– regular infant formula • +/– phototherapy (if bilirubin levels do not ↓)	• Follow up in seven days • Family counseling

Final Dx - Breast-feeding neonatal jaundice

INITIAL MGMT	CONTINUING MGMT	F/U
Office W/U • CBC • Chem 8 • Serum amylase, lipase • Serum *H. pylori* antibody **Rx** • Proton pump inhibitor • Clarithromycin (Biaxin) • Metronidazole		• Follow up in four weeks; patient reports that he is feeling better (if symptoms persist or if *H. pylori* is still present, may proceed to endoscopy) • Patient counseling • Counsel patient to limit alcohol intake • Smoking cessation

Final Dx - Gastritis (*H. pylori* infection)

HIGH-YIELD CASES

CASE 46

HX	PE	DDX
27 yo M presents with malaise, nausea, vomiting, loss of appetite, and fever with chills for the past week. He was in Mexico on an assignment three weeks ago. He has had tea-colored urine for one day. He is married and has a son.	VS: T 38°C (100°F), BP 130/85, HR 90, RR 12 Gen: WD, ill-looking, not in distress Skin: Jaundice HEENT: Sclera icteric Lungs: WNL CV: WNL Abd: Soft, tenderness in the RUQ, liver enlarged about 3 cm below the right costal margin Rectal exam: WNL, guaiac ⊖	• Acute hepatitis A • Autoimmune hepatitis • Cholangitis • Cholecystitis and biliary colic • Cholelithiasis • Drug-induced hepatitis • Gastroenteritis • Liver abscess • Pancreatitis • Small bowel obstruction

CASE 47

HX	PE	DDX
60 yo F G0 presents with a two-month history of ↑ abdominal girth, ↓ appetite, and early satiety. She also has mild shortness of breath.	VS: T 36°C (97°F), BP 140/60, HR 90, RR 23 Gen: Pallor Breast: WNL Lungs: WNL CV: WNL Abd: Distended, nontender, ⊕ BS, no palpable hepatosplenomegaly Pelvic: Solid right adnexal mass Rectal exam: Solid right adnexal mass; no involvement of recto-vaginal septum	• Congestive heart failure • Liver cirrhosis • Ovarian cancer

CASE 48

HX	PE	DDX
32 yo F presents with sudden onset of left lower abdominal pain that radiates to the scapula and back and is associated with vaginal bleeding. Her last menstrual period was five weeks ago. She has a history of pelvic inflammatory disease and unprotected intercourse.	VS: T 37°C (99°F), P 90, BP 120/50, RR 14 Gen: Moderate distress 2° to pain Lungs: WNL CV: WNL Abd: RLQ tenderness, rebound, and guarding Pelvic: Slightly enlarged uterus with small amount of dark bloody discharge from cervix; right adnexal tenderness Rectal exam: WNL Ext: WNL	• Ectopic pregnancy • Ovarian torsion • Pelvic inflammatory disease • Ruptured ovarian cyst • Spontaneous abortion

INITIAL MGMT	CONTINUING MGMT	F/U
Office W/U • CBC • LFTs: ALT 1200, AST 1100 • Serum amylase, lipase • BMP • PT • Hepatitis antibody panel: ⊕ hepatitis A IgG and IgM **Rx** • Bed rest • Strict hand washing • Hepatitis A immune globulin for wife and son	**Office W/U (next day)** • LFTs in three days • PT in three days **Rx** • Advise patient to rest at home • Oral hydration	• Repeat LFTs and PT in seven days • Hepatitis precaution counseling • Avoid alcohol and hepato-toxic drugs • Avoid vigorous activity

Final Dx - Acute hepatitis A

INITIAL MGMT	CONTINUING MGMT	F/U
Office W/U • CBC • Chem 14 • CA-125: 900 • CT—abdomen and pelvis: 10- × 12-cm right complex ovarian cyst; large amounts of ascites • CXR: Right moderate pleural effusion • ECG • Pap smear • Mammogram • Colonoscopy • Gynecology consult	**Ward Rx** • Blood type and crossmatch • PT/PTT, INR • Exploratory laparotomy • TAH-BSO, laparotomy • Staging, laparotomy	• Carboplatin • CA-125 • CBC • Chem 14

Final Dx - Ovarian cancer

INITIAL MGMT	CONTINUING MGMT	F/U
Emergency room W/U • Urinary β-hCG: ⊕ • Quantitative serum β-hCG: 2500 • CBC • Chem 8 • Cervical Gram stain and G&C culture • U/S—transvaginal: 2-cm right adnexal mass, no intrauterine pregnancy, free fluid in cul-de-sac **Rx** • IV normal saline	• Blood type and cross-match • PT/PTT, INR • Gynecology consult • Laparoscopy • Rh IgG (RhoGAM) if Rh- ⊖	• Counsel patient on contraception • Counsel patient on safe sex

Final Dx - Ectopic pregnancy

HIGH-YIELD CASES

CASE 49

HX	PE	DDX
68 yo M presents with LLQ abdominal pain, fever, and chills for the past three days. He also reports recent-onset episodes of alternating diarrhea and constipation. He consumes a low-fiber, high-fat diet.	VS: T 38°C (101°F), BP 130/85, HR 100, RR 22 Gen: Pallor, diaphoresis Lungs: WNL CV: Tachycardia Abd: LLQ tenderness, no peritoneal signs, ⊕ BS Rectal exam: Guaiac ⊖	• Abscess: Diverticular abcess • Crohn's disease • Diverticulitis • Gastroenteritis • Ulcerative colitis

CASE 50

HX	PE	DDX
41 yo F presents with sudden-onset RUQ abdominal pain of six hours' duration. She also reports nausea and emesis. The pain started after lunch and has become more severe and constant. She reports that the pain is exacerbated by deep breathing and that it radiates to her shoulder. She had a similar attack almost one year ago. She is taking OCPs and has three children.	VS: T 39.0°C (102°F), BP 130/82, HR 80, RR 16 Gen: WD, slightly obese, moderate distress Lungs: WNL CV: WNL Abd: Obesity, tenderness and guarding to palpation on RUQ, ⊕ Murphy's sign, ↓ BS Rectal exam: WNL, guaiac ⊖	• Acute appendicitis • Acute cholangitis • Acute cholecystitis • Acute hepatitis • Acute pancreatitis • Acute peptic ulcer disease with or without perforation • Biliary atresia • Cardiac ischemia • Cholelithiasis • Fitz-Hugh–Curtis syndrome (gonococcal perihepatitis) • Gastritis • Renal colic • Right-sided pneumonia • Small bowel obstruction

INITIAL MGMT	CONTINUING MGMT	F/U
Emergency room W/U	**Ward W/U**	days
• CBC: ↑ WBC count	• Urine culture: ⊖	• High-fiber diet
• Chem 14	• Blood culture: ⊖	• Colonoscopy four weeks
• Serum amylase, lipase	**Rx**	after recovery
• UA	• NPO → clear liquid diet	
• Urine culture: Pending	• Surgery consult	
• Blood culture: Pending	• Metronidazole +	
• Stool culture and sensitivity	ciprofloxacin × 7–10 days	
• Stool for ova and parasites	• Discharge home in 3–4	
• CXR		
• KUB		
• CT—abdomen: Diverticulitis		
Rx		
• NPO		
• IV normal saline		
• IV metronidazole + ciprofloxacin		

Final Dx - Diverticulitis

INITIAL MGMT	CONTINUING MGMT	F/U
Emergency room W/U	**Ward W/U**	• Follow up in two weeks
• IV normal saline	• Blood type and cross-	• Patient counseling
• NPO	match	• Counsel patient to limit
• Monitor, continue BP cuff	• PT/PTT, INR	alcohol intake
• ECG	• Surgery consult for chole-	
• CBC	cystectomy	
• Chem 14	• Vitals q 4 h	
• Serum amylase, lipase	• CBC next day	
• LFTs	• Chem 8 next day	
• Blood/urine cultures	**Rx**	
• AXR/CXR	• NPO → advance diet as	
• Pregnancy test—urine	tolerated	
• U/S—abdomen: Gallstones with gallbladder edema	• Continue antibiotic ther- apy	
Rx		
• IM prochlorperazine		
• IV morphine		
• IV cefuroxime		

Final Dx - Acute cholecystitis

CASE 51

HX	PE	DDX
24 yo F presents with bilateral lower abdominal pain that started with the first day of her menstrual period. The pain is associated with fever and a thick, greenish-yellow vaginal discharge. She has had unprotected sex with multiple sexual partners.	VS: T 38°C (100.4°F), P 90, BP 110/50, RR 14 Gen: Moderate distress 2° to pain Lungs: WNL CV: WNL Abd: Diffuse tenderness (greatest in the lower quadrants), no rebound, no distention, ↓ BS Pelvic: Purulent, bloody discharge from cervix; cervical motion and bilateral adnexal tenderness Rectal exam: WNL Ext: WNL	• Dysmenorrhea • Endometriosis • Pelvic inflammatory disease • Pyelonephritis • Vaginitis

CASE 52

HX	PE	DDX
25 yo M is brought to the ER because of abdominal pain and ↓ appetite for four days. This episode was preceded by ↑ urinary frequency, nausea, and vomiting.	VS: T 37°C (98°F), P 120, BP 100/60, RR 25 Gen: Moderate distress Skin: Poor skin turgor HEENT: Dry mucous membranes, "fruity breath" Lungs: WNL CV: Tachycardia Abd: Generalized tenderness Ext: WNL Neuro: WNL **Limited PE**	• Acute intestinal obstruction • Alcoholic ketoacidosis • Appendicitis • Diabetic ketoacidosis • Drug intoxication • Gastroenteritis • Pancreatitis • Pyelonephritis

INITIAL MGMT	CONTINUING MGMT	F/U

Emergency room W/U
- Urinary β-hCG: $\ominus$
- CBC: ↑ WBC count
- Chem 14
- Cervical Gram stain and G&C culture
- U/S—pelvis
- UA and urine culture

Rx
- IV normal saline
- IV cefoxitin or cefotetan + IV doxycycline vs. clindamycin + gentamicin
- Acetaminophen

Ward W/U
Cervical culture: *N. gonorrhoeae*

Rx
- Discontinue IV cefoxitin when symptoms improve (usually in 24–48 hours)
- Switch to doxycycline or clindamycin

- Counsel patient on safe sex practices
- Treat partners

Final Dx - Pelvic inflammatory disease (PID)

INITIAL MGMT	CONTINUING MGMT	F/U

Emergency room STAT
- Glucometer: 400 mg/dL
- IV normal saline

Emergency room W/U
- Continuous monitoring
- Chem 14: ↑ BUN, ↑ K, ↓ Na, ↑ anion gap
- CBC: ↑ WBC count
- Serum amylase, lipase
- UA and urine culture: $\oplus$ glucose, $\oplus$ ketone
- Urine/serum toxicology
- Phosphate: ↓
- ECG
- ABG: Metabolic acidosis (pH = 7.1)
- Quantitative serum ketones: ↑↑↑
- Serum osmolality: ↑
- CXR/AXR

Rx
- IV regular insulin, continue
- Phosphate therapy

ICU W/U
- Continuous monitoring
- Random glucose q 1 h
- Chem 8 q 4 h: ↓ K, glucose < 250

Rx
- Switch IV fluid to D_5W
- IV potassium
- SQ insulin NPH
- SQ insulin regular
- Discontinue IV insulin two hours after starting long-acting insulin (NPH or Lantus)

- Diabetic diet
- Diabetic teaching
- Hb_{A1c} q 3 months
- Follow up in two weeks in the office
- Diabetic foot care
- Ophthalmology consult
- Lipid profile
- Instruct patient in home sugar monitoring
- Home sugar monitoring, glucometer

Final Dx - Diabetic ketoacidosis (DKA)

Constipation/Diarrhea

CASE 53

HX	PE	DDX
67 yo M presents with constipation, ↓ stool caliber, and blood in his stool for the past eight months. He also reports unintentional weight loss. He is on a low-fiber diet and has a family history of colon cancer.	VS: P 85, BP 140/85, RR 14, O_2 sat 98% room air Gen: NAD HEENT: Pale conjunctiva Lungs: WNL CV: WNL Abd: WNL Pelvic: WNL Rectal exam: Hemoccult ⊕	• Angiodysplasia • Colorectal cancer • Diverticulosis • GI parasitic infection (ascariasis, giardiasis) • Hemorrhoids • Hypothyroidism • Inflammatory bowel disease • Irritable bowel syndrome

CASE 54

HX	PE	DDX
28 yo M presents with diffuse abdominal pain, loose stools, perianal pain, mild fever, and weight loss over the past four weeks. He denies any history of travel or recent use of antibiotics.	VS: T 37°C (99°F), BP 130/65, HR 70, RR 14 Gen: NAD Lungs: WNL CV: WNL Abd: WNL Rectal exam: Perianal skin tags, hemoccult ⊕	• Crohn's disease • Diverticulitis • Gastroenteritis • Infectious colitis • Irritable bowel syndrome • Ischemic colitis • Lactose intolerance • Pseudomembranous colitis • Small bowel lymphoma • Ulcerative colitis

CASE 55

HX	PE	DDX
30 yo F presents with periumbilical crampy pain of six months' duration. The pain never awakens her from sleep. It is relieved by defecation and worsens when she is upset. She has alternating constipation and diarrhea but no nausea, vomiting, weight loss, or anorexia.	VS: Afebrile, P 85, BP 130/65, RR 14 Gen: NAD Lungs: WNL CV: WNL Abd: WNL Pelvic: WNL Rectal exam: Guaiac ⊖	• Celiac disease • Chronic pancreatitis • Colorectal cancer • Crohn's disease • Diverticulosis • Endometriosis • GI parasitic infection (ascariasis, giardiasis) • Hypothyroidism • Inflammatory bowel disease • Irritable bowel syndrome

INITIAL MGMT	CONTINUING MGMT	F/U

Office W/U
- CBC: ↓ hematocrit, ↑ RDW, ↓ MCV, ↓ MCHC
- Chem 8
- Ferritin: ↓
- Serum iron: ↓
- TIBC: ↑
- TSH
- Stool for ova and parasites
- ESR: ↑
- Stool guaiac: ⊕

Office W/U
- GI consult
- Colonoscopy: Polyp with adenocarcinoma
- CT—abdomen and pelvis with contrast
- CEA

Rx
- Iron sulfate
- General surgery consult
- Plan partial colectomy

Final Dx - Colorectal cancer

INITIAL MGMT	CONTINUING MGMT	F/U

Office W/U
- CBC
- Chem 14
- Serum amylase, lipase
- Stool for ova and parasites
- Stool C. *difficile*
- AXR
- Colonoscopy: Crohn's disease

Rx
- 5-ASA
- Metronidazole (for perianal abscess or fistula)

- Follow up in two weeks
- Counsel patient re medication compliance and adherence

Final Dx - Crohn's disease

INITIAL MGMT	CONTINUING MGMT	F/U

Office W/U
- CBC
- Chem 14
- TSH
- Stool for ova and parasites
- Stool for WBCs
- Stool culture and sensitivity
- Transglutaminase antibody

Rx
- Educate patient
- Reassurance
- High-fiber diet
- Lactose-free diet

- Follow up in four weeks
- Call with questions

Final Dx - Irritable bowel syndrome

HIGH-YIELD CASES

CASE 56

HX	PE	DDX
8 yo M is brought to the clinic by his mother for intermittent diarrhea alternating with constipation together with vomiting and cramping abdominal pain. His mother also reports that he has had progressive anorexia.	VS: T 37°C (98°F), BP 110/65, HR 90, RR 16 Gen: Pale and dry mucosal membranes; lack of growth Lungs: WNL CV: WNL Abd: WNL Ext: Muscle wasting, especially in gluteal area	• Bacterial gastroenteritis • Celiac disease • Food allergy • Giardiasis • Protein intolerance • Viral gastroenteritis

CASE 57

HX	PE	DDX
28 yo M reports intermittent episodes of vomiting and diarrhea along with cramping abdominal pain for the past two days. He describes his stool as watery. He returned from Mexico three days ago.	VS: T 39°C (101.9°F), BP 135/85, HR 100, RR 22 Gen: Mild dehydration Lungs: WNL CV: WNL Abd: Mild tenderness, no peritoneal signs, hyperactive BS Rectal exam: WNL, guaiac ⊖	• *Campylobacter* infection • Cholera • *C. difficile* colitis • Crohn's disease • Giardiasis • Salmonellosis • Shigellosis • Traveler's diarrhea, *E. coli*

CASE 58

HX	PE	DDX
40 yo F presents with fever, anorexia, nausea, profuse and watery diarrhea, and diffuse abdominal pain. Last week she was on antibiotics for a UTI.	VS: T 38°C (100.4°F), BP 100/50, HR 100, RR 22, orthostatic hypotension Gen: WNL Lungs: WNL CV: Tachycardia Abd: Diffuse tenderness, no peritoneal signs, ⊕ BS Rectal exam: Guaiac ⊕	• Amebiasis • Food poisoning • Gastroenteritis • Giardiasis • Hepatitis A • Infectious diarrhea (bacterial, viral, parasitic, protozoal) • Inflammatory bowel disease • Pseudomembranous (*C. difficile*) colitis • Traveler's diarrhea

INITIAL MGMT	CONTINUING MGMT	F/U
Office W/U • CBC • Chem 14 • UA • Stool for ova and parasites • Stool occult blood • Stool Gram stain • Stool fat stain • Barium enema • CT—abdomen • Ferritin • Serum folate • Serum B_{12} • Serum endomysial antibody: $\oplus$ titers • Serum transglutaminase antibody: $\oplus$ titers	**Ward W/U** • CXR: $\ominus$ • KUB: $\ominus$ • CT—abdomen: $\ominus$ • D-xylose tolerance test: Carbohydrate malabsorption • Peroral duodenal biopsy: Villi are atrophic or absent • Dietary consult **Rx** • Gluten-free diet • Prednisone • Vitamin D • Calcium	• Follow up in one week • Patient counseling • Pneumococcal vaccine

Final Dx - Celiac disease

INITIAL MGMT	CONTINUING MGMT	F/U
Emergency room W/U • CBC • Chem 14 • Stool culture • Fecal leukocyte stain • Stool for *C. difficile* • Stool Gram stain • Stool for ova and parasites • Stool occult blood • Stool fat stain • UA and urine culture	**Emergency room W/U** • Stool culture: $\oplus$ for *E. coli* • Stool Gram stain: $\oplus$ for gram-$\ominus$ rods and $\uparrow$ leukocytes **Rx** • Oral hydration • Ciprofloxacin	• Follow up in one week • Patient counseling • Counsel patient to limit alcohol intake • Smoking cessation

Final Dx - Gastroenteritis

INITIAL MGMT	CONTINUING MGMT	F/U
Emergency room W/U • Stool culture • Stool *Giardia* antigen • Stool for ova and parasites • Stool WBCs: $\oplus$ • Stool for *C. difficile*: $\oplus$ • CBC: $\uparrow$ WBC count • Chem 14 **Rx** • IV normal saline • Metronidazole	**Ward W/U** • No orthostatic hypotension **Rx** • Send home on metronidazole (when diarrhea improves)	• Counsel patient re oral hydration

Final Dx - Pseudomembranous (*C. difficile*) colitis

CASE 59

HX	PE	DDX
33 yo M presents with foul-smelling, watery diarrhea together with diffuse abdominal cramps and bloating that began yesterday. He also vomited once. He was recently in Mexico.	VS: T 37°C (98°F), BP 110/50, HR 85, RR 22, no orthostatic hypotension Gen: WNL Lungs: WNL CV: WNL Abd: No tenderness, no peritoneal signs, ⊕ BS Rectal exam: Guaiac ⊖	• Amebiasis • Food poisoning • Gastroenteritis • Giardiasis • Hepatitis A • Infectious diarrhea (bacterial, viral, parasitic, protozoal) • Inflammatory bowel disease • Pseudomembranous (*C. difficile*) colitis • Traveler's diarrhea

GI Bleeding

CASE 60

HX	PE	DDX
38 yo M presents with intermittent hematemesis of two weeks duration. He has a history of epigastric pain for almost two years that occasionally worsens when he eats food or drinks milk. He also reports melena of three weeks' duration. His social history is ⊕ for alcohol and tobacco use.	VS: T 37°C (98.9°F), BP 90/65, HR 110, RR 24 Gen: Pallor Lungs: WNL CV: WNL Abd: No tenderness, no peritoneal signs, normal BS Rectal exam: WNL, guaiac ⊕ **Limited PE**	• Duodenal ulcers • Esophageal tear • Gastric carcinoma • Gastric ulcer • Portal hypertension

INITIAL MGMT	CONTINUING MGMT	F/U

Office W/U
- Stool culture
- Stool *Giardia* antigen: $\oplus$
- Stool for ova and parasites
- Stool WBCs
- Stool for *C. difficile*
- CBC
- Chem 8

Rx
- Metronidazole

- Counsel patient re oral hydration

Final Dx - Giardiasis

INITIAL MGMT	CONTINUING MGMT	F/U

Emergency room STAT
- IV normal saline
- O_2
- Orthostatic vitals: $\oplus$
- Type and crossmatch

Emergency room W/U
- CBC: Hematocrit 24
- Chem 14
- Upper GI series: Gastric antral lesion with adherent clot
- PT/PTT, INR
- CXR
- ECG

Rx
- NPO
- NG tube, iced saline lavage: Clears with 1 L of normal saline
- IV pantoprazole
- IV cimetidine

ICU W/U
- CBC q 4 h until hematocrit is stable; then frequency can be ↓

Rx
- GI consult
- Combination therapy with epinephrine injection followed by thermal coagulation
- Octreotide
- Advance diet
- Ranitidine
- Pantoprazole
- Transfer to wards if patient remains stable

- Follow up in one week
- Patient counseling
- Counsel patient to cease alcohol intake
- Smoking cessation
- Dietary consult

Final Dx - Bleeding gastric ulcer

CASE 61

HX	PE	DDX
67 yo F presents with acute crampy abdominal pain, weakness, and black stool. She reports diffuse abdominal pain of three months' duration. Eating worsens the pain. She has had a five-pound weight loss over the last three months.	VS: T 37°C (98.9°F), BP 90/65, HR 100, RR 24 Gen: Mild dehydration Lungs: WNL CV: WNL Abd: Tender and mildly distended; no rigidity or rebound tenderness Rectal exam: WNL, guaiac ⊕ **Limited PE**	• Adenocarcinoma of the colon • Appendicitis • Crohn's disease • Diverticulitis • Duodenal ulcers • Infectious colitis • Ischemic colitis • Ulcerative colitis

CASE 62

HX	PE	DDX
30 yo M presents with loose, watery stools that are streaked with blood and mucus. He has also had colicky abdominal pain and weight loss over the past three weeks. He denies any history of travel, radiation, or recent medication use (antibiotics, NSAIDs).	VS: T 37°C (99°F), BP 130/65, HR 70, RR 14 Gen: NAD Lungs: WNL CV: WNL Abd: WNL Rectal exam: Blood-stained stool	• Crohn's disease • Diverticulitis • Gastroenteritis • Infectious colitis • Internal hemorrhoid • Ischemic colitis • Pseudomembranous colitis • Radiation colitis • Ulcerative colitis

INITIAL MGMT	CONTINUING MGMT	F/U

Emergency room STAT
- IV normal saline
- O$_2$

Emergency room W/U
- CBC
- Chem 14
- Serum amylase: ↑
- LDH: ↑
- PT/PTT
- CXR
- ECG
- AXR
- CT—abdomen:
- Blood type and crossmatch

Rx
- NPO
- Surgery consult (for bowel resection)
- Broad-spectrum antibiotics
- NG tube suction

Ward W/U
- Hemoglobin and hematocrit q 4 h

Rx
- Advance diet
- Monitor carefully for persistent fever, leukocytosis, peritoneal irritation, diarrhea, and/or bleeding

- Follow up in four weeks
- Patient counseling
- Counsel patient to cease alcohol intake
- Smoking cessation
- Dietary consult

Final Dx - Ischemic colitis

INITIAL MGMT	CONTINUING MGMT	F/U

Office W/U
- CBC: Mild anemia
- Chem 14
- Serum amylase, lipase
- Stool culture and sensitivity
- Stool for ova and parasites
- Stool WBCs
- PT/PTT
- Flexible sigmoidoscopy and rectal biopsy: Consistent with ulcerative colitis involving rectum and distal sigmoid colon

Rx
- IV steroids (for attack) or
- 5-ASA enema/suppositories
- Sulfasalazine

- Follow up in two weeks
- Counsel patient re medication compliance and adherence

Final Dx - Ulcerative colitis

HIGH-YIELD CASES

CASE 63

HX	PE	DDX
58 yo M presents with painless bright red blood in his stool. He reports that his diet is low in fiber.	VS: T 37°C (98°F), BP 130/85, HR 90, RR 20 Gen: Pallor, diaphoresis Lungs: WNL CV: WNL Abd: Soft, nontender, no peritoneal signs, ⊕ BS Rectal exam: Bloody stool	• Colon cancer • Crohn's disease • Diverticulitis • Diverticulosis • Ulcerative colitis

Hematuria

CASE 64

HX	PE	DDX
71 yo Asian M presents with a three-month history of low back pain that is 3/6 in severity and steady with no radiation. He has BPH and denies any history of trauma.	VS: T 37°C (98.5°F), P 76, BP 140/75, RR 14 Gen: NAD Neck: WNL Back: Tenderness along lumbar spine (L4, L5) Lungs: WNL CV: WNL Abd: WNL Rectal exam: Irregular, enlarged prostate; hemoccult ⊖ Ext: WNL Neuro: WNL	• Disk herniation • Lumbar muscle strain • Muscular spasm • Osteoporosis • Prostate cancer • Sciatic irritation • Spinal stenosis • Tumor in the vertebral canal

CASE 65

HX	PE	DDX
40 yo M complains of a slow-onset dull pain in his left flank and blood in his urine. His father died of a stroke.	VS: T 37°C (98°F), P 98, BP 150/95, RR 18 Gen: WD/WN HEENT: WNL Lungs: WNL CV: WNL (no pericardial rub) Abd: Palpable, nontender mass on both flanks Ext: WNL	• Cystic disease of the kidney • Polycystic kidney disease • Renal cell carcinoma • Renal dysplasia • Simple renal cysts • Tuberous sclerosis • Wilms' tumor

INITIAL MGMT	CONTINUING MGMT	F/U

Emergency room W/U
- NPO
- IV normal saline
- CBC: ↓ hemoglobin
- Chem 14
- PT/PTT
- Serum amylase, lipase
- UA
- CXR
- CT—abdomen: Diverticulosis

Ward W/U
- Colonoscopy: Diverticulosis, no other bleeding source

Rx
- NPO → clear liquid diet
- Surgery consult
- GI consult

- Follow up in four weeks
- Patient counseling
- Counsel patient to cease alcohol intake
- Smoking cessation
- Dietary consult
- High-fiber diet

Final Dx - Diverticulosis

INITIAL MGMT	CONTINUING MGMT	F/U

Office W/U
- CBC
- Chem 14
- UA
- ESR: ↑
- PSA: ↑↑
- XR—back: Metastatic lesions in L4 and L5
- CT—lumbar spine: Mets to L4 and L5
- Echo—rectal: Multinodular enlarged prostate
- Prostate biopsy: Pending

Rx
- Acetaminophen
- Morphine or codeine (if pain persists)

Office W/U
- Bone scan: Diffuse metastases
- Prostate biopsy: Adenocarcinoma
- CT—abdomen and pelvis: ⊕ for lymphatic involvement above aortic bifurcation

Rx
- Flutamide (antiandrogen therapy) or
- Urology consult
- Radiation treatment
- Radiation consult

- Patient counseling

Final Dx - Prostate cancer

INITIAL MGMT	CONTINUING MGMT	F/U

Office W/U
- CBC
- Chem 8
- UA: Hematuria
- U/S—renal or CT—abdomen: Bilateral renal cysts, enlarged kidneys, no liver cysts
- CT—head: No berry aneurysms

Rx
- ACEIs (e.g., captopril, enalapril, lisinopril)

Office W/U
- Nephrology consult (to look for evidence of renal insufficiency—creatinine > 2 mg/dL)
- Urology consult (for nephrectomy, cyst decompression, or unroofing)

- Follow up in eight weeks with blood testing and ultrasound
- Patient counseling
- Counsel patient to cease alcohol intake
- Smoking cessation
- Dietary consult
- Low-sodium diet
- Avoid sports

Final Dx - Polycystic kidney disease

CASE 66

HX	PE	DDX
10 yo M presents with tea-colored urine and periorbital edema. He had a fever and sore throat one week ago. He also complains of malaise, weakness, and anorexia.	VS: T 36°C (97.5°F), BP 140/85, HR 88, RR 18 Gen: Periorbital edema, pallor Lungs: WNL CV: WNL Abd: WNL Ext: Edema around ankles	• Cryoglobulinemia • IgA nephropathy • Membranoproliferative glomerulonephritis • Poststreptococcal glomerulonephritis (PSGN)

Other Urinary Symptoms

CASE 67

HX	PE	DDX
70 yo M complains of waking up 4–5 times a night to urinate. He also has urgency, a weak stream, dribbling, and he needs to strain to initiate urination. He denies any weight loss, fatigue, or bone pain. He also has a sensation of incomplete evacuation of urine from the bladder.	VS: T 37°C (98.5°F), P 78, BP 140/85, RR 14 Gen: NAD Neck: WNL Lungs: WNL CV: WNL Abd: WNL Ext: WNL Rectal exam: Enlarged, nodular, nontender, rubbery prostate gland	• Benign prostatic hypertrophy • Bladder cancer • Bladder stones • Bladder trauma • Chronic pelvic pain • Cystitis • Neurogenic bladder • Prostate cancer • Prostatitis • Urethral strictures • UTI

CASE 68

HX	PE	DDX
39 yo M complains of sudden-onset fever and chills, urgency and burning on urination, and perineal pain. His symptoms started after he underwent urethral dilatation for stricture.	VS: T 37.3°C (99°F), P 65, BP 101/64, RR 16 Gen: No acute distress Lungs: WNL CV: WNL Abd: Suprapubic tenderness GU: Genitalia WNL Rectal exam: Asymmetrically swollen, firm, markedly tender, hot prostate	• Acute cystitis • Anal fistulas and fissures • Epididymitis • Obstructive calculus • Orchitis • Prostatitis • Pyelonephritis • Reiter's syndrome • Urethritis

INITIAL MGMT	CONTINUING MGMT	F/U
Emergency room W/U • CBC • Chem 8 • UA: Hematuria, proteinuria, RBC casts • 24-hour urine protein: Proteinuria • ASO titer: ⊕ • Throat culture: Pending • Total serum complement: ↓ **Rx** • Furosemide • Captopril • Penicillin	**Office W/U** • U/S—renal • Throat culture: ⊕ **Rx** • Furosemide • Captopril • Nephrology consult	• Follow up in three weeks with UA and periodic BP monitoring • Family counseling • Dietary consult • Low-sodium diet • Restrict fluid intake

Final Dx - Acute glomerulonephritis (PSGN)

INITIAL MGMT	CONTINUING MGMT	F/U
Office W/U • CBC • BMP: Creatinine • UA • Urine culture • U/S—prostate • ESR • Total serum PSA • Residual urinary volume **Rx** • Finasteride • Prazosin (selective short-acting α_1-blockers)	**Office W/U** • Urology consult • Urodynamic studies	• Follow up in six months with digital rectal examination and PSA • Patient counseling • Dietary consult

Final Dx - Benign prostatic hypertrophy (BPH)

INITIAL MGMT	CONTINUING MGMT	F/U
Office W/U • UA • Urine Gram stain and culture • CBC • Chem 8 • VDRL **Rx** • TMP-SMX or fluoroquinolone	**Office W/U** • Urology consult • Cystoscopy	• Follow up in four weeks • Patient counseling • Counsel patient to cease alcohol intake • Smoking cessation • Counsel patient re safe sex practices • Treat sexual partner

Final Dx - Prostatitis

HIGH-YIELD CASES

CASE 69

HX	PE	DDX
21 yo M complains of a burning sensation during urination and urethral discharge. He has a history of unprotected sex with a new sexual partner. He denies urinary frequency, urgency, fever, chills, sweats, or nausea.	VS: T 37.3°C (99°F), P 65, BP 101/64, RR 16 Gen: No acute distress Lungs: WNL CV: WNL Abd: Mild suprapubic tenderness GU: Erythema of urethral meatus, no penile lesions, pus expressed from urethra	• Acute cystitis • Epididymitis • Nephrolithiasis • Orchitis • Prostatitis • Pyelonephritis • Reiter's syndrome • Urethritis

CASE 70

HX	PE	DDX
20 yo F presents with a two-day history of dysuria, ↑ urinary frequency, and suprapubic pain. She is sexually active only with her husband. She has no flank pain, fever, or nausea.	VS: P 65, BP 101/64, RR 16 Gen: No acute distress Lungs: WNL CV: WNL Abd: Mild suprapubic tenderness Pelvic: WNL	• Acute cystitis • Nephrolithiasis • PID • Pyelonephritis • Urethritis • Vaginitis

Amenorrhea

CASE 71

HX	PE	DDX
21 yo F complains of irregular menstrual periods once every 3–5 months since menarche at age 15. She also complains of ↑ facial hair.	VS: T 36°C (97°F), BP 120/60, HR 80, RR 16, weight 230 Gen: Obese Skin: Thick hair on face, chest, and buttocks Breast: WNL Lungs: WNL CV: WNL Abd: WNL Pelvic: WNL	• Adrenal neoplasms • Congenital adrenal hyperplasia • Idiopathic hirsutism • Ovarian neoplasm • Polycystic ovarian syndrome

INITIAL MGMT	CONTINUING MGMT	F/U

Office W/U
- UA and urine culture
- Urethral Gram stain: Many WBCs/hpf without bacteria
- Urethral GC culture (for *Neisseria gonorrhoeae* and *Chlamydia trachomatis*)
- CBC
- BMP
- VDRL

Rx
- Azithromycin and doxycycline

- Follow up in four weeks
- Patient counseling
- Counsel patient to cease alcohol intake
- Smoking cessation
- Treat sexual partner
- Counsel patient re safe sex practices

Final Dx - Urethritis

INITIAL MGMT	CONTINUING MGMT	F/U

Office W/U
- UA: ↑↑ WBCs, +4 bacteria, ⊕ nitrites, ⊕ esterase
- Urine culture
- CBC
- Chem 8
- Pregnancy test-urinary

Rx
- TMP-SMX × 3 days

Office W/U
- Urine culture: ⊕ for *E. coli* sensitive to TMP-SMX

Rx
- TMP-SMX

Final Dx - Acute cystitis

INITIAL MGMT	CONTINUING MGMT	F/U

Office W/U
- DHEAS
- Testosterone: ↑
- U/S—pelvis: Ovaries with multiple small cysts
- Serum 17-hydroxyprogesterone
- LH/FSH: ↑
- Prolactin
- TSH

Rx
- Weight loss diet
- Exercise program
- OCPs
- Spironolactone

- Follow up in six months

Final Dx - Polycystic ovarian syndrome (PCOS)

HIGH-YIELD CASES

CASE 72

HX	PE	DDX
50 yo F presents with hot flashes and dyspareunia. Her last menstrual period was six months ago.	VS: T 36°C (97°F), BP 120/60, HR 70, RR 13 Gen: NAD HEENT: WNL Breast: WNL Lungs: WNL CV: WNL Abd: WNL Pelvic: Atrophy of vaginal mucosa	• Hyperthyroidism • Hypothyroidism • Menopause • Pregnancy • Prolactinoma

CASE 73

HX	PE	DDX
14 yo F is brought into the office by her mother. The mother is concerned because her daughter is considerably shorter than her classmates and because her daughter has not yet had her menses. The girl's parents are of normal height, and her sisters had their menses at age 13.	VS: Afebrile, BP 110/70, HR 70, RR 12 Gen: Short stature HEENT: Low posterior hairline, high-arched palate Neck: Short and wide Lungs: Widely spaced nipples CV: Tachycardia, irregular	• Constitutional growth delay • Familial short stature • Hypopituitarism • Hypothyroidism • Turner's syndrome

INITIAL MGMT	CONTINUING MGMT	F/U

Office W/U
- Urine pregnancy test
- Prolactin
- TSH
- FSH: ↑
- Wet mount
- Pap smear
- Mammogram
- DEXA scan

Rx
- Calcium
- Vitamin D
- SSRI (venlafaxine) for hot flashes
- Premarin (vaginal estrogen)
- Vaginal jelly for lubrication

- Follow up in 12 months
- Counsel patient re HRT—not recommended unless only short-term treatment is planned and if the patient has no CHD, breast cancer, or thromboembolic risk factors

Final Dx - Menopause

INITIAL MGMT	CONTINUING MGMT	F/U

Office W/U
- TSH
- FSH: ↑
- LH: ↑
- Karyotyping: Consistent with Turner's syndrome
- Lipid panel
- Fasting glucose

Rx
- Growth hormone therapy
- Estrogen + progestin
- Psychiatry consult for IQ estimation
- Vitamin D
- Calcium

Office W/U
- 2D echocardiography
- U/S—renal
- U/S—pelvis: Streaked ovaries
- Skeletal survey: Short fourth metacarpal
- Chem 13
- CBC
- UA
- Lipid profile
- Hearing test

Rx
- Continue growth hormone therapy until epiphysis is closed
- Combination estrogen and progestin
- Encourage weight-bearing exercises

- Stop growth hormone when bone age > 15 years
- Audiogram every 3–5 years
- Check yearly for hypertension
- Monitor aortic root diameter every 3–5 years

Final Dx - Turner's syndrome

Vaginal Bleeding

CASE 74

HX	PE	DDX
17 yo F presents with prolonged and excessive menstrual bleeding and ↑ menstrual frequency for the past six months.	VS: T 36°C (97°F), BP 120/60, HR 80, RR 14 Gen: WNL HEENT/neck: WNL Lungs: WNL CV: WNL Abd: WNL Pelvic: WNL	• Dysfunctional uterine bleeding • Fibroids • Hyperthyroidism • Hypothyroidism • Pregnancy

CASE 75

HX	PE	DDX
27 yo F whose last menstrual period was seven weeks ago presents with lower abdominal cramping and heavy vaginal bleeding.	VS: T 36°C (97°F), BP 120/60, HR 80, RR 12 Gen: NAD Lungs: WNL CV: WNL Abd: Suprapubic tenderness with no rebound or guarding Pelvic: Active bleeding from cervix, cervical os open, seven-week-size uterus, mildly tender, no cervical motion tenderness, no adnexal masses or tenderness	• Cervical or vaginal pathology (polyp, infection, neoplasia) • Cervical polyp • Ectopic pregnancy • Menstrual period with dysmenorrhea • Spontaneous abortion

CASE 76

HX	PE	DDX
60 yo F G0 who had her last menstrual period 10 years ago presents with mild vaginal bleeding for the last two days. Her medical history is significant for type 2 diabetes, hypertension, and infertility.	VS: T 36°C (97°F), BP 120/60, HR 80, RR 14 Gen: NAD HEENT: WNL Lungs: WNL CV: WNL Abd: WNL Pelvic: WNL	• Atrophic endometritis • Cervical cancer • Endometrial cancer • Endometrial polyp

INITIAL MGMT	CONTINUING MGMT	F/U

Office W/U
- Qualitative urine pregnancy test
- TSH
- CBC: Hypochromic microcytic anemia
- Bleeding time
- PT/PTT, INR
- U/S—pelvis
- Pap smear

Rx
- OCPs
- NSAIDs
- Iron sulfate

		• Follow up in six months
		• Counsel patient re safe sex practices

Final Dx - Dysfunctional uterine bleeding

INITIAL MGMT	CONTINUING MGMT	F/U

Emergency room W/U
- Qualitative urine pregnancy test: ⊕
- Quantitative serum β-hCG: 3000
- CBC: Hemoglobin 9
- Blood type and crossmatch
- Rh factor
- U/S—pelvis: Intrauterine pregnancy sac, fetal pole, no fetal heart tones
- Gynecology consult

Rx
- Fluids, IV normal saline
- D&C

Ward W/U
- CBC

Rx
- Methylergonovine
- Doxycycline
- Counsel patient re birth control
- Grief counseling
- Pelvic rest for two weeks

- Follow up in three weeks

Final Dx - Spontaneous abortion

INITIAL MGMT	CONTINUING MGMT	F/U

Office W/U
- CBC
- Chem 14
- PT/PTT, INR
- Bleeding time
- Pap smear
- Endometrial biopsy: Poorly differentiated endometrioid adenocarcinoma
- U/S—pelvis: 10-mm endometrial stripe
- Gynecology consult

Ward W/U
- CXR
- ECG
- CA-125

Rx
- Exploratory laparotomy
- TAH-BSO
- Depending on staging, patient may benefit from adjuvant therapy (radiation vs. chemo vs. hormonal therapy)

Final Dx - Endometrial cancer

HIGH-YIELD CASES

CASE 77

HX	PE	DDX
32 yo F G2P1011 presents with vaginal bleeding after intercourse for the last month. She has no history of abnormal Pap smears or STDs and has had the same partner for the last eight years. She uses OCPs.	VS: WNL Gen: NAD Abd: WNL Pelvic: Visible cervical lesion Rectal exam: ⊖, guaiac ⊖	• Cervical cancer • Cervical polyp • Cervicitis • Ectropion • Vaginal cancer • Vaginitis

Musculoskeletal Pain

CASE 78

HX	PE	DDX
28 yo F complains of multiple facial and bodily injuries. She claims that she fell on the stairs. She was hospitalized for some physical injuries seven months ago. She denies any abuse.	VS: P 90, BP 120/64, RR 22, O_2 sat 95% room air Gen: Moderate distress with shallow breathing HEENT: 2.5-cm bruise on forehead; 2-cm bruise on left cheek Chest/lungs: Severe tenderness on left fifth and sixth ribs; CTA bilaterally CV: WNL Abd: WNL Ext: WNL Neuro: WNL	• Accident proneness • Domestic violence • Substance abuse

CASE 79

HX	PE	DDX
28 yo F presents with joint pain and swelling along with a butterfly-like rash over her nasal bridge and cheeks that worsens after exposure to the sun. She also reports pleuritic chest pain, shortness of breath, myalgia, and fatigue over the past few months. She says that her joint pain tends to move from joint to joint and primarily involves her hands, wrists, knees, and ankles. She also has weight loss, loss of appetite, and night sweats.	VS: T 38°C (101°F), BP 140/95, HR 80, RR 18 Gen: Pallor, fatigue HEENT: Oral ulcers, malar rash Lungs: CTA, pleural friction rub CV: WNL Abd: WNL Ext: Maculopapular rash over arms and chest; effusion in knees, wrists, and ankles	• Dermatomyositis • Drug reaction • Photosensitivity • Polymyositis • Systemic lupus erythematosus

INITIAL MGMT	CONTINUING MGMT	F/U
Office W/U • UA • Pap smear: HGSIL • Pelvic: Visible cervical lesion • G&C culture or PCR • Wet mount • Gynecology consult	**Office W/U** • Colposcopy • Cervical biopsy: Invasive squamous cell carcinoma of the cervix	• Radical hysterectomy versus radiation therapy • +/− adjuvant chemoradiotherapy • Console patient

Final Dx - Cervical cancer

INITIAL MGMT	CONTINUING MGMT	F/U
Emergency room W/U • XR—ribs: Fracture of left fifth and sixth ribs • Urine toxicology • CT—head • Skeletal survey: Old fracture in forearm **Rx** • Ibuprofen • Oxycodone PRN • Splint • Counsel patient re domestic abuse • Counsel patient re safety plan		• Support group referral • Social work referral

Final Dx - Domestic abuse

INITIAL MGMT	CONTINUING MGMT	F/U
Office W/U • CBC: ↓ hemoglobin • BMP • PT/PTT • ESR: ↑ • Serum ANA: ⊕ • UA: Proteinuria • CXR • Total complement: ↓ C3 and C4 **Rx** • NSAIDs	**Office W/U** • Anti-dsDNA or SLE prep: ⊕ • Bone densitometry **Rx** • Prednisone • NSAIDs • Rheumatology consult • Nephrology consult	• Follow up in four weeks with UA • Patient counseling • Counsel patient to cease alcohol intake • Smoking cessation • Sunblock

Final Dx - Systemic lupus erythematosus (SLE)

HIGH-YIELD CASES

CASE 80

HX	PE	DDX
35 yo M with a history of hypertension presents with pain and swelling in his left knee for the last three days. He was recently started on HCTZ for his hypertension. He is sexually active only with his wife and denies any history of trauma or IV drug abuse.	VS: T 38°C (100.7°F), P 80, BP 130/60, RR 12 Gen: In pain Skin: WNL HEENT: WNL Lungs: WNL CV: WNL Abd: WNL Ext: Left knee is swollen, erythematous, and tender with limited range of motion and effusion	• Bacterial arthritis • Gout • Infective endocarditis • Lyme disease • Pseudogout • Psoriatic arthritis • Reiter's arthritis

CASE 81

HX	PE	DDX
40 yo M with a history of diabetes mellitus presents with pain, swelling, and discoloration of his right leg for the last week. He denies any trauma.	VS: T 38°C (100.5°F), P 70, BP 120/60, RR 12 Gen: NAD Lungs: WNL CV: WNL Abd: WNL Ext: +2 edema in right lower extremity; warmth, erythematous discoloration of skin, 20-cm ulcer	• Calf tear or pull • Cellulitis • Deep venous thrombosis • Lymphedema • Osteomyelitis • Popliteal (Baker's) cyst • Venous insufficiency

CASE 82

HX	PE	DDX
50 yo M complains of a single episode of steady, diffuse, aching pain that affected his skeletal muscles and made it difficult for him to climb stairs. He states that he has never experienced anything like this before and that no one in his family has had a disease similar to his. Because of his ↑ LDL cholesterol, ↓ HDL cholesterol, and ↑ triglycerides, he was started on simvastatin and gemfibrozil about one year ago.	VS: T 37°C (99°F), P 85, BP 127/85, RR 20, O_2 sat 94% room air HEENT and neck: No dysarthria, dysphagia, diplopia, or ptosis; exam WNL Chest: WNL CV: WNL Abd: WNL Ext: Proximal muscle weakness that is more obvious in lower limbs; no evidence of myotonia	• Cocaine abuse • Inclusion body myositis • Myopathy due to drugs/toxins • Myotonic dystrophy • Polymyositis

INITIAL MGMT	CONTINUING MGMT	F/U

Office W/U
- CBC: ↑ WBC count
- Chem 14
- ESR: ↑
- PT/PTT, INR
- XR—left knee
- Joint aspiration fluid analysis: Gram stain ⊖, culture ⊖, ⊖ birefringent and needle-shaped crystals, WBC 8000
- Urethral Gram stain: ⊖

Rx
- NSAIDs or corticosteroids
- Discontinue HCTZ and start losartan

Ward W/U
- Blood culture: ⊖
- Urethral culture: ⊖
- Lyme serology: ⊖
- CBC: WBC is trending down

Rx
- Continue NSAIDs and corticosteroids until patient improves
- Low-purine diet

- Follow up in two weeks in the clinic
- Uric acid ↑
- Low-purine diet
- Start allopurinol or colchicine (to prevent an attack if serum uric acid > 12 or if the patient has tophaceous gout)

Final Dx - Gout

INITIAL MGMT	CONTINUING MGMT	F/U

Emergency room W/U
- CBC: ↑ WBC count
- Chem 14
- PT/PTT
- U/S—left lower extremity: ⊖ for deep venous thrombosis
- ESR
- X-ray
- Blood culture: Pending

Rx
- IV ampicillin-sulbactam
- Surgical consult: Debridement of ulcers

Ward W/U
- Blood culture: ⊖
- Blood glucose: Controlled on insulin regimen
- CBC: WBC is trending down

Rx
- Elevate the leg
- Switch to amoxicillin when patient is afebrile and symptoms improve (usually in 3–5 days)
- Discharge home

- Two weeks later his leg is back to normal
- Amoxicillin is discontinued after a course of 14 days

Final Dx - Cellulitis

INITIAL MGMT	CONTINUING MGMT	F/U

Emergency room W/U
- IV normal saline
- CBC
- BMP
- Serum CPK: ↑
- LDH: ↑
- EMG: Muscle injury
- UA: Myoglobinuria

Rx
- Counsel patient re medication side effects
- NSAIDs

Ward W/U
- CPK, LDH: ↑
- UA: ⊕ for myoglobin

Rx
- Stop the offending simvastatin and gemfibrozil

- Follow up in four weeks
- Patient counseling
- Rest at home
- Counsel patient re medication side effects

Final Dx - Myopathy due to simvastatin and gemfibrozil

CASE 83

HX	PE	DDX
21 yo F stripper complains of hot, swollen, painful knee joints following an asymptomatic dermatitis that progressed from macules to vesicles and pustules. She admits using IV drugs, binge drinking, and having sex with multiple partners. She states that about three weeks ago, during a trip to Mexico, she had dysuria, frequency, and urgency during her menses, followed a few days later by bilateral conjunctivitis.	VS: T 39°C (102°F), P 122, BP 138/82, RR 28, O$_2$ sat 96% room air HEENT and neck: WNL Chest: Four vesicles on thoracic skin CV: WNL Abd: Three vesicles and one pustule on abdominal skin Ext: Knee joints are hot, swollen, and tender; ↓ ROM due to severe pain	• *Chlamydia trachomatis* infection • *Neisseria gonorrhoeae* infection • Reactive arthritis • *S. aureus* infection • *Streptococcus* infection

CASE 84

HX	PE	DDX
25-month-old M is brought to the ER because of sudden respiratory distress. His mother does not remember the boy's immunization, developmental, or nutritional history. She states that her son fell from a sofa a few days ago, and she believes that this accident explains the boy's reluctance to walk. She adds that her son has been exposed to sick children lately and that she has used coin rubbing and cupping as folk medicine practices.	VS: T 37°C (99°F), P 129, BP 82/59, RR 40, O$_2$ sat 89% room air Gen: Undernourished HEENT and neck: Circumferential cord marks around neck; funduscopic exam shows bilateral retinal hemorrhages Chest: Rib fractures CV: WNL Ext: Circumferential burns of both feet and ankles with a smooth, clear-cut border; some light brown bruises; pain on palpation of right lower limb Neuro/psych: Withdrawn, apprehensive child	• Accidental trauma • Child abuse • Deliberate criminal violence (e.g., home invasion)

INITIAL MGMT	CONTINUING MGMT	F/U

Emergency room W/U
- CBC: ↑ WBC count
- GC culture assay: ⊕
- Blood culture: ⊖
- Arthrocentesis
- Joint fluid analysis
- Joint fluid culture: Pending
- Throat culture: Pending
- Anorectal culture: Pending
- Urine β-hCG: ⊖

Rx
- NSAIDs
- Antibiotics: Azithromycin (for *C. trachomatis*), penicillin (if susceptible), ceftriaxone (if not resistant), or fluoroquinolones (if not resistant)

Ward W/U
- Joint fluid analysis and culture: 60,000 leukocytes/mL, ⊕ for *N. gonorrhoeae*
- Throat culture
- Anorectal culture

Rx
- Azithromycin (for *C. trachomatis*), penicillin (if susceptible), ceftriaxone (if not resistant), or fluoroquinolones (if not resistant)
- Joint drainage and irrigation (if indicated)
- Arthroscopy (if indicated)

- Follow up in one week
- Patient counseling
- Counsel patient re safe sex practices
- Treat sexual partner
- Counsel patient to cease illegal drug use
- Counsel patient to cease alcohol intake
- Smoking cessation
- Rest at home

Final Dx - Septic arthritis due to *N. gonorrhoeae* infection

INITIAL MGMT	CONTINUING MGMT	F/U

Emergency room W/U
- CBC
- PT/PTT
- Chem 8
- CT—head: Short-length skull fractures; small subdural hemorrhages
- CXR: Bilateral rib fractures
- XR—femur: Obliquely oriented callus formation in right femur
- CT—lumbar spine: WNL

Rx
- Ventilator (if necessary)
- IV normal saline
- Neurosurgery consult
- Wound dressing

Ward W/U
- CXR: No atelectasis; lungs are expanded

Rx
- Ventilator (if necessary)
- IV normal saline
- Wound dressing

- Child protective services consult

Final Dx - Child abuse

CASE 85

HX	PE	DDX
36 yo F complains of malaise, anorexia, unintended weight loss, and morning stiffness together with swollen and painful wrist, knee, and ankle joints of two years' duration. Initially, she disregarded her symptoms, as they were insidious. However, over time they persisted and ↑ in severity. An acute disabling episode prompted her to visit the office.	VS: T 38°C (100°F), P 95, BP 132/86, RR 20, O_2 sat 95% room air HEENT and neck: Cervical lymphadenopathy Chest: WNL CV: WNL Ext: Symmetric wrist, knee, and ankle joint swelling with tenderness and warmth; subcutaneous nodules over both olecranon prominences; no ulnar deviation of fingers, boutonnière deformity, or swan-neck deformity; no evidence of carpal tunnel syndrome; knee valgus is observed	• Gout • Lyme disease • Osteoarthritis • Paraneoplastic syndrome • Rheumatoid arthritis • Sarcoidosis

CASE 86

HX	PE	DDX
45 yo F bus driver comes to the clinic complaining of pain radiating down the leg that followed back pain. The pain is aggravated by coughing, sneezing, straining, or prolonged sitting.	VS: T 37°C (99°F), P 86, BP 128/86, RR 20, O_2 sat 93% room air Trunk: Lumbar spine mobility ↓ due to pain Ext: ⊕ straight leg raising (Lasègue) sign; ⊕ crossed straight leg sign Neuro: Weak plantar flexion of foot; loss of Achilles tendon reflex	• Cauda equina syndrome • Compression fracture • Facet joint degenerative disease • Lumbar disk herniation • Spinal stenosis • Tumor involving the spine causing radiculopathy

INITIAL MGMT	CONTINUING MGMT	F/U
Office W/U • CBC: Hypochromic normocytic anemia, thrombocytosis • ESR: ↑ • XR—joints: Soft tissue swelling, juxta-articular demineralization, joint space narrowing, erosions in juxta-articular margin • RF: High titer **Rx** • Ibuprofen or celecoxib • Intra-articular triamcinolone (for acute disabling episodes)	**Office W/U** • RF: High titer • Joint fluid analysis: Abnormalities suggesting inflammation **Rx** • Methotrexate (if unresponsive to NSAIDs) • Etanercept (if unresponsive to methotrexate); place PPD • Hydroxychloroquine for mild disease	• Follow up in four weeks • Patient counseling • Physical therapy • Occupational therapy • Rest at home • Exercise program • Splint extremity • Ophthalmologic consult if using hydrochloroquine

Final Dx - Rheumatoid arthritis

INITIAL MGMT	CONTINUING MGMT	F/U
Office W/U • None initially **Rx** • Conservative treatment • Pain control (NSAIDs)	**Office W/U** • MRI—lumbar spine: Disk herniation at L5–S1 level (MRI is not routinely ordered for a disk herniation; it is ordered if conservative treatment fails) **Rx** • Conservative treatment • Orthopedic surgery consult (if conservative treatment fails)	• Follow up in two weeks • Patient counseling • Rest at home

Final Dx - Lumbar disk herniation

Child with Fever

CASE 87

HX	PE	DDX
40-day-old M is brought to the ER because of altered sleep patterns, vomiting, ↓ oral intake, lethargy, and irritability of a few days' duration. Today, the boy had seizures. The baby's weight at delivery was 2500 g, and he was well until last week, when he started to cry more often than usual.	VS: T 39°C (102°F), P 160, BP 77/50, RR 37, O_2 sat 92% room air Lungs: WNL CV: No murmurs or rubs Abd: WNL Ext: Mottled skin color, slow capillary refill, sparse petechiae Neuro: Lethargy, irritability, ↓ responsiveness, bulging fontanelle, seizures, ⊖ Kernig's and Brudzinski's signs	• Bacterial meningitis • CNS fungal infection (in immunocompromised patients) • HIV infection (in immunocompromised patients) • Osteomyelitis of the cervical spine • Viral meningoencephalitis

CASE 88

HX	PE	DDX
12-week-old M is brought to the ER because of apneic episodes following a runny nose, cough, labored breathing, wheezing, and fever of two days' duration. His asthmatic mother was diagnosed with rubella infection during her pregnancy. The baby was delivered prematurely at 28 weeks. The boy has a history of respiratory difficulty and tachycardia; he has missed his doctors' appointments several times.	VS: T 39°C (102°F), P 160, BP 87/58, RR 40, O_2 sat 89% room air Lungs: Tachypnea, intercostal retractions, nasal flaring, hyperresonance to percussion, expiratory wheezing, late inspiratory rales, prolonged expiratory phase CV: Tachycardia; continuous harsh murmur in second left intercostal space Neuro: Irritability	• Asthma • Congestive heart failure • Cystic fibrosis • Pneumonia • RSV bronchiolitis

INITIAL MGMT	CONTINUING MGMT	F/U

Emergency room W/U
- CBC: ↓ platelets
- PT/PTT: ↑
- Random serum glucose: 40 mg/dL
- CSF: Viral PCR pending
- Blood CSF cultures: Pending
- UA: Abnormal osmolality
- ABG and electrolytes: Metabolic acidosis, hyponatremia
- CXR
- CT—head: Small subdural effusion; no evidence of subarachnoid hemorrhage

Rx
- Empiric IV antibiotics
- IV normal saline, glucose
- Fresh frozen plasma
- IV bicarbonate

Ward W/U
- Serum glucose: 60 mg/dL
- DIC screen: ⊖
- Blood and CSF cultures: ⊕ for S. *pneumoniae*

Rx
- IV antibiotics (or antiviral or antifungal medications if appropriate)
- Fluids, $D_{5\,\frac{1}{4}}$ NSS

- Follow up in 48 hours
- Family counseling

Final Dx - Meningitis

INITIAL MGMT	CONTINUING MGMT	F/U

Emergency room W/U
- CBC: WBC 14,000
- Random serum glucose: 70 mg/dL
- CXR: Hyperinflation, bilateral patchy interstitial infiltrates, ↑ pulmonary blood flow, prominent left atrium and ventricle
- ABG: Hypoxemia
- Nasal washing for RSV

Rx
- Frequent suctioning
- IV normal saline
- O_2
- Nebulized albuterol/racemic epinephrine (controversial)
- Ventilatory and hemodynamic support (if necessary)
- Ribavirin aerosol

ICU W/U
- Random serum glucose: 70 mg/dL
- CXR: No change
- ABG: Hypoxemia
- Nasopharynx RSV antigen: ⊕

Rx
- Frequent suctioning
- IV normal saline
- O_2
- Nebulized albuterol/racemic epinephrine (controversial)
- Ventilatory and hemodynamic support
- Ribavirin aerosol

- Follow up in 48 hours
- Family counseling

Final Dx - Bronchiolitis with patent ductus arteriosus (PDA)

HIGH-YIELD CASES

CASE 89

HX	PE	DDX
8-month-old F is brought to the urgent care clinic because of abrupt onset of fever that lasted a couple of days with one seizure episode (the girl and her parents were camping in a remote area). The fever resolved after a rash appeared on the girl's chest and abdomen. Her parents did not notice any lethargy, poor feeding, or vomiting. She has no history of seizures.	VS: T 37°C (100°F); other vital signs WNL HEENT and neck: Bilateral cervical lymphadenopathy, ears WNL, ophthalmologic exam WNL Trunk: Macular rash Neuro: Alert and active; no abnormalities	• Fifth disease • Measles • Meningitis • Roseola infantum • Rubella

CASE 90

HX	PE	DDX
3-day-old M presents to the ER with ↑ temperature, lethargy, respiratory distress, and poor feeding for the past 24 hours. His Apgar scores at birth were 6 and 8. His mother had a prolonged rupture of membranes (30 hours)	VS: T 39°C (102°F), P 170, BP 74/51, RR 70, O$_2$ sat 90% room air Lungs: Grunting respiration, chest indrawing with breathing, ↓ air entry CV: No murmurs or rubs Abd: Distended; ⊖ BS Neuro: Lethargy	• *Bordetella* lung infection • *Chlamydia* lung infection • Complicated congenital lung abnormalities (e.g., sequestration) • Foreign body causing obstruction • Group B streptococcus bacterial pneumonia

Fever

CASE 91

HX	PE	DDX
49 yo F presents to the ER with fever of three days' duration. Since she turned 49 (about seven months ago), she has had recurrent infections that have been treated with antibiotics. She has also been treated with anthracyclines and alkylating agents for another disease for the past 18 months. However, she has not seen a doctor lately. She works in a manufacturing plant that produces cosmetics.	VS: T 39°C (102°F), P 132, BP 108/77, RR 29, O$_2$ sat 88% room air Lungs: No evidence of consolidation CV: WNL Abd: WNL Ext: WNL Neuro: WNL	• Deep abscess (unknown location) • Pneumonia • Pyelonephritis • Sepsis • Severe infection (unknown location)

INITIAL MGMT	CONTINUING MGMT	F/U
Office W/U • CBC: WNL **Rx** • Hydrate • Acetaminophen		• Follow up in seven days or see me as needed • Family counseling

Final Dx - Roseola infantum (exanthem subitum)

INITIAL MGMT	CONTINUING MGMT	F/U
Emergency room W/U • CBC: ↑ WBC count • Random serum glucose: 60 mg/dL • CXR: Patchy infiltrates, pleural effusion, gastric dilation • Blood cultures: Pending • Viral culture • ABG: P_{O_2} 50 mmHg, P_{CO_2} 55 mmHg **Rx** • O_2 • Fluids, D_5 ¼ NSS • Empiric IV antibiotics • Respiratory and hemodynamic support (if necessary)	**Ward W/U** • Random serum glucose: 65 mg/dL • Blood cultures: Group B streptococcus • ABG: P_{O_2} 60 mmHg, P_{CO_2} 50 mmHg **Rx** • Antibiotics • Ventilatory and hemodynamic support (if necessary) • Antiviral drugs (if appropriate) • Bronchoscopy (if indicated)	• Follow up in 48 hours • Family counseling

Final Dx - Pneumonia

INITIAL MGMT	CONTINUING MGMT	F/U
Emergency room W/U • CT—abdomen: WNL • CBC: Neutropenia • CXR: Bilateral infiltrates in both lungs • Sputum cultures: ⊕ for several bacterial species, including *Klebsiella* • Blood cultures: ⊕ for *Klebsiella* • UA: WNL • Urine cultures: ⊖ **Rx** • IV antibiotics (empiric cefepime or quinolone) • Acetaminophen • IV normal saline	**Ward W/U** • Bone marrow biopsy, needle: Low myelogenous progenitor cell lines • CT—chest, spiral: Widespread bilateral infiltrates in both lungs **Rx** • IV antibiotics (appropriate for *Klebsiella*); tailor antibiotics to sensitivies • IV normal saline • G-CSF (for neutropenia)	• Follow up in four weeks • Patient counseling • Counsel patient to cease alcohol intake • Smoking cessation • Chest physical therapy

Final Dx - Lung infection (bilateral pneumonia) in a neutropenic patient

HIGH-YIELD CASES

CASE 92

HX	PE	DDX
43 yo F presents to the ER with fever, fatigue, malaise, and diffuse musculoskeletal pain of two days' duration. She complains of difficulty moving her right eye. The patient has a history of diabetes mellitus and mitral valve prolapse with regurgitation.	VS: T 40°C (104°F), P 134, BP 113/83, RR 31, O_2 sat 93% room air Lungs: WNL CV: Regurgitant murmur Abd: WNL Ext: Petechiae on feet Neuro: CN III palsy Ophthalmology: Visual field defects, conjunctival hemorrhage Funduscopy: Abnormal spots	• Complicated pyelonephritis • Infective endocarditis • Infective process (undetermined location) • Intracranial infection • Sepsis

CASE 93

HX	PE	DDX
60 yo M presents with fever and altered mental status eight hours after undergoing a diverticular abscess drainage.	VS: T 39°C (102°F), P 110, BP 60/35, RR 22, O_2 sat 92% on 2-L NC Gen: Acute distress HEENT: WNL Lungs: WNL CV: Tachycardia Abd: Lower abdominal tenderness Neuro: WNL	• Cardiogenic shock • Hypovolemic shock • Septic shock

INITIAL MGMT	CONTINUING MGMT	F/U

Emergency room W/U
- ESR: 59 mm/hr
- CBC: ↑ WBC
- CXR: Some areas of patchy consolidation
- Blood cultures: Pending
- Echocardiography: Mobile mass attached to a valve
- ECG: RBBB
- UA: Microscopic hematuria

Rx
- IV normal saline
- O_2
- Empiric IV antibiotics (oxacillin and gentamicin)
- Acetaminophen

Ward W/U
- Blood cultures: ⊕ for S. viridans

Rx
- IV antibiotics
- Acetaminophen
- IV normal saline

- Follow up in four weeks
- Patient counseling
- Counsel patient to cease alcohol intake
- Smoking cessation

Final Dx - Infective endocarditis

INITIAL MGMT	CONTINUING MGMT	F/U

Emergency room STAT
- O_2
- IV normal saline/central line
- Blood culture: Pending
- Wound culture
- UA and urine culture

Emergency room W/U
- CBC: ↑ WBC count
- Chem 14
- ABG: Metabolic acidosis
- ECG
- Serum amylase, lipase
- Serum lactate: 6
- Cardiac enzymes
- CXR
- CT—abdomen: Persistent diverticular abscess

Rx
- Ampicillin-gentamicin-metronidazole or piperacillin-tazobactam or ticarcillin-clavulanate

ICU W/U
- Urine output q 1 h
- 2D echocardiography
- Blood culture: ⊕ for E. coli sensitive to gentamicin and ceftriaxone
- Wound culture: ⊕ for E. coli sensitive to gentamicin and ceftriaxone

Rx
- Tailor antibiotics to sensitivities
- Surgery consult

Final Dx - Septic shock

CASE 94

HX	PE	DDX
17 yo F G0 whose last menstrual period was two days ago presents with fever, vomiting, myalgia, and a generalized skin rash.	VS: T 39°C (102°F), BP 75/30, HR 120 Gen: NAD Skin: Diffuse macular erythema; hyperemic mucous membranes Lungs: WNL CV: WNL Pelvic: Menstrual flow; foul-smelling tampon **Limited PE**	• Meningococcemia • Rocky Mountain spotted fever • Streptococcal toxic shock syndrome • Toxic shock syndrome • Typhoid fever

Outpatient Potpourri

CASE 95

HX	PE	DDX
50 yo F presents with a painless lump in her right breast. She first noted this mass one month ago. There is no nipple discharge.	VS: Afebrile, P 70, BP 110/50, RR 12 Gen: NAD Skin: WNL HEENT: WNL Lymph nodes: ⊖ Breast: 3-cm, hard, immobile, non-tender mass with irregular borders; no nipple discharge Lungs: WNL CV: WNL Abd: WNL	• Breast cancer • Fibroadenoma • Fibrocystic disease • Mastitis • Papillomas

CASE 96

HX	PE	DDX
62 yo F complains of vaginal itching, painful intercourse, and a clear discharge.	VS: WNL Gen: NAD Lungs: WNL CV: WNL Pelvic: Vulvar erythema, thin and pale mucosa with areas of erythema, clear discharge, mucosa bleeds easily during exam	• Atrophic vaginitis • Bacterial vaginosis • Candidal vaginitis • Cervicitis (chlamydia, gonorrhea) • Trichomonal vaginitis

INITIAL MGMT	CONTINUING MGMT	F/U

Emergency room STAT
- O_2 inhalation
- IV normal saline
- Tampon removal

Emergency room W/U
- CBC with differential
- Chem 14
- UA
- Blood culture: Pending
- Urine culture: Pending

Rx
- IV clindamycin + vancomycin
- Methylprednisone

ICU W/U
- Blood culture: ⊖
- Urine culture: ⊖

Rx
- Continue IV clindamycin and vancomycin
- Wound care

Final Dx - Toxic shock syndrome

INITIAL MGMT	CONTINUING MGMT	F/U

Office W/U
- Mammography: Suspicious of tumor
- FNA biopsy: Malignancy

Rx
- Surgery consult

Final Dx - Breast cancer

INITIAL MGMT	CONTINUING MGMT	F/U

Office W/U
- Vaginal pH: 6
- Chlamydia PCR
- Gonorrhea PCR
- Wet mount
- Pap smear

Rx
- Vaginal jelly for lubrication
- Counsel patient re local HRT
- Premarin (vaginal estrogen)

- Follow up as needed

Final Dx - Atrophic vaginitis

HIGH-YIELD CASES

CASE 97

HX	PE	DDX
33 yo Rh-negative F who currently lives in a battered-women's shelter calls the on-call physician because she noticed ↓ fetal movements. She is a G1P0 pregnant F at 36 weeks' gestational age. She states that fetal growth has been normal and that her obstetric ultrasound at 18 weeks showed a single normal fetus. The patient has no known preexisting diseases and does not smoke, drink alcohol, or take medications or illicit drugs. She received a dose of anti-D at 28 weeks.	VS: T 37°C (99°F), P 96, BP 141/91, RR 26, O_2 sat 93% room air Gen: No jaundice Eyes: Normal vision Lungs: No rales CV: No gallops or murmurs Pelvic: Fundal height in centimeters is appropriate for gestational age; cephalic presentation; speculum exam reveals unripe cervix, no ferning, nitrazine ⊖ Ext: Slight pedal edema	• Preeclampsia • Pregnancy-induced hypertension

CASE 98

HX	PE	DDX
30 yo F presents for her regular checkup. She denies any complaints but is concerned about her BP, as it has been high on both of her previous visits over the past two months.	VS: P 75, BP 160/90 (no difference in BP between both arms), RR 12 Gen: WNL HEENT: WNL Breast: WNL Lungs: WNL CV: WNL Abd: WNL Pelvic: WNL Ext: WNL Neuro: WNL	• Cushing's disease • Essential hypertension • Hyperaldosteronism • Hyperthyroidism • Pheochromocytoma • Renal artery stenosis • White coat hypertension/anxiety

CASE 99

HX	PE	DDX
6 yo M is brought by his mother with continuous oozing of blood from the site of a tooth extraction he underwent two days ago. The bleeding initially stopped but restarted spontaneously a few hours later. His mother denies any history of epistaxis, easy bruising, petechiae, or bleeding per rectum. The patient's mother has a brother with hemophilia.	VS: Afebrile, P 80, BP 80/50, RR 14 Gen: NAD Skin: WNL HEENT: Blood oozing from site of extracted tooth Lungs: WNL CV: WNL Abd: WNL Ext: WNL	• DIC • Hemophilia • ITP • Liver disease • TTP • Vitamin K deficiency • von Willebrand's disease

INITIAL MGMT	CONTINUING MGMT	F/U
Office W/U • Bun, Creatinine, ALT, AST • CBC • Chem 8 • UA: ⊕ protein • Random serum glucose • Serum uric acid **Rx** • Complete bed rest • Monitor, continue BP cuff • Fetal monitoring	**Ward W/U** • UA: Protein 0.3 g/L/24 hrs; normal sediment • LFTs: WNL **Rx** • Complete bed rest • Monitor, continue BP cuff • Fetal monitoring	• Patient counseling • Counsel patient to cease alcohol intake • Smoking cessation • Admit to labor and delivery for induction of labor • Obstetric consult

Final Dx - Antenatal disorder: Pregnancy-induced hypertension

INITIAL MGMT	CONTINUING MGMT	F/U
Office W/U • Lipid profile • Chem 14 • CBC • UA: +1 protein • ECG: LVH • Echocardiography: LVH • TSH **Rx** • Lisinopril • Exercise program • Low-sodium diet	**Office W/U** • Consider workup for 2° hypertension given the patient's young age (MRI/MRA renal arteries, urine catecholamines, urine cortisol)	• Follow up in one month

Final Dx - Essential hypertension

INITIAL MGMT	CONTINUING MGMT	F/U
Office W/U • CBC • Peripheral smear • Bleeding time • PTT: Prolonged • PT, INR • Plasma factor VIII: 3% • Plasma factor IX **Rx** • Factor VIII therapy • Genetics consult • Consel parents		• Console and reassure patient • Patient counseling • Family counseling

Final Dx - Hemophilia

CASE 100

HX	PE	DDX
27 yo F complains of pain during intercourse. She has a long history of painful periods.	VS: WNL Gen: NAD Lungs: WNL CV: WNL Pelvic: Normal vaginal walls, normal cervix, mild cervical motion tenderness; uterus tender, retroverted, and fixed; right adnexa slightly enlarged and tender	• Endometriosis • PID • Vaginismus • Vaginitis

INITIAL MGMT	CONTINUING MGMT	F/U

Office W/U
- Wet mount
- Chlamydia DNA probe
- Gonorrhea DNA probe
- U/S—pelvis: Retroverted uterus of normal size; 2- × 3-cm cyst on the right adnexa that may represent a hemorrhagic corpus luteum or endometrioma

Rx
- NSAIDs
- OCPs

- If initial treatment with OCPs and NSAIDs does not relieve pain, refer to a gynecologist for a trial of GnRH analogs, progestins, or danazol.
- Follow up as needed

Final Dx - Endometriosis

Acronyms and Abbreviations

Abbreviation	Meaning
5-ASA	5-aminosalicylic acid
5-FU	5-fluorouracil
5-HT	5-hydroxytryptamine (serotonin)
6-MP	6-mercaptopurine
A-a	alveolar-arterial (oxygen gradient)
ABG	arterial blood gas
AC	alternating current
ACEI	angiotensin-converting enzyme inhibitor
ACh	acetylcholine
ACL	anterior cruciate ligament
ACLS	advanced cardiac life support
ACTH	adrenocorticotropic hormone
ADH	antidiuretic hormone
AFB	acid-fast bacillus
AFI	amniotic fluid index
AFP	α-fetoprotein
AHI	apnea-hypopnea index
AICD	automatic implantable cardiac defibrillator
AIDS	acquired immunodeficiency syndrome
ALL	acute lymphocytic leukemia
ALP	alkaline phosphatase
ALS	amyotrophic lateral sclerosis
ALT	alanine transaminase
AMA	antimitochondrial antibody
AML	acute myelogenous leukemia
ANA	antinuclear antibody
ANC	absolute neutrophil count
ANCA	antineutrophil cytoplasmic antibody
ANS	autonomic nervous system
ARB	angiotensin receptor blocker
ARDS	acute respiratory distress syndrome
ARF	acute renal failure
ARR	absolute risk reduction
ASA	acetylsalicylic acid (aspirin)
ASD	atrial septal defect
ASMA	antismooth muscle antibody
ASO	antistreptolysin O
AST	aspartate transaminase
ATN	acute tubular necrosis

Abbreviation	Meaning
AV	arteriovenous, atrioventricular
AVM	arteriovenous malformation
AVN	avascular necrosis
AXR	abdominal x-ray
AZT	azidothymidine (zidovudine)
BAL	British anti-Lewisite (dimercaprol)
BCG	bacille Calmette-Guérin
BID	twice daily
BMP	bone morphogenic protein
BMT	bone marrow transplantation
BP	blood pressure
BPH	benign prostatic hypertrophy
BPP	biophysical profile
BPPV	benign paroxysmal positional vertigo
BS	bowel sounds
BSA	body surface area
BUN	blood urea nitrogen
CAD	coronary artery disease
CALLA	common acute lymphoblastic leukemia antigen
c-ANCA	cytoplasmic antineutrophil cytoplasmic antibody
CAP	community-acquired pneumonia
CBC	complete blood count
CBT	cognitive-behavioral therapy, computer-based test
CCS	Computer-Based Clinical Simulation
CD	cluster of differentiation
CEA	carcinoembryonic antigen
CF	cystic fibrosis
CGD	chronic granulomatous disease
cGMP	cyclic guanosine monophosphate
CHF	congestive heart failure
CI	confidence interval
CIN	Candidate Identification Number, cervical intraepithelial neoplasia
CIS	carcinoma in situ
CK-MB	creatine phosphokinase, MB fraction
CLL	chronic lymphocytic leukemia
CML	chronic myelogenous leukemia
CMT	cervical motion tenderness
CMV	cytomegalovirus

Abbreviation	Meaning
CN	cranial nerve
CNS	central nervous system
COPD	chronic obstructive pulmonary disease
CPAP	continuous positive airway pressure
CPR	cardiopulmonary resuscitation
CPS	child protective services
CrCl	creatinine clearance
CRF	chronic renal failure
CRP	C-reactive protein
CSF	cerebrospinal fluid
CST	contraction stress test
CT	computed tomography
CTA	clear to auscultation
CV	cardiovascular
CVA	cerebrovascular accident
CVS	chorionic villus sampling
CXR	chest x-ray
D&C	dilation and curettage
DA	dopamine
DC	direct current
DCIS	ductal carcinoma in situ
DDAVP	1-deamino-8-D-arginine vasopressin
DES	diethylstilbestrol
DEXA	dual-energy x-ray absorptiometry
DHEA	dehydroepiandrosterone
DHEAS	dehydroepiandrosterone sulfate
DI	diabetes insipidus
DIC	disseminated intravascular coagulation
DIP	distal interphalangeal (joint)
DKA	diabetic ketoacidosis
DL_{CO}	diffusing capacity of carbon monoxide
DM	diabetes mellitus
DNA	deoxyribonucleic acid
DNR	do not resuscitate
DO	doctor of osteopathy
DRE	digital rectal examination
DTaP	diphtheria, tetanus, acellular pertussis (vaccine)
DTRs	deep tendon reflexes
DTs	delirium tremens
DVT	deep venous thrombosis
D_5W	5% dextrose in water
DWI	diffusion-weighted imaging
EBV	Epstein-Barr virus
ECFMG	Educational Commission for Foreign Medical Graduates
ECG	electrocardiography
ECT	electroconvulsive therapy
ED	erectile dysfunction
EDTA	calcium disodium edetate
EEG	electroencephalography
EF	ejection fraction
EGD	esophagogastroduodenoscopy

Abbreviation	Meaning
ELISA	enzyme-linked immunosorbent assay
EM	erythema multiforme
EMG	electromyography
EN	erythema nodosum
ENT	ear, nose, and throat
EPS	extrapyramidal symptoms
ER	emergency room, estrogen receptor
ERCP	endoscopic retrograde cholangiopancreatography
ESR	erythrocyte sedimentation rate
ESWL	extracorporeal shock-wave lithotripsy
ETDIR	estimated total daily insulin requirement
EtOH	ethanol
FAP	familial adenomatous polyposis
Fe_{Na}	fractional excretion of sodium
FEV_1	forced expiratory volume in one second
FFP	fresh frozen plasma
FiO_2	forced inspiratory oxygen
FISH	fluorescent in situ hybridization
FNA	fine-needle aspiration
FSH	follicle-stimulating hormone
FSMB	Federation of State Medical Boards
FT_4	free thyroxine
FTA-ABS	fluorescent treponemal antibody absorption
FUO	fever of unknown origin
FVC	forced vital capacity
GA	gestational age
GAD	generalized anxiety disorder
GBM	glomerular basement membrane
GBS	group B streptococcus
GCS	Glasgow Coma Scale
G-CSF	granulocyte colony-stimulating factor
GERD	gastroesophageal reflux disease
GFR	glomerular filtration rate
GGT	gamma-glutamyl transferase
GI	gastrointestinal
GM-CSF	granulocyte-macrophage colony-stimulating factor
GnRH	gonadotropin-releasing hormone
G6PD	glucose-6-phosphate dehydrogenase
GTC	generalized tonic-clonic (seizure)
GTD	gestational trophoblastic disease
GU	genitourinary
HAART	highly active antiretroviral therapy
HAV	hepatitis A virus
Hb	hemoglobin
HBV	hepatitis B virus
hCG	human chorionic gonadotropin
HCPOA	health care power of attorney
HCTZ	hydrochlorothiazide
HCV	hepatitis C virus
HDL	high-density lipoprotein
HEENT	head, eyes, ears, nose, and throat

Abbreviation	Meaning
HEV	hepatitis E virus
HGSIL	high-grade squamous intraepithelial lesion
HHC	hereditary hemochromatosis
HHNK	hyperglycemic hyperosmolar nonketotic state
Hib	*Haemophilus influenzae* type B
HIDA	hepato-iminodiacetic acid (scan)
HIPAA	Health Insurance Portability and Accountability Act
HIV	human immunodeficiency virus
HLA	human leukocyte antigen
HNPCC	hereditary nonpolyposis colorectal cancer
hpf	high-power field
HPI	history of present illness
HPV	human papillomavirus
HR	heart rate
HRT	hormone replacement therapy
HSV	herpes simplex virus
HUS	hemolytic-uremic syndrome
HVA	homovanillic acid
IBD	inflammatory bowel disease
IBS	irritable bowel syndrome
ICP	intracranial pressure
ICU	intensive care unit
Ig	immunoglobulin
IM	intramuscular
IMG	international medical graduate
INH	isoniazid
INR	International Normalized Ratio
IPV	inactivated polio vaccine
ITP	idiopathic thrombocytopenic purpura
IUD	intrauterine device
IUGR	intrauterine growth restriction
IV	intravenous
IVC	inferior vena cava
IVIG	intravenous immunoglobulin
IVP	intravenous pyelography
JVD	jugular venous distention
JVP	jugular venous pressure
KOH	potassium hydroxide
KUB	kidneys, ureter, bladder
LAP	leukocyte alkaline phosphatase
LBP	low back pain
LCL	lateral collateral ligament
LDH	lactate dehydrogenase
LDL	low-density lipoprotein
LEEP	loop electrocautery excision procedure
LFT	liver function test
LGSIL	low-grade squamous intraepithelial lesion
LH	luteinizing hormone
LKMA	liver-kidney microsomal antibody
LOC	loss of consciousness

Abbreviation	Meaning
LP	lumbar puncture
LTB	latent tuberculosis
LVH	left ventricular hypertrophy
MAOI	monoamine oxidase inhibitor
MCA	middle cerebral artery
MCHC	mean corpuscular hemoglobin concentration
MCL	medial collateral ligament
MCP	metacarpophalangeal (joint)
MCV	mean corpuscular volume
MDI	metered-dose inhaler
MEN	multiple endocrine neoplasia
MGUS	monoclonal gammopathy of undetermined significance
MHA-TP	microhemagglutination assay— *Treponema pallidum*
MI	myocardial infarction
MMR	measles, mumps, rubella (vaccine)
MoM	multiples of the mean
MRA	magnetic resonance angiography
MRCP	magnetic resonance cholangiopancreatography
MRI	magnetic resonance imaging
MRSA	methicillin-resistant *S. aureus*
MSAFP	maternal serum α-fetoprotein
MTP	metatarsophalangeal (joint)
NAD	no active disease
NAFLD	nonalcoholic fatty liver disease
NBME	National Board of Medical Examiners
NBTE	nonbacterial thrombotic endocarditis
NC	nasal cannula
NE	norepinephrine
NG	nasogastric
NHL	non-Hodgkin's lymphoma
NK	natural killer (cell)
NNT	number needed to treat
NPO	nil per os (nothing by mouth)
NPV	negative predictive value
NS	normal saline
NSAID	nonsteroidal anti-inflammatory drugs
NSCLC	non–small cell lung cancer
NST	nonstress test
NSTEMI	non-ST-elevation myocardial infarction
O&P	ova and parasites
OA	osteoarthritis
OCD	obsessive-compulsive disorder
OCP	oral contraceptive pill
OD	overdose
OR	odds ratio, operating room
ORIF	open reduction with internal fixation
OSA	obstructive sleep apnea
P	pulse
PA	posteroanterior
p-ANCA	perinuclear antineutrophil cytoplasmic antibody

Abbreviation	Meaning
PaO$_2$	partial pressure of oxygen in arterial blood
PCL	posterior cruciate ligament
PCO$_2$	partial pressure of carbon dioxide
PCOS	polycystic ovarian syndrome
PCP	phencyclidine hydrochloride, *Pneumocystis carinii* pneumonia
PCR	polymerase chain reaction
P$_{Cr}$	plasma creatinine
PCV	polycythemia vera
PDA	patent ductus arteriosus
PDE	phosphodiesterase
PE	physical examination, pulmonary embolus
PEA	pulseless electrical activity
PEEP	positive end-expiratory pressure
PET	positron emission tomography
PFT	pulmonary function test
PG	prostaglandin
PID	pelvic inflammatory disease
PIP	posterior interphalangeal (joint)
PIV	parainfluenza virus
PMI	point of maximal impulse
PMN	polymorphonuclear (leukocyte)
P$_{Na}$	plasma sodium
PO	per os (by mouth)
PO$_2$	partial pressure of oxygen
P$_{osm}$	plasma osmolarity
PPD	purified protein derivative
PPH	postpartum hemorrhage
PPI	proton pump inhibitor
PPV	positive predictive value
PR	progesterone receptor
PRN	as needed
PROM	premature rupture of membranes
PSA	prostate-specific antigen
PSGN	poststreptococcal glomerulonephritis
PT	physical therapy, prothrombin time
PTH	parathyroid hormone
PTHrP	parathyroid hormone–related peptide
PTSD	post-traumatic stress disorder
PTT	partial thromboplastin time
PTU	propylthiouracil
PUD	peptic ulcer disease
PUVA	psoralen and ultraviolet A
PVS	persistent vegetative state
PWI	perfusion-weighted imaging
RA	rheumatoid arthritis
RAST	radioallergosorbent test
RBC	red blood cell
REM	rapid eye movement
RF	rheumatoid factor
RLQ	right lower quadrant
ROM	rupture of membranes
ROS	review of systems
RPR	rapid plasma reagin

Abbreviation	Meaning
RR	relative risk, respiratory rate
RRR	relative risk reduction
RSV	respiratory syncytial virus
RTA	renal tubular acidosis
RUA	routine urinalysis
RUQ	right upper quadrant
RV	residual volume, right ventricular
RVH	right ventricular hypertrophy
SAAG	serum-ascites albumin gradient
SAH	subarachnoid hemorrhage
SBP	spontaneous bacterial peritonitis
SCID	severe combined immunodeficiency
SCLC	small cell lung cancer
SERM	selective estrogen receptor modulator
SGOT	serum glutamic oxaloacetic transaminase
SGPT	serum glutamic pyruvate transaminase
SIADH	syndrome of inappropriate antidiuretic hormone
SIDS	sudden infant death syndrome
SLE	systemic lupus erythematosus
SMA	superior mesenteric artery
SNRI	selective norepinephrine reuptake inhibitor
SOB	shortness of breath
SPEP	serum protein electrophoresis
SPN	solitary pulmonary nodule
SQ	subcutaneous
SSRI	selective serotonin reuptake inhibitor
STD	sexually transmitted disease
STEMI	ST-elevation myocardial infarction
SVT	supraventricular tachycardia
T	temperature
T$_3$	triiodothyronine
T$_4$	thyroxine
TAH-BSO	total abdominal hysterectomy and bilateral salpingo-oophorectomy
TB	tuberculosis
TBG	thyroxine-binding globulin
TCA	tricyclic antidepressant
Td	tetanus and diphtheria toxoid adsorbed
TD	traveler's diarrhea
TdT	tumor doubling time
TEE	transesophageal echocardiography
TENS	transcutaneous electrical nerve stimulation
TFT	thyroid function test
TGA	transposition of the great arteries
TIA	transient ischemic attack
TIBC	total iron-binding capacity
TID	three times daily
TIG	tetanus immune globulin
TIPS	transjugular intrahepatic portosystemic shunt

Abbreviation	Meaning
TLC	total lung capacity
TMP-SMX	trimethoprim-sulfamethoxazole
TNF	tumor necrosis factor
TNM	tumor, nodes, metastasis (cancer staging system)
tPA	tissue plasminogen activator
TPN	total parenteral nutrition
TPO	thyroid peroxidase
T_3RU	triiodothyronine resin uptake
TSH	thyroid-stimulating hormone
TTP	thrombotic thrombocytopenic purpura
TURP	transurethral resection of the prostate
UA	urinalysis
U_{Cr}	urine creatinine
U_{Na}	urine sodium
U_{osm}	urine osmolarity
UPPP	uvulopalatopharyngoplasty
URI	upper respiratory infection
U/S	ultrasound
USMLE	United States Medical Licensing Examination

Abbreviation	Meaning
UTI	urinary tract infection
UV	ultraviolet
UVA	ultraviolet A
UVB	ultraviolet B
VAP	ventilator-associated pneumonia
VATS	video-assisted thoracoscopy
VDRL	Venereal Disease Research Laboratory
VF	ventricular fibrillation
VMA	vanillylmandelic acid
V/Q	ventilation-perfusion (ratio)
VS	vital signs
VSD	ventricular septal defect
VT	ventricular tachycardia
VZV	varicella-zoster virus
WBC	white blood cell
WD	well developed
WN	well nourished
WNL	within normal limits
W/U	workup
XR	x-ray

Index

hyperkalemia, 157
lower GI bleed, 100
systolic heart failure, 40

Gabapentin, 238
Gadolinium, 173
Gait, 177, 178
Galactorrhea, 30
Galantamine, 180
Gallstones
    diagnosis, 97
    overview, 96
    pancreatitis, acute, 91
    symptoms/exam, 97
    treatment, 97
Gamma-glutamyl transferase (GGT),
    158, 243
Gardnerella vaginalis, 202
Gastric lavage and toxicology, 51
Gastric ulcer
    cases, high-yield CCS mini-, 312,
    313
Gastritis
    cases, high-yield CCS mini-, 300,
    301
    upper GI bleed, 98
Gastroenteritis
    cases, high-yield CCS mini-, 310,
    311
Gastroenterology
    acetaminophen toxicity, 94, 96f
    acute pancreatitis, 91–92
    alcohol abuse, 243
    antitrypsin deficiency, 96
    ascites, 100
    biliary cirrhosis, 97–98
    blood/bleeding
        cases, high-yield CCS mini-,
        312–316
        lower GI bleed, 99
        upper GI bleed, 98–99, 98f
    celiac sprue, 100, 101f
    diarrhea, 90–91
    esophageal dysphagia, 84
    gallstone disease, 96–97
    gastroesophageal reflux disease,
        84–85
    hepatitis, autoimmune, 96
    hepatitis, viral, 92, 94, 95t
    hereditary hemochromatosis, 94
    inflammatory bowel disease, 86–89
    irritable bowel syndrome, 89–90
    liver function tests, 92, 93f
    oncology
        colorectal cancer, 121–122, 122t
        hepatocellular carcinoma, 121
        pancreatic cancer, 120–121
    pediatrics
        intussusception, 223–224
        malrotation/volvulus, 224

Meckel's diverticulum, 225
pyloric stenosis, 223
peptic ulcer disease, 85–86
sclerosing cholangitis, 98
Wilson's disease, 94
Gastroesophageal reflux disease
    (GERD)
    diagnosis, 84
    hoarseness, 20
    risk factors, 84
    symptoms/exam, 84
    treatment, 84–85
Gemfibrozil, 328, 329
Gender
    alcohol abuse, 243
    amyotrophic lateral sclerosis, 179
    anorexia nervosa, 243
    breast cancer, 118
    bulimia nervosa, 244
    cluster headache, 175
    colon cancer, 122
    cystitis, uncomplicated, 134
    erythema nodosum, 23
    fibromyalgia, 148
    generalized anxiety disorder, 232
    hepatitis, autoimmune, 96
    hereditary hemochromatosis, 94
    infertility, 207
    melanoma, 125
    multiple sclerosis, 177
    myocardial infarction, 42
    nephrolithiasis, 163
    pancreatitis, acute, 92
    polycystic ovary syndrome, 204
    polycythemia vera, 108
    polymyositis, 148
    pyloric stenosis, 223
    schizophrenia, 238
    scleroderma, 149
    Sheehan's syndrome, 188
    suicide, 237
    systemic lupus erythematosus, 140
    temporal arteritis, 146
    ulcerative colitis, 87
Generalized anxiety disorder (GAD)
    diagnosis, 232
    differential diagnosis, 232
    symptoms/exam, 232
    treatment, 232
Generalized seizures
    absence, 169
    grand mal, 169
    myoclonic, 169
    status epilepticus, 169
Genetics
    celiac sprue, 100
    cystic fibrosis, 247, 248
    hereditary hemochromatosis, 94
    muscular dystrophy, 178
    psoriasis, 22

recurrent abortion, 196
screening, routine health, 210
See also Family history
Genital herpes
    overview, 135
Genitourinary
    benign prostatic hyperplasia, 30–31
    erectile dysfunction, 29–30
    incontinence, urinary, 28–29
    infectious disease
        cystitis, uncomplicated, 134
        prostatitis, 134
        pyelonephritis, 134
    oncology
        bladder carcinoma, 122–123
        cervical carcinoma, 124
        ovarian carcinoma, 124
        prostate carcinoma, 123
        testicular carcinoma, 123–124
    prostatic nodules and abnormal
        PSA, workup of, 31
    See also Urine/urinalysis
Gentamicin, 63, 157, 215
Gestational trophoblastic disease
    (GTD)
    diagnosis, 190
    hydatidiform mole, 190
    symptoms/exam, 190
    treatment, 191
Giant cell arteritis. *See* Temporal ar-
    teritis
Giardia, 137
Giardiasis
    cases, high-yield CCS mini-, 312,
    313
Gilbert's syndrome, 214
Gingival hyperplasia, 115
Glanzmann's thrombasthenia, 110
Glasgow Coma Scale, 54, 55t
Glatiramer acetate, 177
Gleason score, 123
Gleevec, 116
Glial tumors
    overview, 118
Glitazones, 67
Glomerular filtration rate (GFR)
    acute renal failure, 158, 159
    nephritic syndrome, 162
    overview, 152
Glomerulonephritis, 318, 319
Glucocorticoids, 74
Glucose
    diabetes, 66
    diabetic ketoacidosis, 62
    febrile seizures, 228
    hypercholesterolemia, 35
    hyperkalemia, 157
    hypernatremia, 155
    hyponatremia, 152
    pleural effusion, 252

Polycythemia vera (PCV)
    laboratory features, 109t
    overview, 108
Polydipsia, 69
Polyhydramnios
    oligohydramnios contrasted with,
        192t
Polymerase chain reaction (PCR)
    cervicitis/urethritis, 136
    chronic myelogenous leukemia, 116
    hepatitis, viral, 94
    herpes simplex virus, 128
Polymyalgia rheumatica
    overview, 148
Polymyositis
    diagnosis, 149
    overview, 148
    symptoms/exam, 148
    treatment, 149
Polysomnography, 258
Polyuria, 66, 69, 228
Positive end-expiratory pressure
        (PEEP), 256
Positive predictive value (PPV), 79, 79t
Postnasal drip, 18
Postobstructive pneumonia, 120
Postpartum hemorrhage (PPH), 187
Post-traumatic stress disorder (PTSD)
    diagnosis, 234
    differential diagnosis, 234
    symptoms/exam, 234
    treatment, 234
Potassium, 155, 156, 157, 159
Pott's disease, 172
Prednisone
    acute lymphocytic leukemia, 114
    asthma, 249
    cluster headache, 175
    erythema multiforme, 27
    muscular dystrophy, 178
    Pneumocystis carinii pneumonia,
        133
    polymyalgia rheumatica, 148
    sarcoidosis, 257
    temporal arteritis, 146
Preeclampsia
    defining terms, 184
    diagnosis, 185
    eclampsia vs., 186t
    gestational trophoblastic disease,
        190
    risk factors, 185
Pregnancy
    amenorrhea, 199
    breast cancer, 118
    cesarean section, indications for,
        194, 195t
    complications, medical
        diabetes mellitus, 184, 185t

hyperemesis gravidarum,
        186–187
    hyperthyroidism, maternal,
        185–186
    preeclampsia/eclampsia,
        184–185, 186t
complications, obstetrical, 192
    bleeding, third-trimester, 190,
        191t
    gestational trophoblastic disease,
        190–191
    intrauterine growth retardation,
        190
    oligohydramnios and polyhy-
        dramnios, 192t
    rhesus isoimmunization, 192
ectopic, 205–207, 302, 303
gastroesophageal reflux disease, 84
HIV (human immunodeficiency
    virus), 136
hypercoagulable state, 111
hyperemesis gravidarum, 186
hypertension, pregnancy-induced,
    342, 343
hyperthyroidism, 71
medications during, safe vs. terato-
    genic, 189t
pulmonary embolus, 254
sexual assault, 52
sickle cell anemia, 107
teratogens in, 188
vulvovaginitis, 202
See also Obstetrics
Pregnancy-induced hypertension (PIH)
    cases, high-yield CCS mini-, 342,
        343
Premarin, 198
Premature rupture of membranes
        (PROM)
    diagnosis, 193
    overview, 193
    treatment, 193
Presbycusis, 18
Preterm labor
    diagnosis, 193
    overview, 193
    patent ductus arteriosus, 221
    sepsis, neonatal, 215
    treatment, 193
Prevalence, 79
Priapism, 107
Primum CCS software, 2
    graded, how is CCS, 12
    introduction, 10
    strategies for, high-yield, 12–13
    what is the CCS like
        advancing clock to obtain results,
            11
        finishing the case, 12

interval history or physical exam,
        10
    locations, changing, 11–12
    order sheet format, 10–11
    See also Cases, high-yield CCS
        mini-
Procainamide, 56, 60
Prochlorperazine, 174
Progesterone, 200, 205
Progestin, 202
Prokinetics, 84
Prolactin, 169, 188
Prometric, Inc., 2, 5
Propranolol, 34, 71, 234
Propylthiouracil (PTU), 71, 186
Prostaglandin E (PGE$_1$), 222
Prostate
    benign prostatic hyperplasia, 30–31
    cancer
        cases, high-yield CCS mini-, 316,
            317
        diagnosis, 123
        screening, 31
        symptoms/exam, 123
        treatment, 123
Prostatectomy, 123
Prostate-specific antigen (PSA)
    benign prostatic hyperplasia, 30
    prostate cancer, 123
    workup of prostatic nodules and ab-
        normal, 31
Prostatitis
    cases, high-yield CCS mini-, 318,
        319
    overview, 134
Proteinuria, 162
    acute renal failure, 159
    diagnosis, 161
    nephritic syndrome, 161
    overview, 160
    symptoms/exam, 161
    treatment, 161
Prothrombin/partial thromboplastin
        time (PT/PTT)
    bleeding disorders, 108, 109
    coagulopathies, 110
    preeclampsia/eclampsia, 185
    upper GI bleed, 99
Proton-pump inhibitor (PPI), 84, 86,
        99
Proxy/surrogate, 77
Pruritus, 97, 98, 108
Pseudocyst, 91
Pseudoephedrine, 19
Pseudogout, 143t
Pseudomembranous colitis
    cases, high-yield CCS mini-, 310,
        311
Pseudomonas, 132

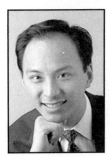
Tao Le, MD

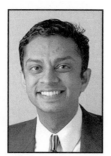
Vikas Bhushan, MD

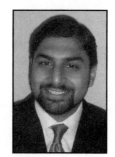
Murtuza Ahmed, MD

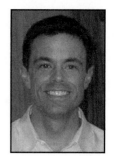
Patrick O'Connell, MD

Tao Le, MD Dr. Le has led multiple medical education projects over the past thirteen years. As a medical student, he was editor-in-chief of the University of California, San Francisco *Synapse,* a university newspaper with a weekly circulation of 9000. Subsequently, he authored *First Aid for the Wards* and *First Aid for the Match* and led the most recent revision of *First Aid for the USMLE Step 2.* At Yale, he was a regular guest lecturer on the USMLE review courses and an adviser to the Yale University School of Medicine curriculum committee. Dr. Le earned his medical degree from the University of California, San Francisco in 1996 and completed his residency training and board certification in internal medicine at Yale–New Haven Hospital. Dr. Le subsequently went on to cofound Medsn and served as its Chief Medical Officer. He is currently pursuing research in asthma education as a fellow in allergy and clinical immunology at the Johns Hopkins Asthma and Allergy Center.

Vikas Bhushan, MD Dr. Bhushan is a world-renowned author, publisher, entrepreneur, and board-certified diagnostic radiologist who resides in Los Angeles, California. Dr. Bhushan conceived and authored the original *First Aid for the USMLE Step 1* in 1992, which, after 11 consecutive editions, has become the most popular medical review book in the world. Following this, he coauthored three additional *First Aid* books as well as developed the highly acclaimed 17-title *Underground Clinical Vignettes* series. He completed his training in diagnostic radiology at the University of California, Los Angeles. Dr. Bhushan has more than 13 years of entrepreneurial experience and started two successful software and publishing companies prior to cofounding Medsn. He has worked directly with dozens of medical school faculty, colleagues, and consultants and corresponded with thousands of medical students from around the world. Dr. Bhushan earned his bachelor's degree in biochemistry from the University of California, Berkeley, and his MD with thesis from the University of California, San Francisco.

Murtuza Ahmed, MD Dr. Ahmed is currently a fellow in Pulmonary, Critical Care, and Sleep Medicine at the University of Pennsylvania. He completed his undergraduate training at Johns Hopkins University and earned his medical degree from West Virginia University. He then went on to residency training in Internal Medicine at Johns Hopkins Bayview Medical Center and served as Assistant Chief of Service there from 2003 to 2004. His interests include medical education, sleep metabolism, and metabolic dysfunction in sleep apnea. He currently resides with his wife Sarah in Philadelphia.

Patrick O'Connell, MD Dr. O'Connell did his medical school training at the University of North Carolina at Chapel Hill. He completed his residency in internal medicine at Johns Hopkins Bayview Medical Center in Baltimore, where he also served as chief resident. Currently, he is a clinician educator at York Hospital in York, Pennsylvania.

ABOUT THE AUTHORS

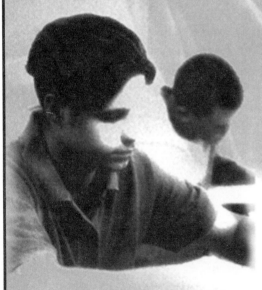